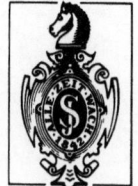

 The Bloomsbury Series in Clinical Science

PARASITIC DISEASE IN CLINICAL PRACTICE

G. C. Cook

With 60 Figures

Springer-Verlag
London Berlin Heidelberg New York
Paris Tokyo Hong Kong

G. C. Cook, MD, DSc, FRCP, FRACP, FLS
Consultant Physician: Hospital for Tropical Diseases, University College
Hospital, St Luke's Hospital for the Clergy and the London School of
Hygiene and Tropical Medicine
Formerly: Medical Specialist, Royal Nigerian Army; Lecturer in
Medicine, Makerere University, Uganda; Professor of Medicine in the
Universities of Zambia, Riyadh and Papua New Guinea

Series Editor
Jack Tinker, BSc, FRCS, FRCP, DIC
Director, Intensive Therapy Unit, The Middlesex Hospital,
London W1N 8AA, UK

ISBN-13:978-1-4471-1771-1   e-ISBN-13:978-1-4471-1769-8
DOI: 10.1007/978-1-4471-1769-8

Cover: Figures 4.2b (background), 11.3 (left), 7.2 (top right)
and 7.3 (bottom right) are taken from the text.

British Library Cataloguing in Publication Data
Cook, G. C. (Gordon Charles)
Parasitic disease in clinical practice.
1. Parasitic diseases
I. Title
616.96
ISBN-13:978-1-4471-1771-1 W. Germany

Library of Congress Cataloging-in-Publication Data
Cook, G. C. (Gordon Charles)
Parasitic disease in clinical practice/G. C. Cook.
p.   cm. – (The Bloomsbury Series in Clinical Science)
Includes bibliographical references.
ISBN-13:978-1-4471-1771-1(alk. paper)   1. Parasitic diseases.   I. Title.   II. Series.
[DNLM: 1. Parasites.   2. Parasitic Diseases.   WC 695 C771p]
RC119.C59 1990 616.9′6 – dc20 DLC
for Library of Congress   90–9639
                                                                       CIP

Typeset by Wilmaset, Birkenhead, Wirral

2128/3916–543210 Printed on acid-free paper

Series Editor's Foreword

Parasitic Disease in Clinical Practice is the sixth monograph to appear in the now established and flourishing Bloomsbury Series in Clinical Science. Written by a distinguished authority in the field, the book gives a comprehensive and detailed description of parasitic infections and their clinical consequences.

Such infections are no longer confined to tropical parts of the world and now have a widespread distribution. Rapid advances are being made in understanding their epidemiology and in diagnosing and treating particular infections. Current literature is largely directed to the parasites, their characteristics and their isolation; a clinical review is clearly needed. This has now been provided, for the author's stated objective is to "inculcate a greater awareness, understanding and appreciation of human parastic disease in the minds of all clinicians".

London, March 1990   Jack Tinker

Preface

Homo sapiens has always existed in a finely balanced equilibrium with a great diversity of infective agents, almost all of them of great antiquity. Many must have exerted a profound effect on the evolution of the human genome. While the average physician is usually aware of potentially pathogenic viruses, bacteria (and rickettsia), and to a lesser extent fungi, his/her knowledge of protozoan and helminthic infections is frequently imperfect and often rudimentary. But the question does get asked from time to time: could this be parasitic? These infections account for morbidity and mortality in the world's developing countries on a vast scale; malaria, schistosomiasis and amoebiasis are perhaps the most important numerically. They are certainly not confined in their geographical distribution to tropical locations, however; they are present in temperate zones too, and in parallel with a huge expansion of overseas travel and tourism has come a rapid increase in their prevalence in northern Europe. They also present a major problem in some members of the immigrant (minor ethnic) groups. Immunosuppression is now a commonplace clinical state (and that induced by chemotherapeutic agents and malignant processes is being rapidly overshadowed by that caused by the HIV-1 and HIV-2 retroviruses) and a greatly enhanced awareness of the relevant parasitic infections (many of them protozoan) is clearly of paramount importance. Zoonotic parasitoses are also widespread in the United Kingdom; *Toxoplasma gondii* infection is important during pregnancy, *Toxocara canis* in infancy and childhood, and *Echinococcus granulosus* (which still exists in western England and Wales), are but three examples. Some parasites are well adapted to the human host and live in an almost symbiotic relationship; others (*Plasmodium falciparum* is an excellent example) have so far failed in this respect and severe morbidity and even death of the infected individual results.

Descriptions of helminthic infections date back thousands of years, but visualization of the protozoa was dependent upon the early microscopists; van Leeuwenhoek visualized *Giardia lamblia* in 1681. It was, however, the great advances in description and taxonomy in the nineteenth century, culminating in the exciting discoveries of man–mosquito cycles by Sir Patrick Manson (*Wuchereria bancrofti*) and Sir Ronald Ross (*Plasmodium* sp), which led to the development of parasitology (the lumping together of protozoology with helminthology is not easily explained) which became a science quite separate from microbiology. In the latter days of Empire and Raj, Great Britain pioneered *clinical* parasitology (a discipline which was closely associated with tropical or 'colonial' medicine). Today, the clinical parasitologist is a very rare breed indeed and is in fact an endangered species.

The last two decades have seen major advances in the understanding, diagnosis, and management of human parasitic disease. Immunological and molecular biological approaches have made significant contributions, although the quest for safe and effective vaccines for protozoan and helminthic infections alike remains a distant dream. A number of the hitherto unknown factors in the host–parasite equation are beginning to reveal their secrets. Serodiagnosis has improved beyond all recognition, and lengthy searches for visual evidence of the parasite itself (adult parasites, larvae, eggs or cysts) is often no longer strictly necessary. Chemotherapy remains difficult in the case of some of the 'exotic' infections with a specific geographical distribution (e.g. trypanosomiasis and leishmaniasis); however in several others (e.g. neurocysticercosis and schistosomiasis) advances have verged on the spectacular. There are very few examples on the other hand of major developments in the eradication of parasitic diseases in either developing or developed countries, even in localized geographical locations.

The resultant diseases encroach into all of the ramifications of general medicine, and also all the clinical specialities. It is therefore essential that not only physicians but all those involved in patient care should develop a high 'index of awareness' for these infections. The major objective of this monograph is therefore to inculcate a greater awareness, understanding and appreciation of human parasitic disease in the minds of all clinicians (and that certainly includes both undergraduate and postgraduate students).

I make no apology for beginning with malaria, which still claims the lives of many unfortunate travellers; the 'opportunistic' infections associated with AIDS are I hope allocated their due amount of space; I have relegated the 'exotic' infections to the last chapter, not because I consider them unimportant but because they form a very small tip of a very large iceberg of parasitoses as seen in northern Europe. For the most part I have used a system-oriented approach.

I thank Miss Andrea Darlow for drawing the parasite life-cycles, the staff of the CT-Scanning Department of University College, London, and that of the Electron-Microscopy Department, London School of Hygiene and Tropical Medicine, for many illustrations, and Mrs Jayne Ball for typing the entire manuscript.

London, September 1989   G. C. Cook

Further Reading

Anderson RM, Facer CA, Rollinson D (eds) (1989) Research developments in the study of parasitic infections. Parasitology 99:S1–S151

Cook GC (1980) Tropical gastroenterology. Oxford University Press, Oxford

Cox FEG (ed) (1982) Modern parasitology: a textbook of parasitology. Blackwell Scientific Publications, Oxford

Despommier DD, Karapelou JW (1987) Parasite life cycles. Springer, Berlin Heidelberg New York

Englund PT, Sher A (eds) (1988) The biology of parasitism. Alan R Liss, New York

Foster WD (1965) A history of parasitology. E & S Livingstone, Edinburgh

Harvey PH, Keymer AE, May RM (1988) Evolving control of diseases. Nature 332:680–681

Katz M, Despommier DD, Gwadz R (1989) Parasitic diseases, 2nd edn. Springer, Berlin Heidelberg New York

Leech JH, Sande MA, Root RK (eds) (1988) Parasitic infections. Churchill Livingstone, New York and Edinburgh

Manson P (1898) Tropical diseases: a manual of the diseases of warm climates. Cassell, London

Mehlhorn H (ed) (1988) Parasitology in focus: facts and trends. Springer, Berlin Heidelberg New York

Piekarski G (1987) Medical parasitology. Springer, Berlin Heidelberg New York

Southwood TRE (1987) The natural environment and disease: an evolutionary perspective. Br Med J 294:1086–1089

Worboys M (1983) The emergence and early development of parasitology. In: Warren KS, Bowers JZ (eds) Parasitology: a global perspective. Springer, Berlin Heidelberg New York, pp 1–18

Contents

Chapter 1

Plasmodium falciparum Infection and the Other Human Malarias

He is so shak'd of a burning quotidian tertian, that it is most lamentable to behold.

William Shakespeare (1564–1616),
Henry V, II,i,123

Introduction

The arthropod-borne protozoan parasitoses caused by *Plasmodium* sp have produced incalculable human misery, morbidity, and mortality since antiquity; it is clear that *Plasmodium* sp is related to the coccidia (Chap. 4) (Bruce-Chwatt 1988a), and that the primate–vector cycle was established around 30 million years ago. It seems certain that early man, in the cradle of civilization of Africa (Stringer 1988; Stringer and Andrews 1988), must have been subjected to this group of infections. 'Malaria', which replaced the older term ague during the eighteenth century and is derived from the Italian description *mal aria* (poisonous air), is not a single disease. Human infection by four separate protozoan parasites belonging to the genus *Plasmodium* (which probably evolved from intestinal coccidia millions of years ago), presents as four diverse and characteristic clinical entities (Spencer and Strickland 1984; Bruce-Chwatt 1985; Haworth 1987; Cook 1989a). That produced by *P falciparum* causes an acute and potentially lethal illness ('malignant tertian' malaria, in the older terminology) while at the opposite end of the spectrum, *P malariae* produces a very chronic infection that may continue, often without serious morbidity, for 50 years or more (Table 1.1.). Diseases with intermediate clinical presentations result from infection with *P vivax* and *P ovale*; though neither is characteristically associated with acute mortality or great chronicity, both result in considerable subacute morbidity.

Numerous eminent individuals have been seriously debilitated or have had their lives cut short by a febrile illness which probably resulted from a *P*

Table 1.1. Clinical manifestations of infection with the four *Plasmodium* species

Plasmodium	Incubation period (d)	Periodicity of fever (h)[a]	Clinical manifestations[b]
falciparum	12 (9–14) (Clinical presentation may be much later)	48	Gastrointestinal symptoms Massive haemolysis Severe anaemia (Phillips et al. 1986a) Jaundice Haemoglobinuria, 'blackwater fever' Shock 'Algid malaria' Cerebral involvement Pulmonary oedema Hypoglycaemia Pregnancy complications Retinal lesions Death
vivax	13 (12–17) Occasionally up to 12 months	48	Chronic anaemia Persisting splenomegaly Rarely splenic rupture
ovale	17 (16–18) or longer	48	Similar to *P vivax*
malariae	28 (18–40) or longer	72	Recrudescences for up to 50 yr or more Persisting splenomegaly Rarely splenic rupture Nephrotic syndrome (most common in African children; rare in non-immunes)

[a]A classical temperature-chart with sharp peaks is unusual in practice, especially in *P falciparum* infections.
[b]With all species hyperreactive malarious splenomegaly is a rare complication.

falciparum infection: Alexander the Great (323 BC), St Augustine (first Archbishop of Canterbury) (604 AD), King James I, King Charles II, Cardinal Wolsey and Oliver Cromwell, to name a handful. The diseases were well known to Chaucer and Shakespeare. For many hundreds of years the Chinese herb *Artemisia annual* has been known to possess antimalarial properties. The medicinal properties of Peruvian bark (the fever-bark tree) were recognized by Jesuit missionaries, and *Cinchona* was first introduced into Rome by Spanish priests in 1632; it was included in the *London Pharmacopoeia* (third edition) in 1677 as *Cortex peruanus* (Bruce-Chwatt 1988b,c). The principal alkaloid of cinchona, quinine, remained the sole chemoprophylactic and chemotherapeutic agent for the malarias until a series of synthetic antimalarial agents was produced in the 1920s and 1930s.

This ancient disease is not only still in our midst, but is responsible for an estimated 100 million cases annually worldwide (World Health Organisation 1987); a high proportion of these infections involve children of less than 5 years old. Even in non-malarious countries the chance of encountering a case has been rising steadily (Phillips-Howard et al. 1988); in the UK, 1986 for example, saw 738 reported cases. A few infections acquired in the UK and other European cities have resulted from the introduction of infected anopheline mosquitoes via air transport (Whitfield et al. 1984). The infection can also be transmitted via blood transfusion, bone-marrow transplantation, 'needle-stick' injury, and across the placenta (Bruce-Chwatt 1985). A further possible route lies in conveyance of an infected mosquito in a suitcase (Rizzo et al. 1989).

We now have at our disposal a wealth of data upon the epidemiology (and micro-epidemiology), parasitology, histopathology, immunology and clinical features of this group of infections (Wernsdorfer and MacGregor 1988). However, diagnosis is still far from being simple (Cook 1989a); there is no short-cut method to examining thick and thin films of peripheral blood (see below). Also, developments in chemoprophylaxis and chemotherapy have largely failed to keep pace with the stealth and craftiness of *Plasmodium* sp and its principal vectors (Cook 1989a). *P falciparum*, a very poorly adapted parasite of man, is the only one to have developed resistance to several of the (formerly) more potent antimalarials: in South America (late 1950s), South-east Asia (early 1960s) and East and Central Africa (early 1980s) (Cook 1988a). Much current interest lies in the rate of development of chloroquine-resistance in West Africa and across the Indian subcontinent. In the former, there is now ample evidence that it is widespread (Cook 1988b); reports from Ghana (Neeguaye 1986), Benin (formerly Dahomey) (Bras et al. 1986), Congo and Gabon (Brandicourt et al. 1986), Nigeria (Jackson et al. 1987), Cameroon (Brasseur et al. 1987a) and Guinea (Brasseur et al. 1987b) document evidence which is convincing. In all areas, evidence of resistance to other antimalarials (including widely used chemoprophylactic and chemotherapeutic agents) is far less complete; however, reduced in vitro sensitivity to mefloquine has now been reported in some strains of *P falciparum* in West Africa, and because it has not previously been used in either prophylaxis or treatment there it must be assumed that these strains are inherently resistant to its action (Oduola et al. 1987; Simet et al. 1988). There is also preliminary evidence of sulfadoxine-pyrimethamine ('Fansidar') resistance in West Africa (Gubler 1988).

Parasitology and Pathogenesis

The malaria parasite was first visualized in Algeria by Laveran on 20 October 1880; he named it *Oscillaria malariae* (Laveran 1881). On 20 August 1897, Ross (working in India) demonstrated Laveran's organism in the stomach of an *Anopheles* mosquito after it had fed on the blood of malaria-infected patients (Ross 1897); he later showed that mosquitos which had fed on malaria-infected birds could infect healthy ones (Ross 1898). This discovery was announced on 28 July 1898 by Manson (on Ross' behalf) at the Edinburgh meeting of the British Medical Association (Cook 1989b). In a classical piece of clinical investigation, Manson (1900) was able to produce *Plasmodium vivax* malaria in his elder son via the bites of infected mosquitos transported from Rome. The pre-erythrocytic (hepatocyte) component in the host was unravelled by Shortt and his colleagues (Shortt and Garnham 1948; Shortt et al. 1948).

Figures 1.1 and 1.2 outline the life-cycles of the *P falciparum* and *P vivax* parasites, respectively. Figure 1.3 shows the developing oocyst (containing sporozoites) in the mosquito mid-gut, and Figure 1.4 an adult *Plasmodium* sp trophozoite.

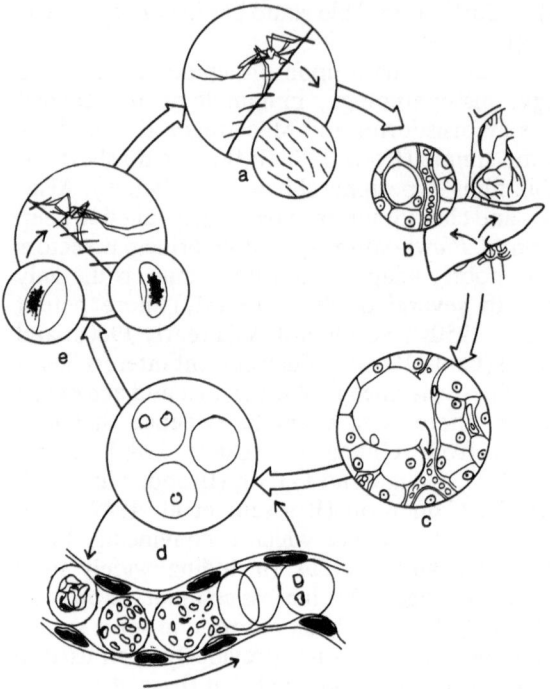

Fig. 1.1. Life-cycle of *Plasmodium falciparum*. (a) Sporozoites (10–14 µm in length) are injected into the cutaneous circulation by an infected female anopheline mosquito; (b) sporozoites become widely dispersed and enter many organs, including an hepatocyte where schizogony (5–7 days) produces numerous intracellular merozoites (the pre-erythrocytic stage); (c) merozoites are liberated from a schizont into the sinusoidal blood-stream, and then (d) enter an erythrocyte where the 48-hour cycle, which depends on the repeated liberation of large numbers of merozoites into the circulation, begins (this is accompanied by fever); (e) gametocytes are ingested by a female mosquito to complete the cycle.

The pathophysiology of *P falciparum* malaria has been reviewed (Warrell 1987; Petersen and Leech 1988). There remain substantial gaps in present knowledge, however; an excellent example is the mechanism(s) which accounts for the major clinical sign – periodic fever – still not being adequately explained (Lumsden 1989; Kwiatkowski and Greenwood 1989). Another vector-borne parasitosis which involves the erythrocytes is babesiosis (Wright et al. 1988) (see below); a greater understanding of the immunopathophysiology of this infection might well elucidate certain deficiencies in the understanding of *P falciparum* malaria. The Bolivian squirrel monkey has emerged as a satisfactory model for the study of the pathological changes of *P falciparum* infection (Whiteley et al. 1987). Many of the complications are associated with sequestration of parasitized erythrocytes, causing microcirculatory obstruction. A similar mechanism has recently been postulated to cause necrosis of skeletal muscle (a rare manifestation of this disease) (DeSilva et al. 1988). Both immune and toxic mechanisms are probably involved; in a study utilizing immunoelectron microscopy, *P falciparum* infected erythrocytes were shown to attach to endothelial cells via electron-dense knobs

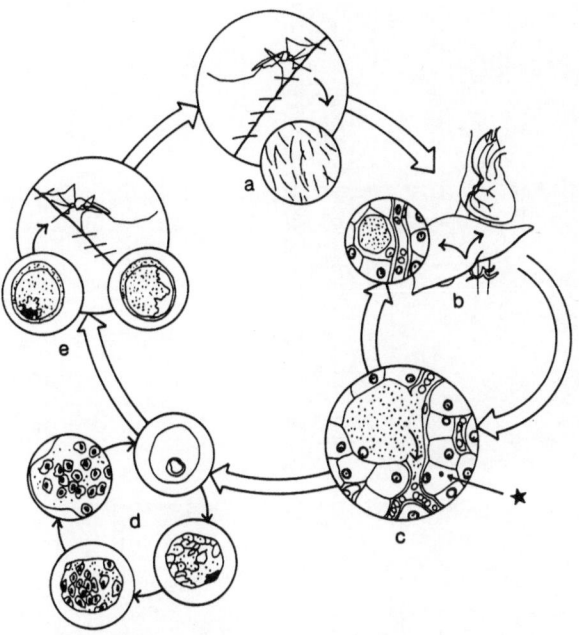

Fig. 1.2. Life-cycle of *Plasmodium vivax*. Stages (a) and (b) are identical to those of *P falciparum* (Fig. 1.1). However, before proceeding to the erythrocyte stage, some merozoites (c) differentiate into a hypnozoite stage (*) (a dormant, non-dividing phase which can result in merozoite formation at a later date – the exo-erythrocytic cycle). The erythrocyte (d) and gametocyte (e) stages are similar to those of *P falciparum*.

(Aikawa 1988; Trager 1989). This latter mechanism has been shown, further-more, to be at least a contributory factor to the development of cerebral malaria (Chap. 8). However, adhesion to endothelial cells is apparently also possible when erythrocytes infected with *P falciparum* parasites are knobless (Udomsang-petch et al. 1989). The role of tumour necrosis factor (TNF) in severe complicated disease remains unclear. Mechanisms of immunity have been reviewed (Hadley and Chulay 1988); both antibody (Nguyen-Dinh et al. 1987b) and cell-mediated factors are involved. The DNA sequence which encodes a major blood-stage antigen of *P falciparum* has recently been determined (Higgins et al. 1989). Absence of an increased susceptibility of individuals suffering from the acquired immune deficiency syndrome (AIDS) to *P falciparum* (Simooya et al. 1988) (Chap. 2) suggests that there is *not* a failure of the immune response to malaria in this infection. In the context of AIDS, an affected patient in Uganda has recently been reported to have had a *P vivax* infection complicated by 'blackwater fever' (Katongole-Mbidde et al. 1988). Whereas monosaccharide absorption from the human small-intestine is probably unaltered in uncomplicated *P falciparum* malaria, it is significantly reduced in severe, complicated disease (Molyneux et al. 1989a); evidence of a reduction of liver blood-flow has also been documented in the latter situation. Changes in hepatic structure and function in malaria have been reviewed (Cook 1990).

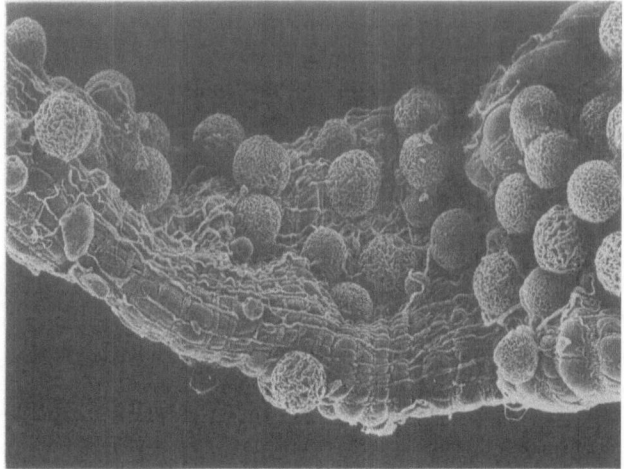

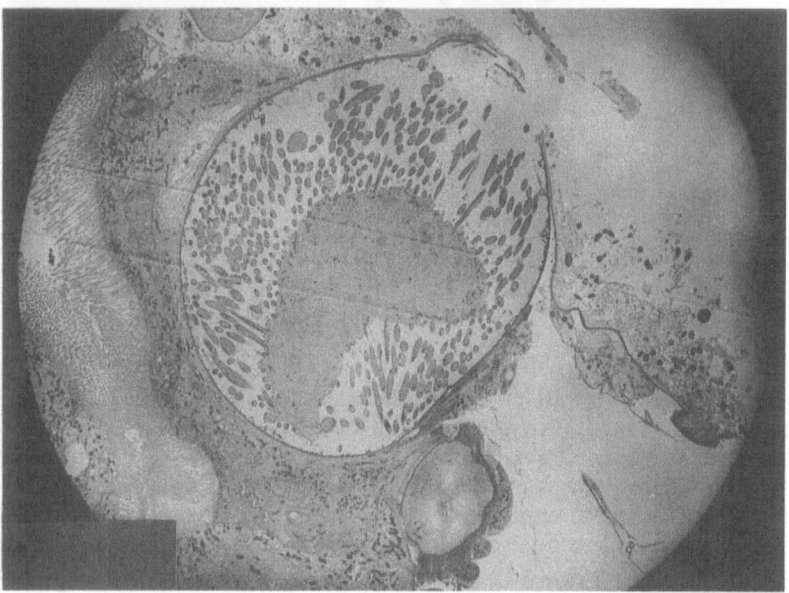

Fig. 1.3a,b. Transmission electron micrographs showing **a** numerous oocysts of *P berghei* in the mid gut of an anopheline mosquito (× 240) and **b** sporozoites developing within an oocyst (× 2100).

Clinical Aspects

Table 1.1 summarizes the major clinical features of the four human malarias. Clinical aspects of *P falciparum* malaria have been reviewed (Cook 1988a; Petersen and Leech 1988). In uncomplicated disease, fever (usually >39°C and sometimes up to 40°C), splenomegaly, and later anaemia (Phillips et al. 1986a) are important clinical findings. Clinical differential diagnoses include all febrile

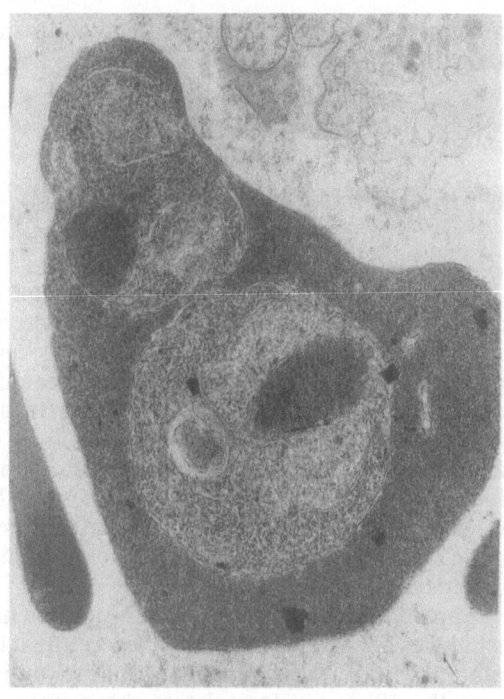

Fig. 1.4. Transmission electron-
micrograph of a mature trophozoite
of *P berghei* (× 24 000).

illnesses acquired in a *P falciparum* infected area, especially when splenomegaly
is concurrently present. Infection with another intra-erythrocytic protozoan
parasite, *Babesia* sp, can produce a comparable illness, with haemolysis and
occasionally renal failure, especially in splenectomized individuals (Ruebush
1984; Manson-Bahr and Bell 1987; Ristic 1988). This organism, which is
transmitted to man by ixodid ticks, and has an animal reservoir in domestic and
wild animals, rarely produces disease in northern America (most cases have been
reported in islands off the coast of New England) and Europe. Because, like the
chronic malarias, parasitaemia may be very prolonged it can be acquired from
infected blood transfusion. (Treatment is with quinine + clindamycin.)

In a severe *P falciparum* infection, multisystem involvement (most importantly
cerebral disease (Chap. 8)) gives rise to substantial morbidity and mortality rates.
Anaemia and jaundice are common (Phillips et al. 1986a). Vasoconstriction may
be present in a shocked or hypoglycaemic patient despite a high cardiac output.
Upper gastrointestinal bleeding is an important complication which has become
less common since the use of corticosteroids for cerebral involvement was
abandoned (Chap. 8). Dehydration is sometimes present, and this depends on
the length of history and degree of gastrointestinal involvement; the skin is often
flushed and dry, comparable with that in heatstroke. Pulmonary oedema and/or
aspiration pneumonia should be sought; the latter can be caused by inhaled
vomitus. Metabolic acidosis should be suspected when there is sustained
hyperventilation in the presence of a normal chest radiograph. Splenic rupture is
a rare event. The intestinal absorptive defect coupled with a reduced hepatic
blood-flow (see above) assumes a practical importance in maintenance of an
adequate plasma concentration of a chemotherapeutic agent (see below). Special

problems relating to malaria infection in infancy and childhood have been summarized (Mashaal 1986).

Diagnosis

Although most patients with a *P falciparum* (and other species also) infection have a peripheral blood parasitaemia (Petersen and Leech 1988), this is not necessarily so, and on rare occasions severe complicated cases have been documented without this finding. Films should always be made at the bedside; a delay can lead to a false-negative result (Brook et al. 1989). Young 'ring' forms (trophozoites) are usually clearly visible in erythrocytes, whilst the 'mature' adherent forms (late trophozoites and later schizonts) are absent from peripheral blood. On rare occasions, *Babesia* sp must be differentiated (Ruebush 1984; Wright et al. 1988); the small ring form may be virtually indistinguishable from a young *P falciparum* trophozoite, although pigment is not produced in the infected erythrocyte.

Improved methods of diagnosis would be highly advantageous. Sophisticated techniques are now available in a few centres; however, it will be a very long time before these are widely applicable in the routine diagnosis of an acute infection. Since the 1960s serological tests have proved to be of value in field studies, epidemiology, the detection of present or past infections, in screening of blood donors, and more recently in the assessment of serological responses to vaccination (Wirth et al. 1986; Bruce-Chwatt 1987a); such techniques can be made species-specific. Malaria-specific antigens and antibodies can now readily be detected (Wirth et al. 1986; Avidor et al. 1987; Campbell et al. 1987; Deloron et al. 1987; Nguyen-Dinh et al. 1987b; Lim 1988; Khusmith et al. 1988); however these tests remain positive often for long after disappearance of the parasitaemia, and it should be stressed that they are of absolutely no value in assessing the presence of a *current* infection. Estimation of the presence and/or size of a parasitaemia in an acute infection is another matter and requires techniques utilizing DNA probes (Bruce-Chwatt 1987a; Holmberg et al. 1987; McLaughlin et al. 1987); using the pPF14 probe for example, a *P falciparum* density of 40 parasites per microlitre of blood can readily be detected (Wirth et al. 1986). Also, a sensitive diagnostic technique, which is species-specific, based on ribosomal RNA and capable of detecting <10 parasites has been developed (Waters and McCutchan 1989). But even when such techniques have been perfected they will obviously not be available in laboratories in the majority of areas where *P falciparum* infection is common. Recently, a rapid diagnostic test based on acridine orange staining of centrifuged parasites in a microhaematocrit tube has given promising results (Rickman et al. 1989a,b; Spielman and Perrone 1989); detection of a parasite count of 2–4 per microlitre of blood is apparently possible.

A severe anaemia without a reticulocytosis is common at presentation; the leucocyte count is usually normal or depressed but occasionally moderately elevated; the platelet count is usually depressed. The plasma fibrinogen concentration is usually raised, and in a minority prothrombin and partial thromboplastic times are prolonged; DIC is a very unusual accompaniment. Blood urea is frequently elevated (usually resulting from dehydration); although some degree of renal impairment is common, oliguric failure (a serious complication), is unusual. Mild hyponatraemia and hypochloraemia are common. Plasma concentrations of hepatic enzymes are usually elevated (haemolysis and release of muscle enzymes often makes interpretation difficult) (Cook 1990). An elevated creatine phosphokinase concentration results also from muscle damage. Serum acute phase proteins are usually elevated whilst the albumin concentration is depressed.

Prevention of Malaria

General Measures

In infected regions of the world, all indigenous individuals are exposed to mosquito bites from the moment of birth onwards; in most, a degree of maternal antibody protection lasts for several months (Udezue 1985). With recurrent antigenic stimulation some inherent immunity is established thereafter, but maintenance of this requires repeated exposure. Such populations are therefore 'partly immune'. The traveller to an infected area from a temperate (uninfected) environment possesses no such immunity and is therefore exceedingly vulnerable. In theory the percutaneous introduction of a single *P falciparum* sporozoite can produce a fatal infection.

Before the modern era of chemoprophylaxis, advice to the traveller was dominated by efforts to avoid a mosquito bite (Nevill et al. 1988). Anopheline mosquitos most often strike between dusk and dawn; thus, by covering all exposed parts and by using an effective mosquito-net during sleep, one can substantially reduce the likelihood of infection (Bruce-Chwatt 1985). Mosquito repellants (e.g., *N,N*-diethyl-*m*-toluamide), impregnation of bed-nets and clothing, and the spraying of living accommodation with an insecticide (e.g., DDT or dieldrin) during the late afternoon constitute additional protective measures. In view of the current difficulties with chemoprophylactic agents (see below), this advice is again being widely offered and is in part effective (Bradley et al. 1986).

In many large towns and cities in malarious areas the potential risk of *P falciparum* infection is exceedingly low, and travellers who will not be venturing into the countryside may be overall safer without chemoprophylaxis. Instead they can carry a small pack of chemotherapeutic agents such as quinine or 'Fansidar' or 'Mefloquine'; however, even self-therapy is not without side-effects (Phillips-Howard et al. 1989).

Chemoprophylaxis

Chemoprophylaxis does not *prevent* infection (Cook 1986a; Warhurst 1986a); it is at best suppressive and limits the blood parasite (schizont) concentration to such an extent that clinical symptoms are absent while the agent is being administered. Therefore no chemoprophylactic regimen can possibly be 100% effective and,

Table 1.2. Chemoprophylactic regimens used against falciparum infection during the past 30 years: adult doses[a]

Agent	Trade name	Oral dose
Proguanil	'Paludrine'	100–200 mg daily
Chlorproguanil	'Lapudrine'	20 mg weekly
Pyrimethamine	'Daraprim'	25 mg weekly
Chloroquine (base)	'Nivaquine'	300 mg weekly
Chloroquine (150 mg) + chlorproguanil (20 mg)	'Lapaquin'	1 tablet weekly
Chloroquine (150 mg) + pyrimethamine (25 mg)	'Darachlor'	1 tablet weekly
Pyrimethamine (12.5 mg) + dapsone (100 mg)	'Maloprim'	1 tablet weekly
Pyrimethamine (25 mg) + sulfadoxine (500 mg)	'Fansidar'	1 tablet weekly
Pyrimethamine (25 mg) + sulphalene (500 mg)	'Metakelfin'[b]	1 tablet weekly
Amodiaquine[c]	'Camoquin'	400 mg weekly
Amodiaquine[c] (150 mg) + primaquine (15 mg)	'Camoprim'	1 tablet weekly
Mefloquine	'Lariam'[b]	250 mg weekly
Mefloquine + 'Fansidar'	'Fansimef'[b]	Equivalent of 1 tablet of each weekly

[a]All regimens must be started at least 1 wk before exposure to infection and continued for 4–6 wk after the last possible mosquito bite.
[b]Not available as a chemoprophylactic agent in UK.
[c]Withdrawn from market for chemoprophylaxis.

Table 1.3. Dosage of chemoprophylactic agents for use in children (Cook 1986)

Body-weight (kg)	Corresponding age (approximate)	Chloroquine or proguanil[a]	'Fansidar' or 'Maloprim'[a]
	0–5 wk	⅛	Not recommended
	6 wk–5 mo	¼	⅛
	6 mo–1 yr	¼	¼
5–20	1–5 yr	½	½
21–40	6–12 yr	¾	¾
>40	>12 yr	Adult dose	Adult dose

[a]Proportion of adult dose.

whenever a suspicion of a *P falciparum* infection exists, chemotherapy must be started immediately. However, whilst the recommended prophylaxis may not be fully effective, it may dampen down an infection sufficiently for it to be readily amenable to a therapeutic regimen that might not itself be regarded as ideal (Peters 1987b). Details of chemoprophylactic agents and regimens have been reviewed (Cook 1986a, 1988a; Lobel and Campbell 1986). Beginning in the 1930s, proquanil and pyrimethamine (dihydrofolate reductase [DHFR] inhibitors or folate antagonists) and chloroquine proved, when wisely used, safe and effective. Tables 1.2 and 1.3 summarize agents which have recently been used, together with their dosage.

The Malaria Global Eradication Campaign, launched by the World Health Organisation in 1957, was associated with much subsequent complacency; efforts to produce new chemoprophylactic agents largely ceased and insecticiding

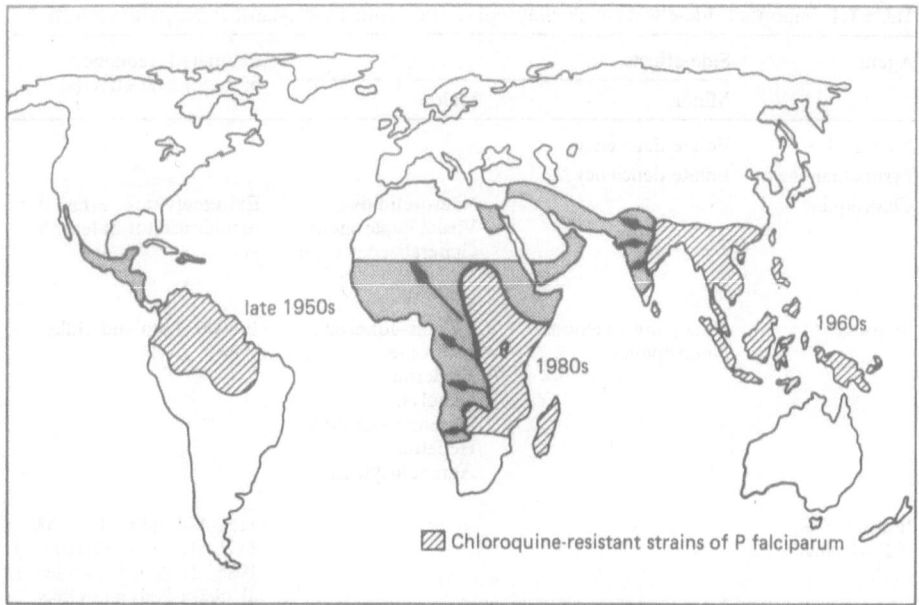

Fig. 1.5. World map which indicates the approximate areas where endemic malaria exists, and those in which good evidence has been provided for resistance of the *P falciparum* parasite to chloroquine. The dates indicate the approximate chronological emergence of resistance in different geographical areas.

became lax. Problems have been compounded during the last decade by the emergence of strains of *P falciparum* which are resistant to most of the widely used synthetic agents (Lobel and Campbell 1986; Cook 1988a, 1988c, 1989a). Figure 1.5 shows the approximate geographical areas where chloroquine resistance (graded from RI to RIII) (World Health Organisation 1973) has become a major problem; resistance to the DHFR inhibitors is also widespread (Saarinen et al. 1987; Watkins et al. 1987; Nahlen et al. 1989) but accurate documentation of the distribution is far less satisfactory. A concurrent problem has been an increasing recognition of side-effects of chemoprophylactic agents (when used alone or in combination) (Table 1.4) some of which are serious (Cook 1986b, 1988a,b). 'Maloprim' (pyrimethamine+dapsone) was shown to be associated, albeit rarely, with bone-marrow depression, which was occasionally fatal. However, this usually followed administration of tablets twice a week rather than once a week (Hutchinson et al. 1986); an idiosyncratic mechanism is probably involved. 'Fansidar' (pyrimethamine+sulfadoxine) was associated with serious side-effects and occasional deaths; however, these seemed to be more common when this combination prophylactic was taken with chloroquine (Stemberger et al. 1984; Miller et al. 1986a,b). Chloroquine had been added because: (i) *P falciparum* strains are rarely completely resistant to its action, and (ii) *P vivax* infection is not prevented by 'Fansidar' alone (see below). In 1985 amodiaquine, which had been used some 20–30 years previously, was resurrected and reintroduced in locations where chloroquine resistance is common (Fig. 1.5.). Although it proved to be moderately effective, neutropenia

Table 1.4. Important side-effects of chemoprophylactic agents used against *P falciparum* infection

Agent	Side-effects		Estimated frequency of major side-effect(s)
	Minor	Major	
Proguanil	Folate deficiency		
Pyrimethamine	Folate deficiency		
Chloroquine		Neuroretinitis Visual impairment Generalized pruritus	Extremely rare, even after regular use for at least 5 yr[a]
'Fansidar'	Cutaneous reactions Neutropenia	Stevens–Johnson syndrome Epidermal necrolysis Systemic vasculitis Hepatitis Agranulocytosis	1:5000 (Peto and Gilks 1986)[b]
'Fansidar' + chloroquine			1:5000–1:8000; 1:18000–1:26000 deaths (Hernborg 1985; Cook 1986; Miller et al 1986[a]; Peto and Gilks 1986)
'Maloprim'	Methaemoglobinaemia Haemolysis	Agranulocytosis	1:10000 (Peto and Gilks 1986) usually associated with high dosage
Amodiaquine	Neutropenia (Rhodes et al. 1986)	Hepatitis	
Amodiaquine + proguanil	Neutropenia	Agranulocytosis Hepatitis	1:2000; 1:8000 deaths (Hatton et al. 1986; Peto and Gilks 1986)
Tetracyclines	Tooth staining in infants and children		Common

[a]After 6 years' administration, 6-monthly screening is sometimes advised; blood concentrations are higher in the presence of renal and hepatic damage.
[b]These rates might vary in different ethnic groups (Cook 1986).

(Hatton et al. 1986; Neftel et al. 1986; Rhodes et al. 1986) and hepatocellular dysfunction (Larrey et al. 1986; Neftel et al. 1986) (which had been recorded when it was previously used) proved troublesome. These seemed more common when it was combined with proguanil; some individuals had also taken 'Fansidar' (Table 1.4). Mefloquine is now commercially available for chemoprophylactic use in Switzerland and France; there is limited suggestive evidence that emergence of resistance is reduced when this agent is combined with 'Fansidar' ('Fansimef') (Win et al. 1985; White 1987); with this regimen, however, the toxicity of 'Fansidar' remains, and it also seems unwise to recommend its use in individuals with evidence of hepatocellular dysfunction (Reisinger et al. 1989). There is much to be said for reserving mefloquine for chemotherapy.

A delicate balance therefore exists between the ill-effects of a *P falciparum* infection and those of the various chemoprophylactic regimens. In travellers to

Kenya from the USA during 1984, for example, the risk of a fatal parasitaemia was about the same as the risk of a fatal 'Fansidar' reaction (Miller et al. 1986b) – presumably resulting from the sulphonamide moiety (Hernborg 1985). Risk-benefit analyses are thus necessary (Peto and Gilks 1986); the likelihood of a fatal *P falciparum* infection is not great, and chemoprophylaxis with potentially toxic agents will often be inadvisable. For the average UK traveller, the actual risk of death from falciparum malaria (when not receiving chemoprophylaxis) has been calculated to be 1 : 10 000 (Peto and Gilks 1986). Even in 1990, only a small minority of strains of *P falciparum* are completely resistant (RIII) (World Health Organisation 1973) to chloroquine and the DHFR inhibitors.

The value of antimicrobial agents in malaria prophylaxis requires further elucidation. Doxycycline has proved more effective than chloroquine in Thailand (Pang et al. 1987; Peters 1987a); however, this agent should not be widely recommended and is contraindicated in young children and pregnant women.

Table 1.5 summarizes the advice, widely offered in 1990, on *P falciparum* chemoprophylaxis (Cook 1988a,c, 1989a); it must be appreciated however, that this errs on the side of safety rather than efficacy. Evidence has now been documented that regimen ii (Table 1.5) is as effective as the formerly recommended one of chloroquine + 'Fansidar' (pyrimethamine 25 mg + sulfadoxine 500 mg) in travellers to East Africa, as well as being significantly safer (Fogh et al. 1988). While recent World Health Organisation recommendations now suggest the abandonment of 'Maloprim' and its substitution with mefloquine in Southeast Asia (and sub-Saharan Africa) (World Health Organisation 1988; Malaria Reference Laboratory 1989), it seems advisable, when possible, to reserve this agent for chemotherapy rather than chemoprophylaxis. Also, there is virtually no evidence of safety of mefloquine when used for prolonged periods of time; acute psychoses have recently been documented when this agent has been used for treatment (Stuiver et al. 1989). Evidence of hepatotoxicity has also been presented (Reisinger et al. 1989). Some would recommend the more widespread use of doxycycline for short-term prophylaxis (see above). However, campylobacter enteritis has now been documented as a complication of this form of prophylaxis (Taylor et al. 1988). Limited evidence indicates that in Papua New Guinea, *P falciparum* is now relatively resistant to the 'Maloprim' + chloroquine

Table 1.5. Current advice on *P falciparum* chemoprophylaxis

Geographical area	Regimen
(i) No evidence of chloroquine (or DHFR inhibitor) resistance	Proguanil 100 or 200 mg daily or chloroquine 300 mg weekly
(ii) Chloroquine resistance commonplace (including East and Central Africa)	Proguanil 200 mg daily plus chloroquine 300 mg weekly[a]
(iii) Chloroquine resistance commonplace and regimen ii apparently ineffective (Southeast Asia and Pacific)[b]	'Maloprim' 1 tablet weekly plus chloroquine 300 mg weekly

[a]Despite widespread use, the safety of this combination regimen has not been formally established (Peters 1987)
[b]Recently, a recommendation that weekly mefloquine (250 mg ≡ 1 tablet) is an acceptable regimen in South-east Asia and sub-Saharan Africa has gained considerable support (Malaria Reference Laboratory 1989).

combination (Edstein et al. 1988). Even when recommended, chemoprophylactic agents are, however, poorly understood and compliance is unsatisfactory (Lobel et al. 1987; Williams and Lewis 1987). The problems associated with chemoprophylaxis for the indigenous population in an endemic area are vast (Slutsker et al. 1988).

Whether or not long-term chemoprophylaxis as currently recommended carries significant risks remains controversial. There is no good evidence that proguanil causes significant problems, although aphthous ulceration certainly seems to be more common (Cook 1988a). The widespread fears that long-term chloroquine causes retinal damage remain but there is absolutely no hard evidence for this. No toxicological studies are available to substantiate the safety of long-term proguanil + chloroquine (Peters 1987b). A recent study has shown a reduced antibody response to human diploid-cell rabies vaccine in those using chloroquine (Pappaioanou et al. 1986). A reduction in serum immunoglobulins IgG and IgM has been documented after long-term 'Maloprim' (Ti et al. 1987); furthermore, an increased rate of non-specific upper respiratory tract infections has been demonstrated in healthy men whilst receiving this prophylactic agent (Lee and Lau 1988).

Chemoprophylaxis for Special Groups

Pregnant women should, when possible, be transferred to a non-malarious area where chemoprophylaxis is unnecessary (Bruce-Chwatt 1983; Editorial 1983; Cook 1986a, 1988a). Abortion, premature labour, and congenital infection can all complicate malaria in pregnancy (Editorial 1983); therefore, in a malarious area effective prophylaxis is safer overall than no prophylaxis. The DHFR inhibitors (proguanil, chlorproguanil, and pyrimethamine) and chloroquine are fairly safe; the former should be supplemented with folic acid at least during the first trimester. Sulphonamide-containing prophylactics in late pregnancy can theoretically produce kernicterus, rarely with damage to the newborn infant; otherwise there are no firm data to contraindicate the use of either 'Fansidar' or 'Maloprim'. Tetracyclines must be avoided.

Infants are vulnerable from birth onwards. 'Fansidar' and 'Maloprim' are contraindicated at less than six weeks, owing to the immaturity of several enzyme systems (Public Health Laboratory Service Malaria Reference Laboratory 1984; Cook 1986a); both of these agents are also excreted in breast milk and should not be given to lactating women during this period. Tetracyclines must be avoided.

Advice for *immunosuppressed* patients is difficult and they should avoid infected areas if at all possible. The fact that *P falciparum* infection does not seem to be more common in individuals with the acquired immunodeficiency syndrome (AIDS) (Nguyen-Dinh et al. 1987a) (Chap. 2) suggests that immunosuppression is not a major risk factor for this infection. In any individual who has been exposed to infection, whether immunosuppressed or not, undiagnosed fever must be treated without delay as though it was caused by *P falciparum*.

A further vulnerable group consists of *Africans and Asians returning home* after two or more years in a temperate climate – e.g., students and their families (Cook 1986a, 1988a). In the absence of recurrent infection partial inherent immunity will have declined rapidly. In intelligent adults the best course is to treat clinical *P falciparum* infections as they arise; some degree of natural immunity will then return (Editorial 1985). In children there is a case for prescribing proguanil for twelve months after their return to the tropics (Table 1.3) and then treating clinical attacks (Udezue 1985).

Malaria Vaccine: A Distant Prospect?

In recent years, the possibility of the introduction of a safe and effective *P falciparum* vaccine in the near future has engendered considerable hope, much of it unjustified. The malaria parasite evades attack as a result of poor immunogenicity of its surface antigens, antigenic variation, mutation, and suppression of the immune response; in this context, protein-heterogeneity within the sporozoite should not be underestimated (Rosenberg et al. 1989). The extent to which false optimism has produced complacency regarding development of new chemoprophylactic agents is impossible to assess. Although work is underway on sporozoite, merozoite and gametocyte vaccines (Miller 1986, 1988; Bruce-Chwatt 1987b; Hadley and Chulay 1988) (each would be stage-specific) there is still a long way to go before any of them has undergone an adequate human trial. Even then they will doubtless only be available, at considerable expense, to travellers; they will be out of reach to the countless millions living in 'Third-world' countries (in whom a take-up rate of at least 95% of the population would be necessary) who most of all require protection against the ravages of malaria, especially the *P falciparum* form. Furthermore, an injectable vaccine in many parts of the tropics, especially Africa, currently carries the risk of introducing an HIV infection.

Most progress has in fact taken place on a sporozoite vaccine (Nussenzweig and Nussenzweig 1986), and initial human trials have yielded generally encouraging but certainly not totally successful results (Ballou et al. 1987; Patarroyo et al. 1988). If protection is not 100% during the 20–30 minutes after infection, one or more sporozoites will enter the hepatocyte pool (Hoffman et al. 1986; Miller 1986). There is evidence that the cellular immune response to sporozoite antigens might be short-lived, and actually suppressed in the event of an acute attack of *P falciparum* malaria (Webster et al. 1988). A gametocyte vaccine (aimed at the sexual stage of the life-cycle) can only protect the community and not the individual. Such vaccines would inevitably be stage-specific therefore (Fig. 1.1), and it is likely that an acceptable vaccine will ultimately contain antigens specific for all three major stages of the parasite's life-cycle (Miller 1986). Recent work suggests that a change of tack in research towards a *P falciparum* vaccine might be beneficial (Schofield et al. 1987; Cox 1988a,b). Immunity against malaria has now been shown to operate against stages of the parasite developing within the hepatocyte; it seems possible that an immunological attack on parasite enzymes (e.g. aldolase) would yield more worthwhile results (Cox 1988b).

Even when a safe and effective *P falciparum* vaccine is available there will still be need for chemoprophylaxis against infections caused by other *Plasmodium* sp. Indeed, Hadley and Chulay (1988) have concluded that the 'control of malaria will probably require a multifaceted approach, involving immunization, chemotherapy, mosquito-eradication, and perhaps even the genetic manipulation of mosquito populations to make them resistant to malaria'.

Management

Treatment of a *P falciparum* infection is in general a less contentious issue than chemoprophylaxis (Cook 1986a, 1988a; Hoffman 1986; Petersen and Leech 1988; White 1988). There can be no doubt that serious and life-threatening *P falciparum* infections are best dealt with by physicians -with considerable experience of this disease, and ideally in intensive therapy units.

Chemotherapy

Advice on chemotherapy is difficult to summarize, but a consensus of opinion is now emerging (Cook 1988a; White 1988). Obviously one must aim for an adequate plasma concentration of the chosen schizonticidal agent, remembering that intestinal absorption is frequently subnormal in a severe infection (see above). In the partly immune individual, management is usually straightforward; in the non-immune, however, treatment must always be started as soon as the diagnosis has been made or even strongly suspected (rapid clinical deterioration can occur within a few hours). The magnitude of the parasite count is an important factor. Table 1.6 summarizes some suitable chemotherapeutic regimens; in most instances quinine (which binds plasmodial DNA) is now the agent of choice (White et al. 1983a; Hoffmann 1986; Wattanagoon et al. 1986), although in some areas (such as Thailand) partial resistance exists. Quinine is a

Table 1.6. Chemotherapeutic regimens that have been used in *P falciparum* infection: adult doses[a]

Agent	Dose during first 4 h	Subsequent dose	Duration course (d)
Quinine (300 mg quinine sulphate/tablet; 300 mg quinine dihydrochloride/ml)	10 mg/kg[b]	10 mg/kg 8-hourly	5–7
Quinidine gluconate	10 mg/kg[b]	10 mg/kg 8-hourly	5–7
Chloroquine[c] (150 mg base/tablet; 40 mg/ml)	10 mg/kg[c]	5 mg/kg after 6 h 5 mg/kg on subsequent 2d	3
'Fansidar'	3 tablets		1
'Fansidar' + mefloquine	3 tablets + 750 mg		1
Mefloquine	0.75g	0.75g	1
Qinghaosu	1.0 g	1.0 g after 24 h	2
Doxycycline[d]	1.5–2 mg/kg	1.5–2 mg/kg 12-hourly	7
Tetracycline[d]	5–6 mg/kg	5–6 mg/kg 6-hourly	7–10
Clindamycin[d]	10 mg/kg	5–10 mg/kg 12 hourly	5

[a]In severely ill patients, the intravenous route should be used when possible. When this route cannot be used, deep intramuscular injections are satisfactory but the oral route can usually be used after 24–48 h.
[b]In severe infections, especially in Thailand, 20 mg/kg is recommended for quinine and 15 mg/kg for quinidine (Chap. 8).
[c]In the partly immune, a single dose is usually effective.
[d]These agents should not be used alone.

safe therapeutic agent when wisely used. Side-effects include [tinnitus], giddiness, tremors, blurred vision, hypotension, urticaria, rashes, cardiac arrhythmias, dysphonia, central nervous system depression, and abdominal pain; high dosage (e.g., in suicide attempts) can cause visual and auditory impairment and cardiac dysfunction. Unusual complications are hypersensitivity reactions, haemolysis, leucopenia, thrombocytopenia, granulomatous hepatitis, and ochronosis. The electrocardiogram may show prolongation of the QT interval and T-wave flattening. Hypoglycaemia (which may also result from *P falciparum* infection *per se*) (White et al. 1983b) and hypotension occasionally follow rapid intravenous infusion. Rate of quinine infusion certainly seems to be an important determinant of drug-induced insulin secretion (Molyneux et al. 1989b). Monitoring of the plasma quinine concentration should be carried out whenever possible. When quinine is not available, quinidine (which should be infused slowly because of its cardiac effects) is an effective alternative (Phillips et al. 1985).

Chloroquine, which has long been the mainstay of chemotherapy, is still valuable (and probably superior to quinine) when the parasite is sensitive to it (Phillips et al, 1986b; White et al. 1987a) and should certainly not be written off (Ellis 1988); since RIII resistance remains infrequent it still has an important place in management. It is also valuable in semi-immune populations. When given by the intramuscular or subcutaneous routes it seldom causes side-effects (Phillips et al. 1986b). Intravenous administration, to achieve a rapidly effective blood concentration, has caused hypotension and other cardiovascular ill-effects, especially in African children (White et al. 1987a). Minor side-effects include gastrointestinal symptoms, dizziness, blurred vision, and generalized pruritus. Severe pruritus is a significant side-effect in some Africans (especially in West Africa) and this can render use of this agent difficult (Burnham et al. 1989; Sowunmi et al. 1989). Extrapyramidal toxicity is rare.

'Fansidar' is slower in action than chloroquine or quinine and should not be used alone in a severe infection; it is usually given in conjunction with quinine. 'Mefloquine' (Jiang et al. 1982; Chanthavanich et al. 1985) is a highly active schizonticide but is moderately slow in action; it is usually combined with 'Fansidar' (Harinasuta et al. 1985; Kofi Ekue et al. 1985) or quinine. Resistance to both of these agents has been recorded, especially in Thailand. Qinghaosu is more rapid in its action (Jiang et al. 1982) and can be given orally or intravenously; side-effects include nausea, vomiting, diarrhoea, dizziness, sinus bradycardia, and acute psychoses. Successful use of a combination regimen of artemether + melfoquine in cerebral malaria has been reported from Burma (Shwe et al. 1989). Several broad-spectrum antibiotics have antiplasmodial properties (Geary and Jensen 1983, 1986; Cook 1986a; Meek et al. 1986; Warhurst 1986a) (Table 1.6): erythromycin (Looareesuwan et al. 1985a), chloramphenicol, clindamycin (Wakeel 1985) and rifampicin are all partly effective (Cook 1986a). In combination with quinine, their action is more rapid than that of either agent alone. The role of both qinghaosu and broad-spectrum antibiotics remains ill-defined. Sulphonamides and co-trimoxazole are also active. Phenanthrene methanols, the most promising of which are halofantrine and enpiroline, are undergoing clinical trial (see below) (Cook 1986a, 1989a; Hoffman 1986).

Severe Infections

Management of a severe *P falciparum* infection (also see Chap. 8) is best entrusted to clinicians experienced with the disease. When the peripheral blood parasitaemia is high (10%–50%) the patient should ideally be cared for in an intensive therapy unit. The first measures should be to record the body-weight, check the airway, collect laboratory specimens (including thick and thin blood films), decide the fluid requirement, and perform a lumbar puncture to exclude meningitis. Table 1.7 summarizes some important aspects of management of a severe or complicated case. In cerebral malaria, a variation in the apparent

Table 1.7. Management of a severe *P falciparum* infection (see also Chap. 8)[a]

Clinical problem	Management
Parasitaemia	Intravenous quinine (see Table 1.6). Exchange blood transfusion hastens reduction of parasitaemia
Hyperpyrexia	Fanning, tepid sponging, cooling blankets, antipyretics. Core temperature should be recorded continuously using a rectal electronic thermometer probe
Pulmonary oedema[b]	Prop up; high inspired O_2 concentration; venesection to induce rapid fall in pulmonary capillary pressure; remove 250 ml blood into donor bag (to be returned as packed cells later); diuretics
Hypoglycaemia	50% glucose intravenously; nasogastric tube with continuous administration sometimes necessary
Cerebral involvement	Maintain airway; phenobarbitone 200 mg intramuscularly for adult (3.5 mg/kg for children) or diazepam (slow intravenous injection)
Severe anaemia (PCV ⩽20%)	Transfusion; beware of pulmonary oedema (see text)
Raised blood nitrogen (>21.4 mmol/l) and serum creatinine (>265 µmol/l) concentration	Maintain urinary output; in 5% of severe cases acute tubular necrosis requires dialysis. An indwelling catheter should be inserted
Shock/hypotension ('algid malaria')	Plasma expanders plus pressor agents (e.g., dopamine). Central venous pressure should be 0–5 cm H_2O. Treat Gram-ve septicaemia
Disseminated intravascular coagulation (DIC)	Infuse fresh whole blood, fresh frozen plasma, red cells, or platelet concentrate; heparin is potentially dangerous
Aspiration pneumonia, and other secondary infections (e.g. Gram-negative septicaemia)	Antimicrobials, oxygen, physiotherapy

[a]Many patients will be comatose, and appropriate nursing procedures (e.g., nursing on the side and light taping of the eyelids to prevent corneal abrasions) must be carefully instituted; in addition, fanning, tepid sponging, cooling blankets and antipyretics should be used to counteract hyperpyrexia.
[b]This is frequently mistaken for a pulmonary infection.

volume of distribution of quinine leads to a higher than expected plasma concentration (White et al. 1983a). Rapid intravenous administration of quinine can also produce hypotension, cardiac arrhythmias, convulsions, and death. Hypoglycaemia is an important complication, especially in late pregnancy (White et al. 1983b); the heavy glucose requirement of the parasite contributes to this. Corticosteroids are *not* indicated in cerebral malaria (Chap. 8) (Warrell et al. 1982; Hoffman 1986). Exchange blood transfusion decreases the level of parasitaemia (Chiodini et al. 1985; Miller et al. 1989) and this procedure is possibly indicated when the peripheral blood parasite concentration is more than 10% in the presence of pulmonary, renal, cerebral, or haemostatic complications, and more than 50% in their absence. Haemodialysis also has a place in the management of severe *P falciparum* infection. Retinoscopy (Looareesuwan et al. 1983) and measurement of CSF lactate (White et al. 1987a) are useful for assessing likely outcome. Problems involved in treatment during infancy and pregnancy (Cook 1986a, 1988a; Hoffman 1986; Mashaal 1986; White 1988) are outlined below.

Management of Special Groups

P falciparum infection is especially dangerous during the last trimester of pregnancy; chloroquine should be used when possible. Quinine occasionally provokes uterine activity, decelerates the foetal heart rate, and causes hypoglycaemia (Looareesuwan et al. 1985b). This agent has not been used as an abortifacient for several centuries without good reason; however, in late pregnancy concern about quinine-induced labour is of secondary importance to the drug's life-saving properties. The physician should always be on the alert for pulmonary oedema immediately before and after delivery. Severe anaemia can be treated by exchange transfusion. Caesarean section, or measures to hasten the second stage of labour, should be considered. Mefloquine has been used successfully in pregnancy and could possibly become the accepted first-line treatment in this situation (Collignon et al. 1989).

In children, parenteral chloroquine seems to produce more severe side-effects than in adults; therefore the dosage should be lower. Hypoglycaemia unrelated to antimalarial treatment can also prove troublesome (White et al. 1987b). The possibility of relapse of a *P vivax* infection after successful treatment of a *P falciparum* infection should be borne in mind (Looareesuwan et al. 1987).

Future Strategies in Chemoprophylaxis and Chemotherapy

Until a *P falciparum* vaccine becomes a reality, much depends on the presently available chemoprophylactic and chemotherapeutic agents, together with the development of newer compounds (Warhurst 1986a, 1987; Peters 1987b; Cook 1988a). Recent advances have been summarized (Cook 1989a). Until relatively recently, the majority of *P falciparum* infections throughout the world were treated with chloroquine (see above); it is a rapidly acting schizonticidal compound and where parasites are sensitive, it remains a superior chemotherapeutic agent to quinine (it also remains the agent of choice for the other three human malaria species). Has chloroquine a future in chemotherapy however? Complete (RIII) resistance is in fact very unusual. Evidence is available, albeit scanty, that resistance of *P falciparum* to this agent decreases as 'drug-pressure' is reduced (Onori and Phan 1986; Thaithong et al. 1988); the latter report refers to the re-emergence of chloroquine-sensitive strains after a brief period of reduced chloroquine usage in Thailand. An interesting possibility in management has recently emerged: i.e., that by adding another therapeutic agent to chloroquine, resistance can be reversed. The calcium antagonist verapamil has been shown to exert just such an action (Martin et al. 1987; Cook 1988b, Jacobs et al. 1988); alteration in calcium homeostasis, lysosomal function, and membrane permeability might all be involved but the mechanism is unclear. These observations have also served to highlight deficiencies in our knowledge of chloroquine-resistance in *P falciparum* (Fitch 1986; Warhurst 1986b, 1988; Krogstad and Schlesinger 1987; Ginsburg 1988). Possible antiplasmodial properties of chloroquine (e.g., monodesethyl-chloroquine) (Gasquet et al. 1987) and other 4-aminoquinoline (e.g., dichlorquinazine) (Bras et al. 1983) derivatives are presently receiving attention.

A new antimalarial agent, pyronaridine, has given encouraging results in China (Childs et al. 1988; Wu et al. 1988). Also, Chinese workers have demonstrated that the tricyclic antihistaminic agent ketotifen, when given with sulfadoxine, exerts schizonticidal activity against *P falciparum* in man. A more potent member of this group is cyproheptadine (which, unlike most antihistaminics, does *not* produce undue drowsiness); Peters et al. (1989) have suggested that a clinical trial of this agent in combination with chloroquine would be justified but emphasize that prior toxicity testing would be necessary. Mefloquine (hydrochloride) (which is not yet commercially available in the UK) is effective both as a chemoprophylactic and chemotherapeutic agent, but resistance is increasingly being reported (Oduola et al. 1987; Simon et al. 1988). Although use in combination with 'Fansidar' has proved successful, objections to this regimen have been made on pharmacodynamic grounds (White 1987).

The sesquiterpene lactone, artemisinin (qinghaosu), which is derived from the wormwood plant *Artemisia annua* L, used in China for many centuries as a febrifuge, has recently received widespread attention and publicity; however, it possesses potentially toxic side-effects and is also only rarely available outside China. Qinghaosu has a unique mode of action and is a more rapidly acting schizonticide than quinine (Warhurst 1986a, 1987; Myint and Shwe 1987; Peters 1987a); its action is potentiated by methoxylated flavones (Elford et al. 1987). In a study using rhesus monkeys infected with *P knowlesi*, artemether (α/β) proved to be a promising agent, which the authors considered warranted clinical trial (Bajpai et al. 1989).

Several broad-spectrum antibiotics and antimicrobial agents possess, albeit relatively weak, antimalarial activity (see above); they should be combined with another antiplasmodial agent (Geary and Jensen 1983; Cook 1986a, 1988a,c; Warhurst 1986a, 1987; Peters 1987b). Doxycycline and tetracycline (neither of which should be used in pregnancy or infancy) have been used successfully in prophylaxis (Pang et al. 1987; Rieckmann 1987). Clindamycin (Wakeel et al. 1985), ciprofloxacin (Krishna et al. 1988) and other quinolones (Midgley et al.

1988), sulphonamides and co-trimoxazole (Warhurst 1986a, 1987; Peters 1987a) also have significant antiplasmodial activity.

The 9-phenanthrenemethanols (halofantrine and enpiroline are the most promising members of this group) (Hoffman 1986; Peters 1987a; Editorial 1989) are also being investigated. Halofantrine has given promising results in clinical trials in imported cases of multi-drug resistant *P falciparum* infection treated in France (Coulaud et al. 1986), and also in Kenya (Watkins et al. 1988) and Malawi (Wirima et al. 1988).

Chronic riboflavin deficiency has been shown to exert an antimalarial effect (Dutta et al. 1985; Cook 1986a, 1988c); work is currently underway to investigate inhibitors of riboflavin metabolism. A riboflavin analog 10-(4'-chlorophenyl)-3-methylflavin exerts significant activity against *P falciparum* in culture (Cowden et al. 1987); 5-deaza-riboflavin has been shown to be active in vitro but not in vivo. Other agents which have been subjected to investigation include emetine and metronidazole (Esposito 1985; James 1985), and cyclosporin A (Nickell et al. 1982).

Infection Caused by *P vivax*, *P ovale* and *P malariae*

Some strains of *P vivax* are resistant to proguanil and pyrimethamine (Peters 1987b) but all except a very small minority are sensitive to chloroquine (Rieckmann et al. 1989). A course of chloroquine (as for *P falciparum* infection) will almost always produce the desired result rapidly and uneventfully (Spencer and Strickland 1984; Bruce-Chwatt 1985; Haworth 1987). When the species is not known with certainty, or a mixed infection is present, the initial treatment should be that for *P falciparum*. The exo-erythrocytic (hypnozoite) cycle (Fig. 1.2) (within the hepatocyte) of *P vivax* and *P ovale* (Shortt and Garnham 1948; Garnham 1988) can only be eradicated with primaquine, 7.5 mg twice a day for 14 days – an agent that does not affect the blood stages of the parasite. In South-east Asia and the Pacific region 25 mg daily is required for a 'radical cure' owing to partial parasite resistance. The main side-effect, arising in patients with glucose-6-phosphate dehydrogenase deficiency (especially the severe Mediterranean and Canton variants) is severe haemolysis. The concentration of this enzyme should therefore be measured before treatment. In patients who are relatively deficient in this enzyme a lower total dose of primaquine (e.g., 45 mg given once weekly for 6 weeks) usually produces a satisfactory cure; careful monitoring is however essential.

Some strains of *P malariae* are also resistant to proguanil and pyrimethamine, but all are sensitive to chloroquine. As with *P falciparum* infection, there is no exo-erythrocytic cycle, and primaquine is therefore not required. In untreated patients the nephrotic syndrome is a serious complication (Kibukamusoke 1984). Figure 1.6 show a young Ugandan patient suffering from this disease. In African children this often presents before 15 years of age and hypertension is common. Some will show *P malariae* in their peripheral blood films whereas affected adults rarely do so. The connection is certainly causal: nephrotic syndrome disappeared from Guyana when *P malariae* was eradicated, and the syndrome can be

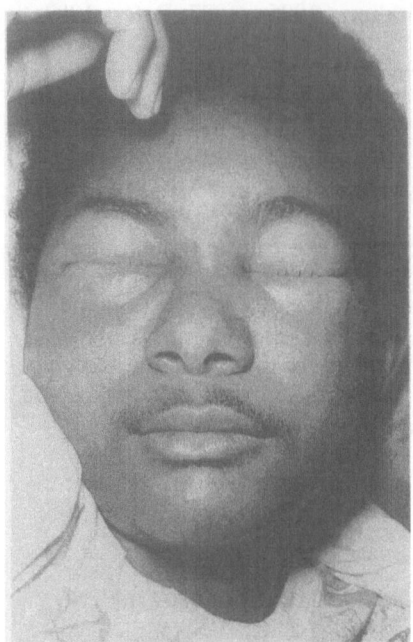

Fig. 1.6. Ugandan boy with a nephrotic syndrome which resulted from a chronic *P malariae* infection.

reproduced by infecting monkeys with this parasite. Antimalarial treatment is not, however, beneficial. Corticosteroids, cyclophosphamide, and azathioprine only occasionally lead to improvement. Remissions are confined to cases with mild proliferative changes.

The best prophylactic regimen for *P vivax*, *P ovale*, and *P malariae* is chloroquine 300 mg weekly.

Hyperreactive Malarious Splenomegaly

In a small minority of individuals infected with any species of human *Plasmodium* (Crane et al. 1977), hyperreactive malarious splenomegaly – an aberrant immunological response formerly known as the tropical splenomegaly syndrome (or simply 'big spleen disease') – is a long-term sequel (Cook 1980; Crane 1986). Figure 1.7 shows a young Papua New Guinean man with proven hyperreactive malarious splenomegaly. It is frequently accompanied by 'hypersplenism': acute haemolytic episodes can occur, especially in infancy, pregnancy, and during lactation. The first step in treatment is a full chemotherapeutic course for the species of *Plasmodium* responsible, followed by lengthy and probably lifelong chemoprophylaxis. The splenomegaly, hepatic sinusoidal lymphocytosis, and raised serum IgM slowly subside. Splenectomy should be avoided, even when splenomegaly is massive, because it will increase the patient's susceptibility to pneumococcal and other bacterial infections in addition to malaria.

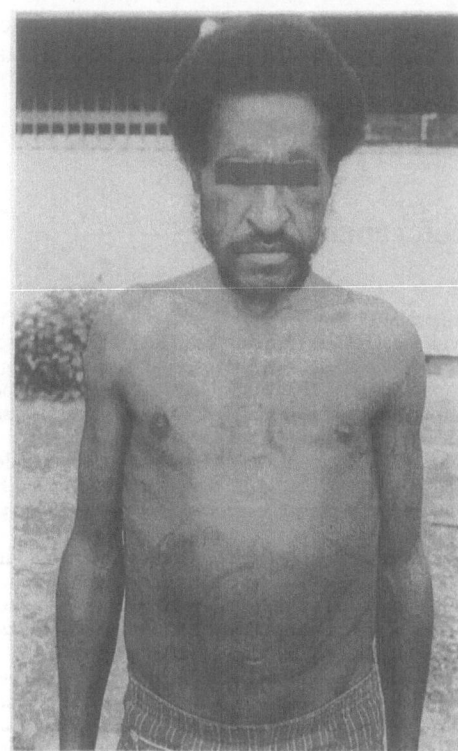

Fig. 1.7. Young Papua New Guinean man with gross splenomegaly (hyperreactive malarious splenomegaly). A needle liver biopsy-specimen showed Kupffer-cell hyperplasia and an intense lymphocytic infiltration in the hepatic sinusoids; serum IgM concentration was greatly elevated.

Conclusions

A vast quantity of work on the human malarias is currently in progress; much of this is designed to simplify diagnosis, and to produce a safe and effective vaccine for *P falciparum* malaria (ideally an oral rather than an injectable one). Meanwhile, the search for alternative antimalarial compounds (for use both in chemoprophylaxis and chemotherapy) continues, and as further resistance to agents currently in use emerges, this is becoming an increasingly urgent matter. Although there must be light at the end of the tunnel it remains distant, and for the average indigenous inhabitant of the rural Third World it is a very long way off indeed. In 1897 Sir Ronald Ross, who had just demonstrated the mosquito component of the mosquito–man cycle of *Plasmodium* sp, wrote (Ross 1988):

> I have found thy secret deeds
> O million-murdering death.
> I know this little thing
> A million men will save.
> O death, where is thy sting?
> Thy victory, O grave?

If he were still alive today, he would be exceedingly disappointed with the lack of progress which has occurred in this crucially important area over the past 100 years!

References

Aikawa M (1988) Human cerebral malaria. Am J Trop Med Hyg 39:3–10

Avidor B, Golenser J, Schutte CHJ, Cox GA, Isaacson M, Sulitzeanu D (1987) A radioimmunoassay for the diagnosis of malaria. Am J Trop Med Hyg 37:225–229

Bajpai R, Dutta GP, Vishwakarma RA (1989) Blood shizontocidal activity of a new antimalarial drug, arteether (α/β), against *Plasmodium knowlesi* in rhesus monkeys. Trans R Soc Trop Med Hyg 83:484

Ballou WR, Hoffman, SL, Sherwood JA, Hollingdale MR, Neva FA, Hockmeyer WT, Gordon DM, Schneider I, Wirtz RA, Young JF, Wasserman GF, Reeve P, Diggs CL, Chulay JD (1987) Safety and efficacy of a recombinant DNA *Plasmodium falciparum* sporozoite vaccine. Lancet i:1277–1281

Bradley AK, Greenwood BM, Greenwood AM, Marsh, K, Byass P, Tulloch S, Hayes R (1986) Bed-nets (mosquito-nets) and morbidity from malaria. Lancet ii:204–207

Brandicourt O, Druilhe P, Brasseur P, Turk P, Diquet B, Datry A, Danis M, Gentilini M (1986) High level of chloroquine resistance in seven *Plasmodium falciparum* malaria cases from the Congo and Gabon. Trans R Soc Trop Med Hyg 80:906–907

Bras J le, Deloron P, Charmot G (1983) Dichlorquinazine (a 4-aminoquinoline) effective in vitro against chloroquine-resistant *Plasmodim falciparum*. Lancet i:73–74

Bras J le, Hatin I, Bouree P, Coco-Cianci O, Garin J-P, Rey M, Charmot G, Roue R (1986) Chloroquine-resistant falciparum malaria in Benin. Lancet ii:1043–1044

Brasseur P, Druilhe P, Kouamouo J, Moyou SR (1987a) Emergence of *Plasmodium falciparum* chloroquine resistance in the Sahel part of West Africa. Trans R Soc Trop Med Hyg 81:162–163

Brasseur P, Pathe-Diallo M, Druilhe P (1987b) Low sensitivity to chloroquine and quinine of *Plasmodium falciparum* isolates from Guinea in March 1986. Am J Trop Med Hyg 37:452–454

Brook MG, Karet F, Lewis DA, Uriel A, Weir WRC (1989) Interpretation of blood films in diagnosis of malaria. Lancet ii:619

Bruce-Chwatt LJ (1983) Malaria and pregnancy. Br Med J 286:1457–1458

Bruce-Chwatt LJ (1985) Essential malariology, 2nd edn. Heinemann, London, pp 51–72, 210–260

Bruce-Chwatt LJ (1987a) From Laveran's discovery to DNA probes: new trends in diagnosis of malaria. Lancet ii:1509–1511

Bruce-Chwatt LJ (1987b) The challenge of malaria vaccine: trials and tribulations. Lancet i:371–373

Bruce-Chwatt LJ (1988a) History of malaria from prehistory to eradication. In: Wernsdorfer WH, McGregor I (eds) Malaria: principles and practice of malariology. Churchill Livingstone, Edinburgh, pp 1–59

Bruce-Chwatt LJ (1988b) Three hundred and fifty years of the Peruvian fever bark. Br Med J 296:1486–1487

Bruce-Chwatt LJ (1988c) Cinchona and its alkaloids: 350 years. NY State J Med 88:318–322

Burnham G, Harries A, Macheso A, Wirima J. Molyneux M (1989) Chloroquine-induced pruritus in Malawi: lack of association with onchocerciasis. Trans R Soc Trop Med Hyg 83:527–528

Campbell GH, Brandling-Bennett AD, Roberts JM, Collins FH, Kaseje DCO, Barber AM, Turner A (1987) Detection of antibodies in human sera to the repeating epitope of the circumsporozoite protein of *Plasmodium falciparum* using the synthetic peptide (NANP)$_3$ in an enzyme-linked immunosorbent assay (ELISA). Am J Trop Med Hyg 37:17–21

Chanthavanich P, Looaressuwan S, White NJ, Warrell DA, Warrell MJ, DiGiovanni JH, Bredow J. von (1985) Intragastric mefloquine is absorbed rapidly in patients with cerebral malaria. Am J Trop Med Hyg 34:1028–1036

Childs GE, Haüsler B, Milhous W, Chen C, Wimonwattrawatee T, Pooyindee N, Boudreau EF (1988) In vitro activity of pyronaridine against field isolates and reference clones of *Plasmodium falciparum*. Am J Trop Med Hyg 38:24–29

Chiodini PL, Somerville M, Salam I, Tubbs HR, Wood MJ, Ellis CJ (1985) Exchange transfusion in severe falciparum malaria. Trans R Soc Tro Med Hyg 79:865–866

Collignon P, Hehir J, Mitchell D (1989) Successful treatment of falciparum malaria in pregnancy with mefloquine. Lancet i:967

Cook GC (1980) The tropical splenomegaly syndrome and other splenic diseases in the tropics. In: Tropical gastroenterology. Oxford University Press, Oxford, pp 205–221

Cook GC (1986a) *Plasmodium falciparum* infection: problems in prophylaxis and treatment in 1986. Q J Med 61:1091–1115

Cook GC (1986b) Serious problems with antimalarial drugs. J Infect 13:1–4

Cook GC (1988a) Prevention and treatment of malaria. Lancet i:32–37

Cook GC (1988b) Chemotherapy of parasitic infections. Curr Opin Infect Dis 1:423–438

Cook GC (1988c) Malaria prophylaxis and treatment: present and future. Curr Med Lit: Infect Dis 2:1–5

Cook GC (1989a) The great malaria problem: where is the light at the end of the tunnel? J Infect 18:1–10

Cook GC (1989b) The great malaria problem. Natl Med J India 2:57

Cook GC (1990) Hepatic structure and function in experimental and human malaria. In: Bianchi L (ed) Infectious diseases of the liver. MTP Press Lancaster (in press)

Coulaud JP, Bras J le, Matheron S, Morinière B, Saimot AG, Rossignol JF (1986) Treatment of imported cases of falciparum malaria in France with halofantrine. Trans R Soc Trop Med Hyg 80:615–617

Cowden WB, Butcher GA, Hunt NH, Clark IA, Yoneda F (1987) Antimalarial activity of a riboflavin analog against *Plasmodium vinckei* in vivo and *Plasmodium falciparum* in vitro. Am J Trop Med Hyg 37:495–500

Cox FEG (1988a) Vaccine development: which way for malaria? Nature 331:486–487

Cox FEG (1988b) Malaria vaccines: the shape of things to come. Nature 333:702

Crane GG (1986) Hyperreactive malarious splenomegaly (tropical splenomegaly syndrome). Parasitol Today 2:4–9

Crane GG, Gardner A, Hudson P, Hudson B, Voller A (1977) Malarial antibodies in tropical splenomegaly syndrome in Papua New Guinea. Trans R Soc Trop Med Hyg 71:308–314

Deloron P, Le Bras J, Savel J, Coulaud JP (1987) Antibodies to the PF155 antigen of *Plasmodium falciparum*: measurement by cell-ELISA and correlation with expected immune protection. Am J Trop Med Hyg 37:22–26

DeSilva HJ, Goonetilleke AKE, Senaratna N, Ramesh N, Jayawickrama US, Jayasinghe KSA, Amarasekera LR (1988) Skeletal muscle necrosis in severe falciparum malaria. Br Med J 296:1039

Dutta P, Pinto J, Rivlin R (1985) Antimalarial effects of riboflavin deficiency. Lancet ii:1040–1043

Editorial (1983) Malaria in pregnancy. Lancet ii:84–85

Editorial (1985) *Plasmodium falciparum*: a major health hazard to Africans and Asians returning home. Lancet ii:871–872

Editorial (1989) Halofantrine in the treatment of malaria. Lancet ii:537–538

Edstein MD, Veenendaal JR, Rieckmann KH, O'Donoghue M (1988) Failure of dapsone/pyrimethamine plus chloroquine against falciparum malaria in Papua New Guinea. Lancet i:237

Elford BC, Roberts MF, Phillipson JD, Wilson RJM (1987) Potentiation of the antimalarial activity of qinghaosu by methoxylated flavones. Trans R Soc Trop Med Hyg 81:434–436

Ellis CJ (1988) Death despite malaria prophylaxis. Br Med J 296:952

Esposito R (1985) Emetine and metronidazole as antimalarial drugs. Lancet ii:784

Fitch CD (1986) Antimalarial schizontocides: ferriprotoporphyrin IX interaction hypothesis. Parasitol Today 2:330–331

Fogh S, Schapira A, Bygbjerg IC, Jepsen S, Mordhorst CH, Kuijlen K, Ravn P, Rønn A, Gøtzsche PC (1988) Malaria chemoprophylaxis in travellers to east Africa: a comparative prospective study of chloroquine plus proguanil with chloroquine plus sulfadoxine-pyrimethamine. Br Med J 296:820–822

Garnham PCC (1988) Hypnozoites and 'relapses' in *Plasmodium vivax* and in vivax-like malaria. Trop Geog Med 40:187–195

Gasquet M, Atouk A, Samat A, Timon-David P, Viala A (1987) In vitro chemosensitivity of *Plasmodium falciparum* to four chloroquine derivatives. Ann Trop Med Parasitol 81:355–358

Geary TG, Jensen JB (1983) Effects of antibiotics on *Plasmodium falciparum* in vitro. Am J Trop Med Hyg 32:221–225

Geary TG, Jensen JB (1986) Protozoan infections of man: malaria. In: Campbell WC, Rew RS (eds) Chemotherapy of parasitic diseases. Plenum Press, New York, pp 87–114

Ginsburg H (1988) Effect of calcium antagonists on malaria susceptibility to chloroquine. Parasitol Today 4:209–211

Gubler J (1988) Sulfadoxine-pyrimethamine resistant malaria from west or central Africa. Br Med J 296:433

Hadley TJ, Chulay JD (1988) Perspectives on immunization against malaria. In: Leech JH, Sande MA, Root RK (eds) Parasitic infections. Churchill Livingstone, New York and Edinburgh, pp 285–310

Harinasuta T, Bunnag D, Lasserre R, Leimer R, Vinijanont S (1985) Trials of mefloquine in vivax and of mefloquine plus 'Fansidar' in falciparum malaria. Lancet i:885–888

Hatton CSR, Peto TEA, Bunch C, Pasvol G, Russell SJ, Singer CRJ, Edwards G, Winstanley P (1986) Frequency of severe neutropenia associated with amodiaquine prophylaxis against malaria. Lancet i:411–414

Haworth J (1987) Malaria in man: its epidemiology, clinical aspects and control. Trop Dis Bull 84:R1–R51

Hernborg A (1985) Stevens–Johnson syndrome after mass prophylaxis with sulfadoxine for cholera in Mozambique. Lancet ii:1072–1073

Higgins DG, McConnell DJ, Sharp PM (1989) Malarial proteinase? Nature 340:604

Hoffman SL (1986) Treatment of malaria. In: Strickland GT (ed) Clinics in tropical medicine and communicable diseases, vol 1. Saunders, Philadelphia, pp 171–224

Hoffman SL, Wistar R, Ballou WR, Hollingdale MR, Wirtz RA, Schneider I, Marwoto HA, Hockmeyer WT (1986) Immunity of malaria and naturally acquired antibodies to the circumsporozoite protein of *Plasmodium falciparum*. N Engl J Med 315:601–606

Holmberg M, Shenton FC, Franzén L, Janneh K, Snow RW, Pettersson U, Wigzell H, Greenwood BM (1987) Use of a DNA hybridization assay for the detection of *Plasmodium falciparum* in field trials. Am J Trop Med Hyg 37:230–234

Hutchinson DBA, Whiteman PD, Farquhar JA (1986) Agranulocytosis associated with Maloprim: a review of cases. Hum Toxicol 5:221–227

Jackson DV, Marcarelli P, Segal G (1987) Chloroquine-resistant *Plasmodium falciparum* malaria in West Africa. MMWR 36:13–14

Jacobs GH, Oduola AMJ, Kyle DE, Milhous WK, Martin SK, Aikawa M (1988) Ultrastructural study of the effects of chloroquine and verapamil on *Plasmodium falciparum*. Am J Trop Med Hyg 39:15–20

James RF (1985) Malaria treated with emetine or metronidazole. Lancet ii:498

Jiang J-B, Li G-Q, Guo X-B, Kong YC, Arnold K (1982) Antimalarial activity of mefloquine and qinghaosu. Lancet ii:285–288

Katongole-Mbidde E, Banura C, Kizito A (1988) Blackwater fever caused by *Plasmodium vivax* infection in the acquired immune deficiency syndrome. Br Med J 296:827

Khusmith S, Tharavanij S, Chongsa-Nguan M, Vejvongvarn C, Kasemsuth R (1988) Field applications of an immunoradiometric assay for the detection of *Plasmodium falciparum* antigen in a population in a malaria endemic area in Thailand. Am J Trop Med Hyg 38:1–6

Kibukamusoke JW (1984) Quartan malaria nephropathy. In: Kibukamusoke JW (ed) Tropical nephrology. Citforge, Canberra, pp 58–75

Kofi Ekue JM, Simooya OO, Sheth UK, Wernsdorfer WH, Njelesani EK (1985) A double-blind clinical trial of a combination of mefloquine, sulfadoxine and pyrimethamine in symptomatic falciparum malaria. Bull WHO 63:339–343

Krishna S, Davis TME, Chan PCY, Wells RA, Robson KJH (1988) Ciprofloxacin and malaria. Lancet i:1231–1232

Krogstad DJ, Schlesinger PH (1987) The basis of antimalarial action: non-weak base effects of chloroquine on acid vesicle pH. Am J Trop Med Hyg 36:213–220

Kwiatkowski D, Greenwood BM (1989) Why is malaria fever periodic? A hypothesis. Parasitol Today 5:264–266

Larrey D, Castot A, Pessayre D, Merigot P, Machayekhy J-P, Feldmann G, Lenoir A, Rueff B, Benhamou J-P (1986) Amodiaquine-induced hepatitis: a report of seven cases. Ann Intern Med 104:801–803

Laveran A (1881) Un nouveau parasite trouvé dans le sang des malades atteints de fièvre palustre. Bull Soc Med Hop Paris (Mem) 17:158–164

Lee PS, Lau EYL (1988) Risk of acute non-specific upper respiratory tract infections in healthy men taking dapsone-pyrimethamine for prophylaxis against malaria. Br Med J 296:893–895

Lim TS (1988) A sensitive malaria immunoperoxidase assay for the detection of *Plasmodium falciparum* antibody. Am J Trop Med Hyg 38:255–257

Lobel HO, Campbell CC (1986) Malaria prophylaxis and distribution of drug resistance. In:

Strickland GT (ed) Clinics in tropical medicine and communicable diseases, vol 1. Saunders, Philadelphia, pp 225–242

Lobel HO, Campbell CC, Pappaioanou M, Huong AY (1987) Use of prophylaxis for malaria by American travelers to Africa and Haiti. JAMA 257:2626–2627

Looareesuwan S, Warrell DA, White NJ, Chanthavanich P, Warrell MJ, Chantaratherakitti S, Changswek S, Chongmankongcheep L, Kanchanaranya C (1983) Retinal haemorrhage, a common sign of prognostic significance in cerebral malaria. Am J Trop Med Hyg 32:911–915

Looareesuwan S, Phillips RE, White NJ, Karbwang J, Benjasurat Y, Attanath P, Warrell DA (1985a) Intravenous amodiaquine and oral amodiaquine/erythromycin in the treatment of chloroquine-resistant falciparum malaria. Lancet ii:805–808

Looareesuwan S, Phillips RE, White NJ, Kietinun S. Karbwang J, Rackow C, Turner RC, Warrell DA (1985b) Quinine and severe falciparum malaria in late pregnancy. Lancet ii:4–8

Looareesuwan S, White NJ, Chittamas S, Bunnag D, Harinasuta T (1987) High rate of *Plasmodium vivax* relapse following treatment of falciparum malaria in Thailand. Lancet ii:1052–1055

Lumsden WHR (1989) Sweating it out. Br Med J 299:1341

Malaria Reference Laboratory (1989) Prophylaxis against malaria for travellers from the United Kingdom. Br Med J 299:1087–1089

Manson P (1900) Experimental proof of the mosquito-malaria theory. Br Med J ii:949–951

Manson-Bahr PEC, Bell DR (1987) Malaria and babesiosis. In: Manson's tropical diseases, 19th edn. Baillière, Tindall, London, 3–51

Martin SK, Oduola AMJ, Milhous WK (1987) Reversal of chloroquine resistance in *Plasmodium falciparum* by verapamil. Science 235:899–901

Mashaal H (1986) Malaria in infants and children. In: Clinical malariology 1986. Japan: Southeast Asian Medical Information Center, Japan, 126–40

McLaughlin GL, Breman JG, Collins FH, Schwartz IK, Brandling-Bennett AD, Sulzer AJ, Collins WE, Skinner JC, Ruth JL, Andrysiak PM, Kaseje DCO, Campbell GH (1987) Assessment of a synthetic DNA probe for *Plasmodium falciparum* in African blood specimens. Am J Trop Med Hyg 37:27–36

Meek SR, Doberstyn EB, Gaüzère BA, Thanapanich C, Nordlander E, Phuphaisan S (1986) Treatment of falciparum malaria with quinine and tetracycline or combined mefloquine/sulfadoxine/pyrimethamine on the Thai–Kampuchean border. Am J Trop Med Hyg 35:246–250

Midgley JM, Keter DW, Phillipson JD, Grant S, Warhurst DC (1988) Quinolones and multiresistant *Plasmodium falciparum*. Lancet ii:281

Miller KD, Lobel HO, Pappaioanou M, Patchen LC, Churchill FC (1986a) Failures of combined chloroquine and Fansidar prophylaxis in American travellers to East Africa. J Infect Dis 154:689–691

Miller KD, Lobel HO, Satriale RF, Kuritsky JN, Stern R, Campbell CC (1986b) Severe cutaneous reactions among American travelers using pyrimethamine-sulfadoxine (Fansidar) for malaria prophylaxis. Am J Trop Med Hyg 35:451–458

Miller KD, Greenberg AE, Campbell CC (1989) Treatment of severe malaria in the United States with a continuous infusion of quinidine gluconate and exchange transfusion. N Engl J Med 321:65–70

Miller LH (1986) Research in malaria vaccines. N Eng J Med 315:640–641

Miller LH (1988) Malaria: effective vaccine for humans? Nature 332:109–110

Molyneux ME, Looareesuwan S, Menzies IS, Grainger SL, Phillips RE, Wattanagoon Y, Thompson RPH, Warrell DA (1989a) Reduced hepatic blood flow and intestinal malabsorption in severe falciparum malaria. Am J Trop Med Hyg 40:470–476

Molyneux ME, Taylor TE, Wirima JJ, Harper G (1986b) Effect of rate of infusion of quinine on insulin and glucose responses in Malawian children with falciparum malaria. Br Med J 299:602–603

Myint PT, Shwe T (1987) A controlled clinical trial of artemether (qinghaosu derivative) versus quinine in complicated and severe falciparum malaria. Trans R Soc Trop Med Hyg 81:559–561

Nahlen BL, Akintunde A, Alakija T, Ngugen-Dinh P, Ogunbode O, Edungbola LD, Adetoro O, Breman JG (1989) Lack of efficacy of pyrimethamine prophylaxis in pregnant Nigerian women. Lancet ii:830–834

Neeguaye J (1986) In vivo chloroquine-resistant falciparum malaria in western Africa. Lancet i:153

Neftel KA, Woodtly W, Schmid M, Frick PG, Fehr J (1986) Amodiaquine induced agranulocytosis and liver damage. Br Med J 292:721–723

Nevill CG, Watkins WM, Carter JY, Munafu CG (1988) Comparison of mosquito nets, proguanil hydrochloride, and placebo to prevent malaria. Br Med J 297:401–403

Nguyen-Dinh P, Greenberg AE, Ryder RW, Mann JM (1987a) Absence of association between HIV seropositivity and *Plasmodium falciparum* malaria in Kinshasa, Zaire. Abstracts of Third International Conference on AIDS, Washington, DC, p 22

Nguyen-Dinh P, Berzins K, Collins WE, Wahlgren M, Udomsangpetch R, Perlmann P (1987b) Antibodies to PF155, a major antigen of *Plasmodium falciparum*: longitudinal studies in humans. Am J Trop Med Hyg 37:501–505

Nickell SP, Scheibel LW, Cole GA (1982) Inhibition by cyclosporin A of rodent malaria in vivo and human malaria in vitro. Infect Immunol 37:1093–1100

Nussenzweig V, Nussenzweig RS (1986) Development of a sporozoite malaria vaccine. Am J Trop Med Hyg 35:678–688

Oduola AMJ, Milhous WK, Salako LA, Walker O, Desjardins RE (1987) Reduced in-vitro susceptibility to mefloquine in west African isolates of *Plasmodium falciparum*. Lancet ii:1304–1305

Onori E, Phan VT (1986) Is *Plasmodium falciparum* resistance to chloroquine reversible in absence of drug pressure? Lancet i:319

Pang LW, Linsomwong N, Boudreau EF, Singharaj P (1987) Doxycycline prophylaxis for falciparum malaria. Lancet i:1161–1164

Pappaioanou M, Fishbein DB, Dreesen DW, Schwartz IK, Campbell GH, Sumner JW, Patchen LC, Brown WJ (1986) Antibody response to preexposure human diploid-cell rabies vaccine given concurrently with chloroquine. N Engl J Med 314:280–284

Patarroyo ME, Amador R, Clavijo P, Moreno A, Guzman F, Romero P, Tascon R, Franco A, Murillo LA, Ponton G, Trujillo G (1988) A synthetic vaccine protects humans against challenge with asexual blood stages of *Plasmodium falciparum* malaria. Nature 332:158–161

Peters W (1987a) Chemotherapy and drug resistance in malaria, 2nd edn. Academic Press, Orlando and London, p 1100

Peters W (1987b) How to prevent malaria. Trop Doct 17:1–3

Peters W, Ekong R, Robinson BL, Warhurst DC, Pan X-Q (1989) Antihistaminic drugs that reverse chloroquine resistance in *Plasmodium falciparum*. Lancet ii:334–335

Petersén C, Leech JH (1988) Diagnosis, treatment, and prevention of malaria due to *Plasmodium falciparum*. In: Leech JH, Sande MA, Root RK (eds) Parasitic infections. Churchill Livingstone, New York and Edinburgh, pp 311–326

Peto TEA, Gilks CF (1986) Strategies for the prevention of malaria in travellers: comparison of drug regimens by means of risk–benefit analysis. Lancet i:1256–1261

Phillips RE, Warrell DA, White NJ, Looareesuwan S, Karbwang J (1985) Intravenous quinidine for the treatment of severe falciparum malaria: clinical and pharmacokinetic studies. N Engl J Med 312:1273–1278

Phillips RE, Looareesuwan S, Warrell DA, Lee SH, Karbwang J, Warrell MJ, White NJ, Swasdichai C, Weatherall DJ (1986a) The importance of anaemia in cerebral and uncomplicated falciparum malaria: role of complications, dyserythropoiesis and iron sequestration. Q J Med 58:305–323

Phillips RE, Warrell DA, Edwards G, Galagedera Y, Theakstone RDG, Abeysekera DTDJ, Dissanayaka P (1986b) Divided dose intramuscular regimen and single dose subcutaneous regimen for chloroquine: plasma concentrations and toxicity in patients with malaria. Br Med J 293:13–16

Phillips-Howard PA, Bradley DJ, Blaze M, Hurn M (1988) Malaria in Britain: 1977–86. Br Med J 296:245–248

Phillips-Howard PA, Behrens RH, Dunlop J (1989) Stevens–Johnson Syndrome due to pyrimethamine/sulfadoxine during presumptive self-therapy of malaria. Lancet ii:803–804

Public Health Laboratory Service Malaria Reference Laboratory (1984) Prevention of malaria in pregnancy and early childhood. Br Med J 289:1296–1297

Reisinger EC, Horstmann RD, Dietrich M (1989) Tolerance of mefloquine alone and in combination with sulfadoxine-pyrimethamine in the prophylaxis of malaria. Trans R Soc Trop Med Hyg 83:474–477

Rhodes EGH, Ball J, Franklin IM (1986) Amodiaquine induced agranulocytosis: inhibition of colony growth in bone marrow by antimalarial agents. Br Med J 292:717–718

Rieckmann KH (1987) Tetracycline prophylaxis for malaria. Lancet ii:507–508

Rieckmann KH, Davis DR, Hutton DC (1989) *Plasmodium vivax* resistance to chloroquine? Lancet ii:1183–1184

Rickman LS, Long GW, Hoffman SL (1989a) Rapid diagnosis of malaria. Lancet i:1271

Rickman LS, Long GW, Oberst R, Cabanban A, Sangalang R, Smith JI, Chulay JD, Hoffman SL (1989b) Rapid diagnosis of malaria by acridine orange staining of centrifuged parasites. Lancet i:68–71

Ristic M (ed) (1988) Babesiosis of domestic animals and man. CRC Press, Boca Raton, Florida, p 255

Rizzo F, Morandi N, Riccio G, Ghiazza G, Caravelli P (1989) Unusual transmission of falciparum malaria in Italy. Lancet i:555–556

Rosenberg R, Wirtz RA, Lanar DE, Sattabongkot J, Hall T, Waters AP, Prasittisuk C (1989) Circumsporozoite protein heterogeneity in the human malaria parasite *Plasmodium vivax*. Science 245:973–976

Ross R (1897) On some peculiar pigmented cells found in two mosquitos fed on malarial blood. Br Med J ii:1786–1788

Ross (1898) The rôle of the mosquito in the evolution of the malarial parasite. Lancet ii:488–489

Ross R (1988) The great malaria problem and its solution: from the memoirs of Ronald Ross. Keynes Press, London, p 236

Ruebush TK (1984) Babesiosis. In: Strickland GT (ed) Hunter's tropical medicine, 6th edn. Saunders, Philadelphia, pp 608–611

Saarinen M, Thoren E, Iyambo N, Carlstedt A, Shinyafa L, Fernanda M, Paajanen H, Paajanen K, Indongo I, Rombo L (1987) Mass proguanil prophylaxis. Lancet i:985–986

Schofield L, Villaquiran J, Ferreira A, Schellekens H, Nussenzweig R, Nussenzweig V (1987) Interferon, $CD8^+$ T cells and antibodies required for immunity to malaria sporozoites. Nature 330:664–666

Shortt HE, Garnham PCC (1948) Demonstration of a persisting exo-erythrocytic cycle in *Plasmodium cynomolgi* and its bearing on the production of relapses. Br Med J i:1225–1228

Shortt HE, Garnham PCC, Covell G, Shute PG (1948) The pre-erythrocytic stage of human malaria. *Plasmodium vivax*. Br Med J i:547

Shwe T, Myint PT, Myint W, Htut Y, Soe L, Thwe M (1989) Clinical studies on treatment of cerebral malaria with artemether and mefloquine. Trans R Soc Trop Med Hyg 83:489

Simon F, Bras J le, Gaudebout C, Girard PM (1988) Reduced sensitivity of *Plasmodium falciparum* to mefloquine in west Africa. Lancet i:467–468

Simooya OO, Mwendapole RM, Siziya S, Fleming AF (1988) Relation between falciparum malaria and HIV seropositivity in Ndola, Zambia. Br Med J 297:30–31

Slutsker L, Breman JG, Campbell CC (1988) Strategies for control of malaria in Africa. Lancet ii:283

Sowunmi A, Walker O, Salako LA (1989) Pruritus and antimalarial drugs in Africans. Lancet ii:213

Spencer HC, Strickland GT (1984) Malaria. In: Strickland GT (ed) Hunter's tropical medicine, 6th edn. Saunders, Philadelphia, pp 516–552

Spielman A, Perrone JB (1989) Rapid diagnosis of malaria. Lancet i:727

Stemberger H, Leimer R, Wiedermann G (1984) Tolerability of long-term prophylaxis with Fansidar: a randomized double-blind study in Nigeria. Acta Trop (Basel) 41:391–399

Stringer C (1988) The dates of Eden. Nature 331:565–566

Stringer CB, Andrews P (1988) Genetic and fossil evidence for the origin of modern humans. Science 239:1263–1268

Stuiver PC, Ligthelm RJ, Goud TJLM (1989) Acute psychosis after mefloquine. Lancet ii:282

Taylor DN, Pitarangsi C, Echeverria P, Diniega BM (1988) *Campylobacter* enteritis during doxycycline prophylaxis for malaria in Thailand. Lancet ii:578–579

Thaithong S, Suebsaeng L, Rooney W, Beale GH (1988) Evidence of increased chloroquine sensitivity in Thai isolates of *Plasmodium falciparum*. Trans R Soc Trop Med Hyg 82:37–38

Ti T-Y, Jacob E, Wee YJ (1987) The effect of dapsone-pyrimethamine on immunoglobulin concentrations in malaria chemoprophylaxis. Trans R Soc Trop Med Hyg 81:245–246

Trager W (1989) Erythrocyte knobs and malaria. Nature 340:352

Udezue EO (1985) Persistence of malarial antibody in Nigerian children born in the UK and its clinical relevance. Trans R Soc Trop Med Hyg 79:427–429

Udomsangpetch R, Aikawa M, Berzins K, Wahlgren M, Perlmann P (1989) Cytoadherence of knobless *Plasmodium falciparum*-infected erythrocytes and its inhibition by a human monoclonal antibody. Nature 338:763–765

Wakeel El S El, Homeida MMA, Ali HM, Geary TG, Jensen JB (1985) Clindamycin for the treatment of falciparum malaria in Sudan. Am J Trop Med Hyg 34:1065–1068

Warhurst DC (1986a) Antimalarial drugs: mode of action and resistance. J Antimicrob Chemother 18 [suppl B]:51–59

Warhurst DC (1986b) Antimalarial schizontocides: why a permease is necessary. Parasitol Today 2:331–334

Warhurst DC (1987) Antimalarial drugs: an update. Drugs 33:50–65

Warhurst DC (1988) Mechanism of chloroquine resistance in malaria. Parasitol Today 4:211–213

Warrell DA (1987) Pathophysiology of severe falciparum malaria in man. Parasitology 94:S53–S76

Warrell DA, Looareesuwan S, Warrell MJ, Kasemsarn P, Intaraprasert R, Bunnag D, Harinasuta T (1982) Dexamethasone proves deleterious in cerebral malaria: a double-blind trial in 100 comatose patients. N Engl J Med 306:313–319

Waters AP, McCutchan TF (1989) Rapid, sensitive diagnosis of malaria based on ribosomal DNA. Lancet i:1343–1346

Watkins WM, Branding-Bennett AD, Oloo AJ, Howells RE, Gilles HM, Koech DK (1987) Inadequacy of chlorproguanil 20 mg per week as chemoprophylaxis for falciparum malaria in Kenya. Lancet i:125–128

Watkins WM, Oloo JA, Lury JD, Mosoba M, Kariuki D, Mjomba M, Koech DK, Gilles HM (1988) Efficacy of multiple-dose halofantrine in treatment of chloroquine-resistant falciparum malaria in children in Kenya. Lancet ii:247–250

Wattanagoon Y, Phillips RE, Warrell DA, Silamut K, Looareesuwan S, Nagachinta B, Back DJ (1986) Intramuscular loading dose of quinine for falciparum malaria: pharmacokinetics and toxicity. Br Med J 293:11–13

Webster HK, Ho M, Looareesuwan S, Pavanand K, Wattanagoon Y, Warrell DA, Hockmeyer WT (1988) Lymphocyte responsiveness to a candidate malaria sporozoite vaccine (R32$_{tet32}$) of individuals with naturally acquired Plasmodium falciparum malaria. Am J Trop Med Hyg 38:37–41

Wernsdorfer WH, MacGregor I (eds) (1988) Malaria: principles and practice of malariology (2 vols). Churchill Livingstone, Edinburgh, p 1818

White NJ (1987) Combination treatment for falciparum prophylaxis. Lancet i:680–681

White NJ (1988) The treatment of falciparum malaria. Parasitol Today 4:10–14

White NJ, Looareesuwan S, Warrell DA, Warrell MJ, Chanthavanich P, Bunnag D, Harinasuta T (1983a) Quinine loading dose in cerebral malaria. Am J Trop Med Hyg 32:1–5

White NJ, Warrell DA, Chanthavanich P, Looareesuwan S, Warrell MJ, Krishna S, Williamson DH, Turner RC (1983b) Severe hypoglycemia and hyperinsulinemia in falciparum malaria. N Engl J Med 309:61–66

White NJ, Miller KD, Brown J, Marsh K, Greenwood B (1987a) Prognostic value of CSF lactate in cerebral malaria. Lancet i:1261

White NJ, Miller KD, Marsh K, Berry CD, Turner RC, Williamson DH, Brown J (1987b) Hypoglycaemia in African children with severe malaria. Lancet i:708–711

White NJ, Watt G, Bergqvist Y, Njelesani EK (1987c) Parenteral chloroquine for treating falciparum malaria. J Infect Dis 155:192–201

Whiteley HE, Everitt JI, Kakoma I, James MA, Ristic M (1987) Pathologic changes associated with fatal Plasmodium falciparum infection in the Bolivian squirrel monkey (Saimiri sciureus bolivien-sis). Am J Trop Med Hyg 37:1–8

Whitfield D, Curtis CF, White GB, Targett GAT, Warhurst DC, Bradley DJ (1984) Two cases of falciparum malaria acquired in Britain. Br Med J 289:1607–1609

Williams A, Lewis DJM (1987) Malaria prophylaxis: postal questionnaire survey of general practitioners in south-east Wales. Br Med J 295:1449–1452

Win K, Thwe Y, Lwin TT, Win K (1985) Combination of mefloquine with sulfadoxine-pyrimetha-mine compared with two sulfadoxine-pyrimethamine combinations in malaria chemoprophylaxis. Lancet ii:694–695

Wirima J, Khoromana C, Molyneux ME, Gilles HM (1988) Clinical trials with halofantrine hydrochloride in Malawi. Lancet ii:250–252

Wirth DF, Rogers WO, Barker R, Dourado H, Suesebang L, Albuquerque B (1986) Leishmaniasis and malaria: new tools for epidemiologic analysis. Science 234:975–979

World Health Organisation (1973) Chemotherapy of malaria and resistance to antimalarials. World Health Organisation, Geneva, pp 30–54 (WHO Tech Rep Ser 529)

World Health Organisation (1987) World malaria situation, 1985. World Health Stat Q 40:142–170

World Health Organisation (1988) Vaccination certificate requirements and health advice for international travel. WHO, Geneva, p 85

Wright IG, Goodger BV, Clark IA (1988) Immunopathophysiology of Babesia bovis and Plasmodium falciparum infections. Parasitol Today 4:214–218

Wu L-J, Rabbege JR, Nagasawa H, Jacobs G, Aikawa M (1988) Morphological effects of pyronaridine on malarial parasites. Am J Trop Med Hyg 38:30–36

Chapter 2

'Opportunistic' and Other Parasitic Infections in Relation to the Acquired Immune Deficiency Syndrome (AIDS)*

Patients rarely die of the disease from which they suffer; secondary or terminal infections are the real cause of death.

Sir William Osler (1849–1919),
St Bartholomew's Hospital Reports 1916, 52:39

Introduction

The acquired immune deficiency syndrome (AIDS) is generally considered to be caused by the HIV-1 and HIV-2 retroviruses, despite a minority viewpoint that the close correlation between infection with these agents and the clinical syndrome does not necessarily establish beyond doubt a causative role (Duesberg 1989). The origin of these viruses is the subject of much conjecture (Penny 1988; Sharp and Li 1988; McClure and Schulz 1989; Seale 1989). Although extremely important in 'Western' countries, the brunt of the pandemic is being felt in developing ones, especially those in Africa (De Cock et al. 1989; Reeve 1989) where the impact on human population growth and structure over the next few decades is likely to be massive (Anderson et al. 1988). With the prospect of an effective vaccine merely a distant dream (Newmark 1988; Ada 1989), these infections (and their associated diseases) are likely to constitute a dominant theme in health care in a world context for many generations to come.

Initial awareness of the existence of AIDS resulted largely from the recognition of an unusually high incidence of 'opportunistic' infections and Kaposi's sarcoma in groups of individuals in the USA now known to be at 'high risk' for this disease (Pape et al. 1983). Notable amongst these infections is the protozoan parasite

---

*NB Chapters 4 and 9 should be read in conjunction with this one.

Pneumocystis carinii (Blaser and Cohn 1986). In addition, several other such infections, including *Cryptosporidium* sp and various other small-intestinal coccidia (Chap. 4), and *Toxoplasma gondii* (Chap. 9) have been shown to be important in shaping the course of disease in AIDS, both in the Western world (Pape et al. 1983; Blaser and Cohn 1986; Tuazon and Labriola 1987) and in Africa (Bureau of Hygiene and Tropical Diseases 1985; Quinn et al. 1986; Sewankambo et al. 1987). Infection of the respiratory tract (with *P carinii*) and central nervous system (with *T gondii*) gives rise to significant morbidity and mortality, and the gastrointestinal infections – *Cryptosporidium* sp, *Isospora belli*, *Sarcocystis hominis* and *Microsporidium* sp – by producing severe diarrhoea and malabsorption (Pape et al. 1983) are important contributors to the gross weight-loss which is a major clinical feature of AIDS (Malebranche et al. 1983; Modigliani et al. 1985; Gelb and Miller 1986) and is especially important in Africa (Quinn et al. 1986; Sewankambo et al. 1987). It seems likely that the relative prevalence of these infections in individuals harbouring the major human immunodeficiency virus (HIV-1) and related retroviruses including HIV-2, is dependent in part at least upon geographical factors and the prevalence of these organisms in the population group under consideration (Cook 1987a). All of them are usually self-limiting in the immune-competent individual. Overall, diagnosis of an opportunistic parasitic infection does not usually present insuperable difficulty (although there are some problems with toxoplasmosis); however, treatment is extremely unsatisfactory (Bureau of Hygiene and Tropical Diseases 1985). Until satisfactory treatment of the causative retroviruses is forthcoming (Editorial 1989; Ezzell 1989), accurate diagnosis and treatment of the opportunistic infections, when possible, constitutes the major thrust of management strategies in sufferers from AIDS (Cook 1987a).

Pneumocystis carinii

Introduction

P carinii is a cosmopolitan organism which was first recognized early this century (it was first identified in guinea-pig lung tissue by Chagas in 1909, and human lung tissue in 1911 (Hopewell 1988)), and which usually infects individuals early in life. Most normal children have demonstrable antibody to this organism by 4 years of age (Hughes 1984); lymphocytes from 78% of normal adults proliferate when exposed to *P carinii* antigens (Blaser and Cohn 1986). Pneumonia caused by *P carinii* in the immunocompromised adult usually results, therefore, from reactivation of a latent infection (Hopewell 1988). In the United Kingdom and the USA some 85% of pulmonary infections in AIDS sufferers are caused by this organism; other systems are not usually affected. In Africa, however, *P carinii* infections seem to be overall less common than in Europe and North America in AIDS patients (Blaser and Cohn 1986), although there is considerable variation in different parts of that continent (Piot et al. 1984; Perre et al. 1984; Lucas et al. 1988, 1989; Elvin et al. 1989; Kayembe et al. 1989; McLeod et al. 1989).

Parasitology and Pathogenesis

The natural habitat of *P carinii* and the mode of transmission of infection are largely unknown (Hughes 1984; Kovacs and Masur 1988); the organism is distributed throughout the world and there is some evidence of epidemic spread. Recent work utilizing DNA probes has suggested that *P carinii* belongs strictly to the fungi rather than protozoa (*Lancet* 1988); however, in the absence of well-defined and generally accepted criteria for the classification of protozoa and fungi (Hughes and Gigliotti 1988), many protozoologists and mycologists prefer for the present, at least, to leave it where it has rested for many years. It should be recalled that there is enormous variation within the protozoa; *Plasmodium* sp, is, for example, a *very* long way from *Trypanosoma* sp! (It is perhaps no exaggeration to say that variations amongst protozoa are as marked as those between man and a cabbage.) Many mammalian species in addition to man are infected (Kovacs and Masur 1988); although the organism obtained from different sources is identical on morphological, ultrastructural and histochemical grounds, antigenic differences have recently been confirmed (Tanabe et al. 1987); it seems likely therefore that *P carinii* in the rat belongs to a different species from that of man. In infected tissue, it is present as cystic and extracystic forms. The cysts measure 4–6 μm in diameter and contain up to eight intracystic cells (sporozoites) measuring 1–2 μm in diameter; the extracystic form (the trophozoite) is thin-walled, nucleated, round to crescentic in shape, and measures 1.5–4 μm in diameter. Humoral responses to *P carinii* in infected AIDS patients have been compared with those in immunocompromised homosexual men (Hofmann et al. 1985); a striking reduction in IgG and IgM antibodies was demonstrated in them.

Clinical Aspects

Pneumonia resulting from *P carinii* infection, which is virtually confined to those with impaired cell-mediated immunity (Hopewell 1988) – the debilitated, the malnourished and immunocompromised, including AIDS patients (Kovacs et al. 1984) – frequently but not always has a sudden onset which is sometimes preceded by diarrhoea. Presentation is with dyspnoea (inability to take a deep inspiration is common), a dry unproductive cough and pyrexia. At presentation, which is often several weeks after onset of disease, symptoms have usually progressed rapidly, and massive involvement of pulmonary tissue is already present. Compared with patients with a compromised immune response from other causes, presentation of this form of pneumonia in AIDS sufferers may be subtle and uncharacteristic (Kovacs et al. 1984). Although widespread disseminated *P carinii* in AIDS is clinically very unusual, infection at extrapulmonary sites has been recorded (Pilon et al. 1987), and longstanding persistence of such foci may in part explain recurrent episodes of pneumonia after treatment.

Diagnosis

Diagnostically, it is essential to identify *P carinii* positively; whereas sputum and bronchial secretions sometimes yield the organism, these techniques are not entirely dependable. Sputum induction by inhalation of nebulized hypertonic saline has recently given an excellent result (Leigh et al. 1989). Fibreoptic bronchoscopy with bronchoalveolar lavage and transbronchial biopsy or needle-aspiration are frequently necessary (Hopewell 1988); there are few indications for an open lung biopsy. Histological preparations should be stained with the Gomori–Grocott methenamine-silver nitrate, or toluidine-blue O techniques (Nielsen et al. 1986); Giemsa staining is also of value. If Gram, methylene-blue, or Ziehl–Neelsen techniques are used, results should always be confirmed using the more specific methods. Improved detection by indirect immunofluorescence using monoclonal antibodies has been recorded (Elvin et al. 1988; Kovacs et al. 1988). Serological (either an indirect immunofluorescent antibody (IIFT) or complement fixation (CFT)) tests are of only limited value because a high percentage of 'normal' people have detectable antibody. Furthermore, isolation and culture of the organism is fraught with difficulties (Kovacs and Masur 1988). Early in the disease, chest radiography may give a normal result; however, later on a perihilar haze gives rise to diffuse symmetrical shadowing in the mid- and lower zones, usually with peripheral sparing (Hopewell 1988). Figure 2.1 shows a chest radiograph in a patient with *P carinii* pneumonia. While arterial oxygen tension is reduced, and CO_2 concentration is either normal or reduced (Hopewell 1988), arterial pH is normal or increased. The combined use of gallium-67 scintigraphy and bronchial washings, obtained by fibreoptic bronchoscopy, for diagnosis and assessment of response to treatment has recently been evaluated (Tuazon et al. 1985); this approach to diagnosis gives far more positive results than those obtained by radiology and transbronchial biopsy.

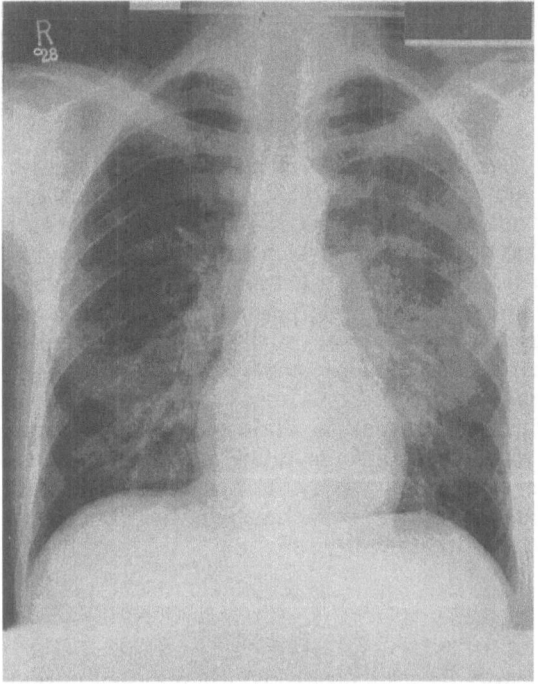

Fig. 2.1. Chest radiograph of a homosexual man with the fully developed acquired immune deficiency syndrome (AIDS) (Cook 1987a). Bilateral diffuse 'ground glass' appearances are most marked in the middle zones; these were shown to be caused by *Pneumocystis carinii*.

Management

Treatment consists first and foremost of supportive measures, which include oxygen to maintain the PaO_2 above 70 mmHg. Efforts should be made to diagnose and treat any co-existent viral, bacterial or fungal infection. Table 2.1 summarizes some of the therapeutic regimens which have been used to combat a *P carinii* pneumonia (Mitsuyasu et al. 1983; Gordin et al. 1984; Haverkos 1984; Hughes and Smith 1984; Kovacs et al. 1984; Farthing et al. 1985; Tuazon et al. 1985; Leoung et al. 1986; Wharton et al. 1986; Macfadden et al. 1987; Millar 1987; Tuazon and Labriola 1987; Weller 1987); those currently used have been reviewed by Hopewell (1988).

Table 2.1. Some therapeutic regimens which have been used against *Pneumocystis carinii* infections in immunocompromised (including AIDS) patients (Cook 1987a; Hopewell 1988)

Chemotherapeutic agent (Millar 1987; Tuazon and Labriola 1987; Weller 1987)	Suggested dose regimen (often continued indefinitely)	Side-effects
Trimethoprim + sulphamethoxazole ('co-trimoxazole')[a,b]	20 mg + 100 mg/kg daily oral for minimum of 3 weeks	(See text)
Pentamidine isethionate[a,b]	4 mg/kg daily; intravenous for minimum of 3 weeks	(See text)
Dapsone (diaminodiphenylsulfone) Dapsone + trimethoprim	100 mg daily 100 mg + 200 mg/kg daily	} Haemolysis (especially in G-6-PD deficiency), methaemoglobinaemia, leucopenia, agranulocytosis, dermatitis, infectious mononucleosis syndrome, hepatotoxicity, peripheral neuropathy, gastrointestinal symptoms, renal papillary necrosis, etc.
Trimetrexate (TMX)	—	Mucosal lesions, mild marrow depression, dermatitis, anorexia, mild abdominal cramps
α-Difluoromethylornithine (DFMO, eflornithine, MDL 71782)	75–100 mg qds intravenously	Thrombocytopenia, leucopenia, anaemia, reversible hearing loss, alopecia, gastrointestinal symptoms

[a]An intravenous preparation is also available (Millar 1987).
[b]Of established value with minimal toxicity in *P carinii* infection in the immunointact (Tuazon et al. 1985, Tuazon and Labriola 1987).

Although there is some evidence that in AIDS, pentamidine gives better results than trimethoprim-sulphamethoxazole ('co-trimoxazole') (both are very effective in the immune-intact individual), the latter combination regimen is usually preferred initially, owing to its relative lack of toxicity (which results from the sulphonamide component). However, fever, rashes, hepatotoxicity, marrow depression and gastrointestinal symptoms occur in up to 6%–8% and are more common in AIDS than in non-AIDS patients (Kovacs et al. 1984; Tuazon et al. 1985; Tuazon and Labriola 1987). Intravenous folinic acid (15 mg either daily or on alternate days) can be given to reduce the incidence of leucopenia and thrombocytopenia (Millar 1987; Weller 1987). The most frequent side-effects associated with pentamidine isethionate (up to 38%) are nephrotoxicity, hepatotoxicity, hypotension, marrow depression, hyperkalaemia, hypocalcaemia, sterile abcesses and hypo- (Lingenfelser et al. 1989) and hyperglycaemia (Tuazon et al. 1985). Acute renal failure has been reported after nebulized pentamidine (see below) (Miller et al. 1989). In a controlled prospective study, however, there was no significant difference in the incidence of side-effects between 'co-trimoxazole' and pentamidine when one or other of those agents was used for the initial treatment of a *P carinii* infection in AIDS patients (Wharton et al. 1986), despite previous suggestions to the contrary (Mitsuyasu et al. 1983; Gordin et al. 1984). No data are available on the incidence of side-effects when 'co-trimoxazole' and pentamidine are administered simultaneously (Haverkos 1984). Aerosolized pentamidine, inhaled for 20 minutes daily for 21 days, is probably of value in first episodes of *P carinii* pneumonia associated with AIDS (Montgomery et al. 1987), and is widely used. In the event of failure of response to inhaled pentamidine, use of the intravenous route remains effective (Pierone et al. 1989); this probably reflects drug dosage or distribution within the lung.

A combination regimen of trimethoprim + dapsone has been claimed to be at least as effective and better tolerated than the two established lines of treatment, and to carry a lower incidence of side-effects (Leoung et al. 1986). Clindamycin + primaquine was also shown to be of value in a limited study (Toma et al. 1989). In another study in which *P carinii* was the sole respiratory pathogen, the addition of intravenous methylprednisolone (40 mg four times daily for 7 days) to the therapeutic regimen produced a marked improvement in 10 AIDS patients whose respiratory function was deteriorating rapidly (Macfadden et al. 1987). The addition of a corticosteroid to the therapeutic regimen in patients with *severe P carinii* pneumonia (Macfadden et al. 1987) has also been shown to be valuable (Mottin et al. 1987).

Table 2.1 summarizes some other chemotherapeutic agents which have been used against *P carinii* pneumonia in AIDS patients. α-Difluoromethylornithine (DFMO) acts by inhibiting ornithine decarboxylase, thereby decreasing polyamine synthesis. Trimetrexate (TMX) acts by inhibiting dihydrofolate reductase and possesses excellent cellular membrane penetration due to its lipid solubility. Neither DFMO nor TMX has an established role in treatment however (Hopewell 1988). It is clear that new anti-pneumocystis agents are urgently required.

In an experimental study, diaminodiphenylsulphone proved at least as effective as 'co-trimoxazole' in *P carinii* pneumonia in dexamethasone-immuno-compromised rats (Hughes and Smith 1984); in that study the following therapeutic agents were shown to be ineffective: allopurinol, ketoconazole, α-difluoromethylornithine, diloxanide furoate, nifurtimox, suramin, melarsoprol, gentian violet, primaquine, and chloroquine.

Untreated, the mortality rate for *P carinii* pneumonia in AIDS sufferers is 100%. The mortality rate after treatment is around 30%–50%; the survival rate at 90 days after starting chemotherapy is similar in this group of individuals to that in patients with *P carinii* pneumonia who are immunodeficient for other reasons (Haverkos 1984; Tuazon and Labriola 1987). Overall, life expectancy after diagnosis of a *P carinii* infection is 12.5 months in the United Kingdom and nine months in the USA (Millar 1987); 2-year survival is uncommon.

Prophylactically, several strategies have been used. 'Co-trimoxazole' (2–4 tablets daily), 'Fansidar' (pyrimethamine + sulfadoxine) (1 tablet weekly), and 'Maloprim' (pyrimethamine + dapsone) have been used, but with only limited success (Farthing et al. 1985; Fischl and Dickinson 1986; Millar 1987; Weller 1987). A combination of primaquine + clindamycin has also received attention, but seems ineffective (Girard et al. 1989a). Monthly intramuscular pentamidine has also been suggested to be of value (Weller 1987). The efficacy of pentamidine has been confirmed both in patients receiving zidovudine (Girard et al. 1989b), and those not so treated (Golden et al. 1989); inhalation of this agent fortnightly or monthly in the prevention of relapse and reduction in severity of *P carinii* infection has been documented (Thomas et al 1990). Opportunistic infections, *P carinii* included, have been shown to be reduced in patients receiving zidovudine alone (Fischl et al. 1987).

Visceral Leishmaniasis (Kala-azar)

This chronic protozoan infection, which is caused by *Leishmania donovani* (a facultative intracellular pathogen) (Chap. 12) is widely distributed in Africa, Asia and the Mediterranean littoral; much of the affected territory coincides with that in which African AIDS is now a commonplace infection. The disease is normally characterized by irregular fever, hepatosplenomegaly, weight-loss, leucopenia and a grossly elevated serum IgG concentration.

Diagnosis is by demonstration of Leishman–Donovan bodies in bone-marrow or splenic aspirate; in Indian cases, amastigotes can be demonstrated in buffy-coat smears. Serology using the ELISA technique is of value in diagnosis, approximately 95% being positive (Chap. 12). Kala-azar has been recorded, and is probably more common, as an opportunistic infection in immunosuppressed individuals (Aguado et al. 1983; Badaró et al. 1986; Letona et al. 1986; Fernández-Guerrero et al. 1987). It is not surprising therefore, that it has now been described on a number of occasions in the presence of AIDS; at least 25 cases (several of them from Spain, Portugal, Italy and southern France) have now been recorded of visceral leishmaniasis in association with HIV infection (Clauvel et al. 1986; Gonzalez et al. 1986; Medrano-Gonzáles et al, 1986; Senaldi et al. 1986; Antunes et al. 1987; Alvar et al. 1987; Blázquez et al. 1987; Franco-Vicario et al. 1987; Montalban et al. 1987; Verdejo et al. 1987; Bernard et al. 1988; Falk et al. 1988; Fuzibet et al. 1988; Rizzi et al. 1988; Yebra et al. 1988; Alvar et al. 1989; Berenguer et al. 1989; Smith et al. 1989). Montalban et al. (1989) consider that in endemic areas it should be considered an 'indicator disease' for the diagnosis of AIDS. Presentation is often with atypical features, and splenomegaly (which is a usual accompaniment in immunointact individuals) is frequently absent; this is presumably a result of a failure of macrophage response. Also, serological tests for *L donovani* are usually negative; this seems likely to result from polyclonal B-cell activation after acquisition of the HIV infection (Lane et al. 1983). In addition, response to chemotherapy (Chap. 12) is poor and rapid death, usually resulting from respiratory disease (*L donovani* has been demonstrated in lung tissue at post-mortem) the usual sequel; this can presumably be explained on the basis of a severe cell-mediated immunity (CMI) impairment. It seems likely that by stimulating activation of CD4$^+$ lymphocytes and macrophages, *L donovani* increases HIV replication within them thus accelerating the resultant immunodeficiency.

Explanation for the Increased Prevalence of Some Protozoan Infection in AIDS

The nature of the immunological defect which allows the proliferation of these opportunistic organisms has been the subject of much recent investigation (Siegel et al. 1986; Eales et al. 1987; Weissman 1988). There is a selective dysfunction of CMI. A subset of large granular lymphocytes (LGL) is seriously affected by HIV-1 and other retroviruses; this, combined with a failure of T-cell function, allows these infections (which are usually latent), to reactivate and become established. Total T-lymphocyte numbers, most strikingly the Leu-3a T-cell subset, have been shown to be strikingly reduced in small-intestinal mucosa (Rodgers et al. 1986); furthermore, AIDS patients with diarrhoea have been shown to have lower mean numbers of helper-inducer (OKT 4) lymphocytes than those without diarrhoea (Smith et al. 1988). There are undoubted differences in prevalence rates for these infections in differing geographical locations (Perre et al. 1984; Piot et al. 1984; Lucas et al. 1988; Kayembe et al. 1989). Why for example is *P carinii* infection a less common opportunistic infection in AIDS patients in Africa than in Europe and North America (Elvin et al. 1989)? One obvious explanation is that the causative organism is either absent, or is less common in the local environment (see above) (Cook 1987a; Lucas et al. 1990); however, Lucas (1990) has stressed that *P carinii* infection has been clearly documented in malnourished children in Uganda, for example. An alternative possibility lies in the fact that *P carinii* is an opportunistic pathogen of relatively low virulence (Lucas 1990); in this case infection would emerge later in the evolution of AIDS, while more virulent pathogens (e.g. *Mycobacterium tuberculosis* and *Toxoplasma gondii*) would already have caused significant mortality before *P carinii* had had time to gain a foothold. No published data exist on circulating T-helper-cell ($CD4^+$) numbers in AIDS patients in Africa; the possibility has been raised that associated lymphopenia is overall less common than in European and North American cases (Lucas 1990), and this obviously requires investigation.

Protozoan Infections *Without* an Increased Prevalence in AIDS

An important question which must be asked is: why are certain protozoan and helminthic infections *not* more common in AIDS sufferers (Cook 1987a; Lucas 1990).

Entamoeba histolytica, and 'Non-pathogenic' and 'Free-Living' Amoebae

Entamoeba histolytica is a common intestinal parasite of homosexual men (Chap. 6); however, present evidence indicates that the strains (zymodemes) involved are rarely invasive ones (Allason-Jones et al. 1986). In addition there does not seem to be an increased incidence of amoebic liver 'abscess' in AIDS patients either in the United Kingdom, USA, or Africa; one case of liver 'abscess' associated with an HIV infection was recorded by Perre et al. (1984). There is no evidence either of amoebic proctocolitis in symptomatic HIV-infected individuals (Sewankambo et al. 1987; Colebunders et al. 1988). Although the immunology of amoebiasis is complex (Denis and Chadee 1988; Salata and Ravdin 1988), depressed CMI, malnutrition, pregnancy and corticosteroid therapy are known to increase the prevalence and severity of this infection. It is surprising on *a priori* grounds therefore that HIV infection of CD4$^+$ lymphocytes and macrophages does *not* impair the host defence mechanism agent *E histolytica*; lymphokine-activated macrophages and T-cytotoxic lymphocytes both have a cidal action on trophozoites in vitro. Interestingly, *E histolytica* secretes a lectin which stimulates T-cell replication (Petri and Ravdin 1987); if the lectin gained access to mucosal lymphocytes, this might *increase* HIV replication. Lucas (1990) has suggested that in vivo factors, such as defensive properties of mucus, complement-dependent lysis of parasites (which is inhibited by the parasites themselves), and modulation of the parasite-strain, might be important but they have not been studied in the context of immunodepression; in fact, in vitro events probably do not reflect the highly complex in vivo situation when dealing with large extracellular protozoa. Overall, therefore, it seems unlikely that this organism is of any great significance in AIDS patients. But similarly, there are insufficient data available to suggest a protective effect of HIV infection against invasive amoebiasis (Lucas 1990).

Limited data suggest, however, that some of the 'non-pathogenic' amoebae (*Entamoeba hartmanni*, *E coli*, *Endolimax nana* and *Iodamoeba bütschlii*) (Chap. 6) might be responsible for chronic diarrhoea and weight-loss in AIDS patients when present at high intra-luminal concentration; five patients (who did not harbour other intestinal pathogens) who were infected responded to a 10-day course of metronidazole; however, two of them subsequently suffered a relapse 4 and 8 weeks later (Rolston et al. 1986).

Fatal meningoencephalitis (Chap. 8) caused by *Acanthamoeba culbertsoni* has been documented in a 34-year-old man with AIDS (Wiley et al. 1987). This organism which is a 'free-living' amoeba can be inhaled; diagnosis is made from wet or dry CSF smears. It seems likely that in this case infection occurred via chronically infected nasal sinuses. This route of infection also seemed likely in another patient suffering from AIDS who developed an *A castellani* infection and subsequently died (Gonzalez et al. 1986). Amphotericin B + flucytosine in combination seems to form the best approach to chemotherapy (Wiley et al. 1987); rifampicin and ketoconazole were administered to the second of these two patients (Gonzalez et al. 1986). As things stand, there is no good evidence therefore for an increased prevalence of 'free-living' amoebic infections in AIDS sufferers.

Giardia lamblia

G lamblia infections are common in homosexual men. Although *G lamblia* has been reported in patients with AIDS (Sewankambo et al. 1987), frequently in association with other luminal protozoa (and other 'opportunistic' organisms also), there is no good evidence that this protozoon is unduly common or abnormally virulent in this situation.

Plasmodium falciparum

P falciparum infections are extremely common in some geographical areas where African AIDS is a major problem (Chap. 1). Immunity to *P falciparum*, although the subject of considerable controversy (see below) is generally considered to be largely T-cell mediated and it might therefore be anticipated that this protozoan infection would be more common in AIDS sufferers. However, present evidence, though limited, indicates that there is no such increase in frequency (Nguyen-Dinh et al. 1987; Simooya et al. 1988); in studies carried out at Kinshasa, Zaire, and Ndola, Zambia, respectively, no evidence of an increase in *P falciparum* infection rate in HIV-1 positive individuals could be demonstrated. Furthermore, severity and response to antimalarial chemotherapy did not seem to differ from those in HIV-negative children and adults (Greenberg 1989). The sole difference between these groups was that children who had received a blood transfusion for severe *P falciparum* malaria were more often HIV-positive.

In experimental studies of immunity, T-lymphocytes and splenic macrophages are important; $CD4^+$ and $CD8^+$ T-cells are required for protection (Liew 1989), while $CD8^+$ cells kill intra-hepatic parasites by direct lysis or via lymphokine α-interferon, and $CD4^+$ lymphocytes activate macrophages to kill intra-erythrocytic organisms – possibly by involving tumour necrosis factor (TNF) (Clark 1987; Good and Miller 1989). Because $CD4^+$ lymphocytes are depleted, and macrophages are infected by HIV, a high parasitaemia would on *a priori* grounds be anticipated in an HIV-positive individual. Lucas (1990) has summarized some possible explanations for this seeming paradox in HIV-infected individuals: (i) the establishment of a new equilibrium in the host immune response(s), (ii) maintenance of relatively competent macrophage function in the presence of a reduced T-helper cell population, and largely unaffected T-suppressor (cytotoxic) population, and (iii) unresolved complexities in TNF production (and circulating-concentration) in the presence of HIV infection.

Trichomonas vaginalis

Trichomonas vaginalis is a flagellated protozoon which infects both female and male genitourinary tracts (Simpson 1984). It is widely distributed geographically, being common in many tropical countries, and its major clinical manifestation is vaginal discharge; cystitis in women, and urethritis, prostatitis and epididymitis in men are other sequelae. In the immunointact individual it rapidly responds to one of the 5-nitroimidazole compounds. The magnitude of the problem in homosexual men, HIV-infected individuals, and those with AIDS is poorly defined; however there is no good evidence that this is an unusually common protozoan infection in any of these groups.

Intestinal Helminthic Infections in AIDS

Strongyloides stercoralis

S stercoralis can produce a severe overwhelming infection ('hyperinfection syndrome') in immunocompromised individuals (Chap. 5) (Cook 1987b; Grove 1989); multisystem infection is often accompanied by a Gram-negative septicaemia, and the condition carries a high mortality rate. Although extra-intestinal strongyloidiasis has been considered by some to constitute an 'opportunistic' infection in HIV-1 positive individuals, there is no good evidence for this (Petithory and Derouin 1987); larvae have not been conclusively demonstrated outside the gastrointestinal tract in this disease. Also *S stercoralis* infection does not seem to be unusually common in African AIDS in geographical areas where this is a common intestinal parasite (Bureau of Hygiene and Tropical Diseases 1985; Quinn et al. 1986; Sewankambo et al. 1987). The explanation for this remains unclear because HIV-induced depression of CMI would be expected to predispose to a severe *S stercoralis* infection wherever this helminth is endemic (Petithory and Derouin 1987; Lucas 1990); indeed, early definitions of AIDS included extra-intestinal strongyloidiasis as one of the major criteria for diagnosis (World Health Organisation 1986). Whilst a small number of HIV-infected patients with diarrhoea in Africa have had a small-intestinal *S stercoralis* infection (Colebunders et al. 1988; Lucas 1989), there are only 6 recorded cases of disseminated strongyloidiasis in the presence of HIV infection (Piot et al. 1984; Maayan et al. 1987; Lucas 1990). In some HIV-negative patients with strongyloidiasis, the circulating T-helper (CD4$^+$) to T-suppressor/cytoxic (CD8$^+$) ratio is inverted; however, whether this is parasite-induced, is an underlying condition, or is caused by corticosteroid administration is unknown (Genta 1989). In AIDS, evidence points to the fact that neither a reduction in T-helper cells in the small-intestinal mucosa and submucosa, nor HIV infection of local macrophages, increases the potential of *S stercoralis* to rapidly multiply and disseminate; in AIDS the small-intestinal CD4$^+$: CD8$^+$ T-lymphocyte ratio is inverted and parallels events in peripheral blood (Ellekany et al. 1987). Corticosteroids on the other hand, influence mast cells, composition of the surface mucus layer, local antibody responses, and turnover of crypt enterocytes in addition to their effect on CMI (Lucas 1990). It is also worth noting that patients with disseminated strongyloidiasis who have an absence of IgE antibody and no peripheral eosinophilia have a less favourable outcome than those in whom one or both of these mechanisms are in operation.

Lucas (1990) has drawn attention to the fact that observations on the course of *Capillaria philippinensis* infection – which is the only other helminth to have an autoinfection-cycle – in AIDS patients will be of great interest. In AIDS, the impairment of intestinal CMI (Rodgers et al. 1986) therefore seems to favour protozoan (especially coccidian) rather than helminthic infection.

Conclusions

Certain protozoan infections undoubtedly cause important 'opportunistic' events in the presence of infection with HIV-1 and the related retroviruses, which have a profound effect on the cellular immune response (Rodgers et al. 1986; Siegal et al. 1986); these are dominated by *Pneumocystis carinii*, the intestinal coccidia, and *Toxoplasma gondii*. However, *Entamoeba histolytica* (many zymodemes of which are invasive) does not present a major problem; it is unlikely that T-cell immunity represents an important defence mechanism against this organism, and the possibility exists that the luminal milieu of the male homosexual colorectum is unfavourable to pathogenic zymodemes of this organism. *Plasmodium* sp, which is closely related to intestinal coccidia taxonomically, is also not unduly common in AIDS patients; cellular immunity is obviously important here, but this presumably involves a different T-cell function. Despite the fact that it causes a serious hyperinfection syndrome in the presence of immunosuppression, there is no existing evidence that the small-intestinal nematode *S stercoralis* is either more common or produces more severe disease in HIV-infected individuals.

It seems impossible at present to find a common denominator amongst those protozoa which produce important 'opportunistic' infections in AIDS. All are very common and widely spread in the environment; furthermore they usually infect the majority of individuals in infancy or childhood. It seems possible that they all exist as latent infections which can be reactivated by the severe immune deficiency produced by AIDS (Siegal et al. 1986). With the intestinal coccidia, however, a latent focus or foci of infection has not been positively identified (or excluded). Diagnosis poses certain problems but these are not usually insuperable. Treatment, however, is grossly unsatisfactory; in none of these infections is there an adequate answer, and diagnosis of their presence currently carries a grave prognostic significance, usually amounting to a 'death sentence'.

From another viewpoint, the AIDS pandemic has brought with it recognition of the enormous prevalence of several 'opportunistic' organisms in the environment, and has emphasized their vast potential for causing serious, often fatal human disease and suffering.

References

Ada G (1989) Prospects for a vaccine against HIV. Nature 339:331–332

Aguado JM, Gómez Berne J, Figuera A, Villalobos E de, Fernández-Guerrero ML, Sanchez Fayos J (1983) Visceral leishmaniasis (Kala-azar) complicating acute leukaemia. J Infect 7:272–274

Allason-Jones E, Mindel A, Sargeaunt P, Williams P (1986) *Entamoeba histolytica* as a commensal intestinal parasite in homosexual men. N Engl J Med 315:353–356

Alvar J, Verdejo J, Osuna A, Nájera R (1987) Visceral leishmaniasis in a patient seropositive for HIV, Eur J Clin Microbiol 6:604–606

Alvar J, Blazquez J, Najera R (1989) Association of visceral leishmaniasis and human immunodeficiency virus infections. J Infect Dis 160:560–561

Anderson RM, May RM, McLean AR (1988) Possible demographic consequences of AIDS in developing countries. Nature 332:228–234

Antunes F, Carvalho C, Tavares L, Botas J, Forte M, Rio AM del, Dutschmann L, Costa A, Abranches P, Pereira CS, Paiva JED, Araujo FC, Baptista A (1987) Visceral leishmaniasis recrudescence in a patient with AIDS. Trans R Soc Trop Med Hyg 81:595

Badaró R, Carvalho EM, Rocha H, Queiroz AC, Jones TC (1986) *Leishmania donovani*: an opportunistic microbe associated with progressive disease in three immunocompromised patients. Lancet i:647–649

Berenguer J, Moreno S, Cercenado E, Bernaldo de Quirós JC, García de la Fuente A, Bouza E (1989) Visceral leishmaniasis in patients infected with human immunodeficiency virus (HIV). Ann Intern Med 111:129–132

Bernard E, Rodot S, Michiels JF, Politano S, le Fichoux Y, Dellamonica P (1988) Visceral leishmaniasis in acquired immunodeficiency syndrome. Presse Méd 17:872

Blaser MJ, Cohn DL (1986) Opportunistic infections in patients with AIDS: clues to the epidemiology of AIDS and the relative virulence of pathogens. Rev Infect Dis 8:21–30

Blázquez J, Alvar J, Nájera R (1987) Leishmaniasis in an HIV (LAV/HTLV III) serologically positive patient. J Infect 14:89–90

Bureau of Hygiene and Tropical Diseases (1985) African AIDS: a bibliography. Bureau of Hygiene and Tropical Diseases, London, pp 1–15

Clark IA (1987) Cell-mediated immunity in protection of pathology of malaria. Parasitol Today 3:300–305

Clauvel JP, Couderc LJ, Belmin J, Daniel MT, Rabian C, Seligmann M (1986) Visceral leishmaniasis complicating acquired immunodeficiency syndrome (AIDS). Trans R Soc Trop Med Hyg 80:1010–1011

Colebunders R, Lusakumuni K, Nelson AM, Gigase P, Lebughe I, Marck E van, Kapita B, Francis H, Salaun J-J, Quinn TC, Piot P (1988) Persistent diarrhoea in Zairian AIDS patients: an endoscopic and histological study. Gut 29:1687–1691

Cook GC (1987a) Opportunistic parasitic infections associated with the acquired immune deficiency syndrome (AIDS); parasitology, clinical presentation, diagnosis and management. Q J Med 65:967–983

Cook GC (1987b) *Strongyloides stercoralis* hyperinfection syndrome: how often is it missed? Q J Med 64:625–629

De Cock KM, Porter A, Odehouri K, Barrere B, Moreau J, Diaby L, Kouadio JC, Heyward WL (1989) Rapid emergence of AIDS in Abidjan, Ivory Coast. Lancet ii:408–411

Denis M, Chadee K (1988) Immunopathology of *Entamoeba histolytica* infections. Parasitol Today 4:247–252

Duesberg PH (1989) Human immunodeficiency virus and acquired immunodeficiency syndrome: correlation but not causation. Proc Natl Acad Sci USA 86:755–764

Eales L-J, Moshtael O, Pinching AJ (1987) Microbicidal activity of monocyte derived macrophages in AIDS and related disorders. Clin Exp Immunol 67:227–235

Editoral (1989) Aids now a tractable disease? Nature 340:663

Ellakany S, Whiteside TL, Schade RR, Thiel DH van (1987) Analysis of intestinal lymphocyte subpopulations in patients with acquired immunodeficiency syndrome (AIDS) and AIDS-related complex. Am J Clin Pathol 87:356–364

Elvin KM, Björkman A, Linder E, Heurlin N, Hjerpe A (1988) *Pneumocystis carinii* pneumonia: detection of parasites in sputum and bronchoalveolar lavage fluid by monoclonal antibodies. Br Med J 297:381–384

Elvin KM, Lumbwe CM, Luo NP, Björkman A, Källenius G, Linder E (1989) *Pneumocystis carinii* is not a major cause of pneumonia in HIV infected patients in Lusaka, Zambia. Trans R Soc Trop Med Hyg 83: 553–555

Ezzell C (1989) Aids closer to becoming a treatable disease. Nature 340:581

Falk S, Helm EB, Hübner K, Stutte HJ (1988) Disseminated visceral leishmaniasis (Kala-azar) in acquired immunodeficiency syndrome (AIDS). Pathol Res Pract 183:253–255

Farthing CF, Shanson DC, Gazzard BG (1985) The acquired immune deficiency syndrome: problems associated with the management of *Pneumocystis carinii* pneumonia. J Infect 11:103–108

Fernández-Guerrero ML, Aguado JM, Buzón L, Barros C, Montalbán C, Martín T, Bouza E (1987) Visceral leishmaniasis in immuncompromised hosts. Am J Med 83:1098–1102

Fischl MA, Dickinson GM (1986) Fansidar prophylaxis of pneumocystis pneumonia in the acquired immunodeficiency syndrome. Ann Intern Med 105:629

Fischl MA, Richman DD, Grieco MH, Gottlieb MS, Volberding PA, Laskin OL, Leedom JM, Groopman JE, Midvan D, Schooley RT, Jackson GG, Durack DT, King D, AZT Collaborative Working Group (1987) The efficacy of azidothymidine (AZT) in the treatment of patients with AIDS and AIDS-related complex. N Engl J Med 317:185–191

Franco-Vicario R, Beltran de Heredia JM, Rojo P, Hermosa C (1987) Leishmaniasis associated with the acquired immunodeficiency syndrome. Med Clin (Barc) 88:565–566

Fuzibet JG, Marty P, Taillan B, Bertrand F, Pras P, Pesce A, LeFichoux Y, Dujarin P (1988) Is *Leishmania infantum* an opportunistic parasite in patients with anti-human immunodeficiency virus antibodies? Arch Intern Med 148:1228

Gelb A, Miller S (1986) AIDS and gastroenterology. Am J Gastroenterology 81:619–622

Genta RM (1989) Immunology. In: Grove DI (ed) Strongyloidiasis: a major roundworm infection of man. Taylor and Francis, London, pp 133–153

Girard P-M, Lepretre A, Detruchis P, Matheron S, Coulaud J-P (1989a) Failure of pyrimethamine–clindamycin combination for prophylaxis of *Pneumocystis carinii* pneumonia. Lancet i:1459

Girard P-M, Landman R, Gaudebout C, Lepretre A, Lottin P, Michon C, Truchis P de, Matheron S, Camus F, Farinotti R, Marche C, Coulaud J-P, Saimot AG (1989b) Prevention of *Pneumocystis carinii* pneumonia relapse by pentamidine aerosol in zidovudine-treated AIDS patients. Lancet i:1348–1353

Golden JA, Chernoff D, Hollander H, Feigal D, Conte JE (1989) Prevention of *Pneumocystis carinii* pneumonia by inhaled pentamidine. Lancet i:654–657

Gonzales FM, Lorenzo AA, Perez JL (1986) Visceral leishmaniasis that proved fatal associated with HTLV-III infection. Med Clin (Barc) 87:730–731

Gonzalez MM, Gould E, Dickinson G, Martinez AJ, Visvesvara G, Cleary TJ, Hensley GT (1986) Acquired immunodeficiency syndrome associated with *Acanthamoeba* infection and other opportunistic organisms. Arch Pathol Lab Med 110:749–751

Good MF, Miller LH (1989) Involvement of T cells in malaria immunity: implications for vaccine development. Vaccine 7:3–9

Gordin FM, Simon GL, Wofsy CB, Mills J (1984) Adverse reactions to trimethoprim-sulfamethoxazole in patients with the acquired immunodeficiency syndrome. Ann Intern Med 100:495–499

Greenberg AE (1989) Studies of the relationship between *Plasmodium falciparum* malaria and HIV infection in Africa. Vth International Conference on AIDS. Montreal, Canada, Abstract WGO7, p 983

Grove DI (1989) Clinical manifestations. In: Grove DI (ed) Strongyloidiasis: a major roundworm infection of man. Taylor and Francis, London, pp 155–173

Haverkos HW (1984) Assessment of therapy for *Pneumocystis carinii* pneumonia: PCP therapy project group. Am J Med 76:501–508

Hofmann B, Ødum N, Platz P, Ryder LP, Svejgaard A, Nielsen PB, Holten-Andersen W, Gerstoft J, Nielson JO, Mojon M (1985) Humoral responses to *Pneumocystis carinii* in patients with acquired immunodeficiency syndrome and in immunocompromised homosexual men. J Infect Dis 152:838–840

Hopewell PC (1988) Diagnosis and treatment of *Pneumocystis carinii* pneumonia. In: Leech JH, Sande MA, Root RK (eds) Parasitic infections. Churchill Livingstone, New York and Edinburgh, pp 195–220

Hughes WT (1984) Pneumocystosis. In: Strickland GT (ed) Hunter's tropical medicine, 6th edn. Saunders, Philadelphia, pp 605–608

Hughes WT, Gigliotti F (1988) Nomenclature for *Pneumocystis carinii*. J Infect Dis 157:432–433

Hughes WT, Smith BL (1984) Efficacy of diaminodiphenylsulfone and other drugs in murine *Pneumocystis carinii* pneumonitis. Antimicrob Agents Chemother 26:436–440

Kayembe N, Nelson AM, Ilunga N, Angritt P, Kalengay HM (1989) Pathology of HIV infection in Zaire. Vth International Conference on AIDS. Montreal, Canada, Abstract Th Go 32, p 994

Kovacs JA, Masur H (1988) Advances in the biology and immunology of *Pneumocystis carinii*. In: Leech JH, Sande MA, Root RK (eds) Parasitic infections. Churchill Livingstone, New York and Edinburgh, pp 177–193

Kovacs JA, Hiemenz JW, Macher AM, Stover D, Murray HW, Shelhamer J, Lane C, Urmacher C, Honig C, Longo DL, Parker MM, Natanson C, Parrillo JE, Fauci AS, Pizzo PA, Masur H (1984) *Pneumocystis carinii* pneumonia: a comparison between patients with the acquired immunodeficiency syndrome and patients with other immunodeficiencies. Ann Intern Med 100:663–671

Kovacs JA, Ng VL, Masur H, Leoung G, Hadley WK, Evans G, Lane HC, Ognibene FP, Shelhamer J, Parrillo JE, Gill VJ (1988) Diagnosis of *Pneumocystis carinii* pneumonia: improved detection in sputum with use of monoclonal antibodies. N Engl J Med 318:589–593

Lancet, (1988) *Pneumocystis carinii* finds its identity. Lancet ii:522

Lane HC, Masur H, Edgar LC, Whalen G, Rook AH, Fauci AS (1983) Abnormalities of B-cell activation and immunoregulation in patients with the acquired immunodeficiency syndrome. N Engl J Med 309:453–458

Leigh TR, Parsons P, Hume C, Husain OAN, Gazzard B, Collins JV (1989) Sputum induction for diagnosis of *Pneumocystis carinii* pneumonia. Lancet ii:205–207

Leoung GS, Mills J, Hopewell PC, Hughes W, Wofsy C (1986) Dapsone-trimethoprim for *Pneumocystis carinii* pneumonia in the acquired immunodeficiency syndrome. Ann Intern Med 105:45–48

Letona JML de, Vázquez CM, Maestu RP (1986) Visceral leishmaniasis as an opportunistic infection. Lancet i:1094

Liew FY (1989) Immunity to protozoa. Current Opin Immunol 1:441–447

Lingenfelser T, Glück T, Scheurlen M, Overkamp D, Jakober B (1989) Pentamidine and hypoglycaemia. Lancet ii:458

Lucas SB (1990) Missing infections in AIDS. Trans R Soc Trop Med Hyg 84 (suppl 1): 34–38

Lucas S, Sewankambo N, Nambuya A, Nsubuga P, Goodgame R, Mugerwa J, Carswell JW (1988) The morbid anatomy of African AIDS. In: Giraldo G, Beth-Giraldo E, Clumeck N, Gharbi M-R, Kyalwazi SK, The G de (eds) AIDS and associated cancers in Africa. Karger, Basel, pp 124–133

Lucas S, Goodgame R, Kocjan G, Serwadda D (1989) Absence of pneumocystosis in Ugandan AIDS patients. AIDS 3:47–48

Macfadden WT, Edelson JD, Hyland RH, Rodriguez CH, Inouye T, Rebuck AS (1987) Corticosteroids as adjunctive therapy in treatment of *Pneumocystis carinii* pneumonia in patients with acquired immunodeficiency syndrome. Lancet i:1477–1479

Malebranche R, Arnoux E, Guérin JM, Pierre GD, Laroche AC, Péan-Guichard C, Elie R, Morisset PH, Spira T, Mandeville R, Drotman P, Seemayer T, Dupuy J-M (1983) Acquired immunodeficiency syndrome with severe gastrointestinal manifestations in Haiti. Lancet ii:873–878

Maayan S, Wormser GP, Widerhorn J, Sy ER, Kim YH, Ernst JA (1987) *Strongyloides stercoralis* hyperinfection in a patient with the acquired immune deficiency syndrome. Am J Med 83:945–948

McClure MO, Schulz TF (1989) Origin of HIV. Br Med J 298:1267–1268

McLeod D, Neill P, Robertson VJ, Latif AS, Emmanuel J, Els JE, Gwanzura LKZ, Trijssenaar FEJ, Nziramasanga P, Jongeling GR, Katzenstein DA, Nkanza N, Lucas SB (1989) Pulmonary diseases in patients infected with the human immunodeficiency virus in Zimbabwe, Central Africa. Trans R Soc Trop Med Hyg 83:694–697

Medrano-González F, Alemán-Lorenzo A, Beato-Pérez JL (1986) Visceral leishmaniasis of fatal outcome associated with HTLV-III infection. Med Clin Barcelona 87:780-781

Millar A (1987) AIDS and the lung. Br Med J 294:1334–1337

Miller RF, Delaney S, Semple SJG (1989) Acute renal failure after nebulised pentamidine. Lancet i:1271–1272

Mitsuyasu R, Groupman J, Volberding P (1983) Cutaneous reaction to trimethoprim-sulfamethoxazole in patients with AIDS and Kaposi's sarcoma. N Engl J Med 308:1535-1536

Modigliani R, Bories C, Charpentier Y le, Salmeron M, Messing B, Galian A, Rambaud JC, Lavergne A, Cochand-Priollet B, Desportes I (1985) Diarrhoea and malabsorption in acquired immune deficiency syndrome: a study of four cases with special emphasis on opportunistic protozoan infestations. Gut 26:179–187

Montalban C, Sevilla F, Moreno A, Nash R, Celma ML, Muñoz RF (1987) Visceral leishmaniasis as an opportunistic infection in the acquired immunodeficiency syndrome. J Infect 15:247–250

Montalban C, Martinez-Fernandez R, Calleja JL, Garcia-Diaz J de D, Rubio R, Dronda F, Moreno S, Yebra M, Barros C, Cobo J, Martinez MC, Ruiz F, Costa JR (1989) Visceral leishmaniasis (Kala-azar) as an opportunistic infection in patients infected with The Human Immunodeficiency Virus in Spain. Rev Infect Dis 11:655–660

Montgomery AB, Debs RJ, Luce JM, Corkery KJ, Turner J, Brunette EN, Lin ET, Hopewell PC (1987) Aerosolised pentamidine as sole therapy for *Pneumocystis carinii* pneumonia in patients with acquired immunodeficiency syndrome. Lancet ii:480–483

Mottin D, Denis M, Dombret H, Rossert J, Mayaud C, Akoun G (1987) Role for steroids in treatment of *Pneumocystis carinii* pneumonia in AIDS. Lancet ii:519

Newmark P (1988) Receding hopes of AIDS vaccines. Nature 333:699

Nguyen-Dinh P, Greenberg AE, Ryder RW, Mann JM (1987) Absence of association between HIV seropositivity and *Plasmodium falciparum* malaria in Kinshasa, Zaire. 3rd International Conference on AIDS, Washington DC, Abstracts, p 22

Nielsen PB, Goyot P, Mojon M (1986) The microscopic diagnosis of *Pneumocystis carinii*: an evaluation of the Gram, the Methylene Blue, and the Ziehl-Neelsen procedures. Acta Pathol Microbiol Scand [B] 94:19–23

Pape JW, Liautaud B, Thomas F, Mathurin J-R, Amand M-M A St, Boncy M, Pean V, Pamphile M, Laroche AC, Johnson WD (1983) Characteristics of the acquired immunodeficiency syndrome (AIDS) in Haiti. N Engl J Med 309:945–950

Penny D (1988) Origins of the AIDS virus. Nature 333:494–495

Perre P van de, Rouvroy D, LePage P, Bogaerts J, Kestelyn P, Kayihigi J, Hekker AC, Butzler J-P, Clumeck N (1984) Acquired immunodeficiency syndrome in Rwanda. Lancet ii:62–65
Petithory JC, Derouin F (1987) AIDS and strongyloidiasis in Africa. Lancet i:921
Petri WA, Ravdin JI (1987) Treatment of homosexual men infected with *Entamoeba histolytica*. N Engl J Med 315:393
Pierone G, Turett G, Masci JR, Nicholas P (1989) Inhaled pentamidine in *Pneumocystis carinii* pneumonia. Lancet ii:559
Pilon VA, Echols RM, Celo JS, Elmendorf SL (1987) Disseminated *Pneumocystis carinii* infection in AIDS. N Engl J Med 316:1410–1411
Piot P, Taelman H, Minlangu KB, Mbendi N, Ndangi K, Kalambayi K, Bridts C, Quinn TC, Feinsod FM, Wobin O, Mazebo P, Stevens W, Mitchell S, McCormick JB (1984) Acquired immuno deficiency syndrome in a heterosexual population in Zaire. Lancet ii:65–69
Quinn TC, Mann JM, Curran JW, Piot P (1986) AIDS in Africa: an epidemiological paradigm. Science 234:955–963
Reeve PA (1989) HIV infection in patients admitted to a general hospital in Malawi. Br Med J 298:1567–1568
Rizzi M, Arici C, Bonaccorso C, Gavazzeni G (1988) Visceral leishmaniasis in a patient with human immunodeficiency virus. Trans R Soc Trop Med Hyg 82:565
Rodgers VD, Fassett R, Kagnoff MF (1986) Abnormalities in intestinal mucosal T cells in homosexual populations including those with the lymphadenopathy syndrome and acquired immunodeficiency syndrome. Gastroenterology 90:552–558
Rolston KVI, Hoy J, Mansell PWA (1986) Diarrhea caused by 'non-pathogenic amebae' in patients with AIDS. N Engl J Med 315:192
Salata RA, Ravdin JI (1988) Human cell-mediated immune mechanisms directed against *Entamoeba histolytica*. In: Ravdin JI (ed) Amebiasis: human infection by *Entamoeba histolytica*. John Wiley, New York, pp 471–479
Seale J (1989) Crossing the species barrier – viruses and the origins of AIDS in perspective. J R Soc Med 82:519–523
Senaldi G, Cadeo G, Carnevale G, Perri G di, Carosi G (1986) Visceral leishmaniasis as an opportunistic infection. Lancet i:1094
Sewankambo N, Mugerwa RD, Goodgame R, Carswell JW, Moody A, Lloyd G, Lucas SB (1987) Enteropathic AIDS in Uganda. An endoscopic, histological and microbiological study. AIDS 1:9–13
Sharp PM, Li W-H (1988) Understanding the origins of AIDS viruses. Nature 336:315
Siegal FP, Lopez C, Fitzgerald PA, Shah K, Baron P, Leiderman IZ, Imperato D, Landesman S (1986) Opportunistic infections in acquired immune deficiency syndrome result from synergistic defects of both the natural and adaptive components of cellular immunity. J Clin Invest 78:115–123
Simooya OO, Mwendapole RM, Siziya S, Fleming AF (1988) Relation between falciparum malaria and HIV seropositivity in Ndola, Zambia. Br Med J 297:30–31
Simpson TW (1984) Trichomoniasis. In: Strickland GT (ed). Hunter's tropical medicine, 6th edn. Saunders, Philadelphia, pp 499–502
Smith D, Gazzard B, Lindley RP, Darwish A, Reed C, Bryceson ADM, Evans DA (1989) Visceral leishmaniasis (Kala-azar) in a patient with AIDS. AIDS 3:41–43
Smith PD, Lane CL, Gill VJ, Manischewitz JF, Quinnan GV, Fauci AS, Masur H (1988) Intestinal infections in patients with the acquired immunodeficiency syndrome (AIDS): etiology and response to therapy. Ann Intern Med 108:328–333
Tanabe K, Fuchimoto M, Egawa K, Nakamura Y (1987) Use of *Pneumocystis carinii* genomic DNA clones for DNA hybridization analysis of infected human lungs. J Infect Dis 157:593–596
Thomas S, O'Doherty M, Bateman N (1990) *Pneumocystis carinii* pneumonia: aerosolised pentamidine gives effective prophylaxis. Br Med J 300:211–212
Toma E, Fournier S, Poisson M, Morisset R, Phaneuf D, Vega C (1989) Clindamycin with primaquine for *Pneumocystis carinii* pneumonia. Lancet i:1046–1048
Tuazon CU, Labriola AM (1987) Management of infectious and immunological complications of acquired immunodeficiency syndrome (AIDS): current and future prospects. Drugs 33:66–84
Tuazon CU, Delaney MD, Simon GL, Witorsch P, Varma VM (1985) Utility of gallium[67] scintigraphy and bronchial washings in the diagnosis and treatment of *Pneumocystis carinii* pneumonia in patients with the acquired immune deficiency syndrome. Am Rev Resp Dis 132:1087–1092
Verdejo J, Alvar J, Polo RM, González-Lahoz JM (1987) Visceral leishmaniasis associated with positive anti-HTLV-III antibody. Rev Clin Esp 180:221

Weissman I (1988) Approaches to an understanding of pathogenic mechanisms in AIDS. Rev Infect
    Dis 10:385–398
Weller IVD (1987) Treatment of infections and antiviral agents. Br Med J 295:200–203
Wharton JM, Coleman DL, Wofsy CB, Luce M, Blumenfeld W, Hadley WK, Ingram-Drake L,
    Volberding PA, Hopewell PC (1986) Trimethoprim-sulfamethoxazole or pentamidine for *Pneumo-
    cystis carinii* pneumonia in the acquired immunodeficiency syndrome: a prospective randomized
    trial. Ann Intern Med 105:37–44
World Health Organisation (1986) Acquired immunodeficiency syndrome (AIDS): WHO/CDC case
    definition for AIDS. Weekly Epidemiol Rec 61:69–76
Wiley CA, Safrin RE, Davis CE, Lampert PW, Braude AI, Martinez AJ, Visvesvara GS (1987)
    Acanthameba meningoencephalitis in a patient with AIDS. J Infect Dis 155:130–133
Yebra M, Segovia J, Manzano L, Vargas J, Bernaldo-de-Quirós L (1988) Disseminated-to-skin kala-
    azar and the acquired immunodeficiency syndrome. Ann Intern Med 108:490–491

considerable clinical importance in the indigenous population of some tropical countries. Multiple infections too are common in the Third World, the common 'trinity' being ascariasis, hookworm infection and trichuriasis. The degree to which individual parasites influence each other requires more investigation.

At a clinical level, host defence mechanisms are clearly important (Allardyce and Bienenstock 1984; Walker 1984). Whereas immunological mechanisms probably play a part (Keymer and Bundy 1989), and there is some evidence that undernutrition interferes with this (Greenwood and Whittle 1981), hypochlor-hydria (which is a relatively common problem in developing Third World countries) has probably been underestimated (Cook 1985b). Reasonable evidence exists that *Strongyloides stercoralis* (Chap. 5), for example, is more common in hypochlorhydrics. Statistically, the anatomical site of infection is usually the proximal small-intestine, where clearly the luminal milieu is acceptable to nematodes, trematodes and cestodes alike. Larvae of *Anisakis* sp (see below) sometimes involve the stomach.

Epidemiological aspects of this group of infections has received extensive coverage (Akogun 1989; Cook 1988, 1989; Fashuyi 1988). Although present throughout the world, low standards of sanitation (Feachem et al. 1983) and poor socioeconomic conditions are obvious predisposing factors to infection. Direct or indirect (e.g. as night soil) deposition of faecal material on to the ground is the major factor responsible for infection. Figure 3.1 shows human night soil being distributed as a vegetable fertilizer in West Africa. Therefore, rates of infection are usually much higher in tropical compared with non-tropical countries. Climatic influences – heat and humidity – *per se* are also relevant. Effect on working capacity is difficult to assess; many of the heaviest infections are in children. Management can be summarized: (i) environmental, including

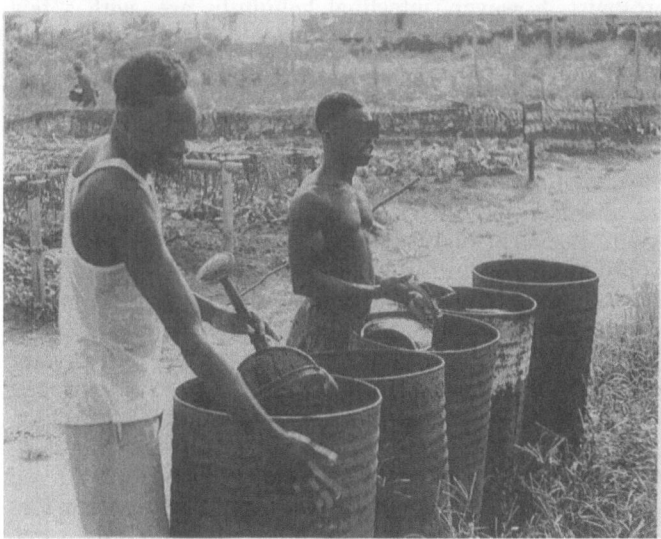

Fig. 3.1. Human night-soil being used as a crop-fertilizer in West Africa; this is obviously an important cause of *A lumbricoides* (and other orally transmitted helminthic) infections.

Chapter 3

Some Small-Intestinal and Biliary Parasites*

For indeed there is no goodness in the worm.

William Shakespeare (1564–1616),
Antony and Cleopatra V, ii, 266

Introduction

Whilst helminths seem to enjoy the small-intestinal *milieu intérieur*, protozoa by and large find the colorectal environment more to their liking (Cook 1986). To the clinical gastroenterologist, however, intestinal helminths are, with a few notable exceptions, of less than outstanding interest when compared with their protozoan counterparts. Of those involving the small-intestine, the more interesting are associated with absorptive disturbances; numerically, however, hookworm disease and ascariasis dominate the scene.

Most reviews of this subject are orientated around taxonomic parasitological classifications (World Health Organisation 1981; Gilles 1984; Goldsmith and Markell 1984; Variyam and Banwell 1984). In common with several recent reviews (Cook 1980, 1981, 1985a, b, c, 1986) the *clinical* importance of these helminths will be the dominant theme in this chapter. Clearly their importance varies and emphases are quite different in developing 'Third World' compared with 'Westernized' countries. Whereas hypochromic, iron-deficient anaemia is numerically extremely important in hookworm infections in the former (Keymer and Bundy 1989) it rarely causes major problems in expatriates, who have usually been infected during either brief or prolonged exposure to tropical conditions; the magnitude of infection and underlying nutritional status are therefore important. Similarly, epilepsy resulting from neurocysticercosis (Chap. 10) and large-duct biliary or pancreatic duct obstruction caused by *Ascaris lumbricoides* are rarities in European travellers who have become infected, but often assume

---

*NB Chapters 4 and 5 should be read in conjunction with this one.

sanitation – use of soil disinfectants etc., (ii) health education, (iii) chemo-therapy, which can be separated into treatment of an individual or of the community (mass treatment, selective chemotherapy, and targeted population chemotherapy), and (iv) awareness and participation in control by the local community (Warren 1988; Latham 1989). An example of a control strategy for hookworm infection (and the consequent hypochromic anaemia) has been outlined (Gilles 1985). Although these aspects of control are important and must be applied concurrently (especially in the Third World), this chapter focuses on clinical aspects, including chemotherapy of the individual.

Significance of Intestinal Helminths in the Third World

The more important intestinal helminthic infections cause major human illness in the Third World (Hall et al. 1982; Udonsi 1983; Elkins 1984; Farag 1985; Bundy 1989). Only rarely are accurate figures of infection rate(s) available. One estimate of world incidence rates for infection is: hookworm one billion, and roundworm 1.3 billion (Janssens 1985). This estimate for the world prevalence of hookworm infection is precisely the same as that arrived at 75 years ago (Keymer and Bundy 1989). Host susceptibility and the number of reinfections per unit time are obviously important in pathogenicity. Repeated and intensive infection is of paramount importance in determining clinical significance, e.g. in hookworm anaemia (Latham et al. 1982); although most individuals have light infections only, a minority harbour heavy loads. Intestinal capillariasis caused a major problem in the late 1960s in the Philippines after the infection had been newly introduced there.

Significance of Intestinal Helminths in the Western World

Although infection with some helminths (e.g. hookworm and *A lumbricoides*) is not uncommon in UK travellers to the tropics, intensity of infection is usually not sufficiently high to produce significant clinical symptoms and signs. Infections are usually revealed by routine screening tests. Immigrant populations, however, not infrequently harbour intestinal helminths, many of which are nematodes. Over the last few years the importance of parasitic infections – including helminths – has become apparent in the presence of immunosuppression (Wong 1984; Cook 1987) (Chap. 5). Although intestinal parasitoses are important in human HIV infections, helminths are of minor importance compared with protozoa.

Helminthic Infections *Not* Associated with Malabsorption

Table 3.1 summarizes the small-intestinal helminthic infections of man which are numerically most important. Whereas most are of limited clinical importance, several assume major significance, especially in Third World countries.

Table 3.1. Helminths of small-intestine for which no good evidence exists for a role in an absorption defect

	Major clinical importance	Minor clinical importance
Nematodes	*Ancylostoma duodenale* *Necator americanus* *Ascaris lumbricoides* *Anisakis* sp (?)	*Gnathostoma spinigerum* *Angiostrongylus costaricensis* *Ternidens deminutus* *Trichinella spiralis* *Trichostrongylus orientalis*
Cestodes	*Taenia solium* [*Cysticercus cellulosae*[a] (Chap. 10)] *T saginata*	*Dipylidium caninum* *Hymenolepis diminuta* *H nana*
Trematodes	*Heterophyes heterophyes* *Fasciolopsis buski* (?)	*Echinostoma* sp *Gastrodiscoides hominis*

[a]Term which is still occasionally used for the cystic *larval* stage of *T solium*.

Hookworm

Hookworm disease in man is caused by *Ancylostoma duodenale* and *Necator americanus*, at least one of which occurs in nearly all tropical and subtropical countries. Whereas *N americanus* is predominant in much of Asia, the Pacific, the Central Americas and southern Africa, *A duodenale* is present in most other areas; there is frequently an overlap (Hira and Patel 1984). In parts of India and the Philippines, *A ceylanicum* infection is also a problem. Filariform larvae penetrate intact skin with the occasional production of 'ground itch' – usually on the feet of children (oral infection is also possible); larvae are easily killed by freezing and desiccation, and therefore significant rainfall (usually >125 cm per year) is required for their survival.

Parasitology and Pathogenesis

The human component of the hookworm life-cycle of the parasite results in the development of mature adult worms in the duodenum and jejunum some four to five weeks after initial infection; they may still be present some five years or more later. Figure 3.2 summarizes the life-cycle of *A duodenale* and *N americanus*. A recent report documented a *N americanus* infection which continued for over 18 years (Beaver 1988). During this initial phase systemic manifestations are occasionally encountered during tissue penetration (see below). Individuals can be divided into (i) those with a few adult worms and no symptoms ('the carrier state'), and (ii) those with many worms and severe symptoms and signs of hookworm *disease*. One estimate of symptomatology is as follows: a worm load of one to 25, nil; 25 to 100, mild; 100 to 500, moderate; 500 to 1000, severe; >1000, extreme (Janssens 1985). Current knowledge of many factors involved in the host–parasite equilibrium contains many deficiencies; the role of immunity in reinfection is unknown.

Clinical Aspects

Clinical manifestations include 'ground itch' (pruritus) at the site of the initial infection (which is rare); secondary infection of the localized lesion (oedema,

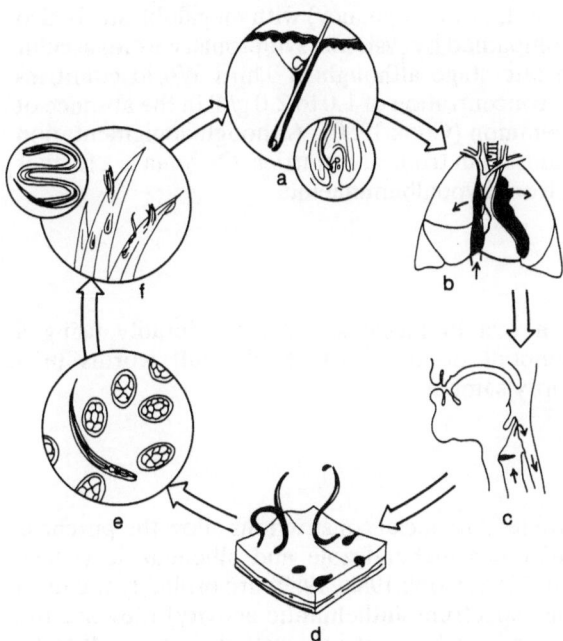

Fig. 3.2. Life-cycle of the hookworm (*Ancylostoma duodenale* and *Necator americanus*). (a) A filariform larva enters the cutaneous circulation at the base of a hair follicle; (b) haematogenous transmission to the heart and pulmonary circulation takes place, and this is followed by penetration of an alveolar capillary into an alveolar space; (c) movement occurs up the respiratory tree to the pharynx, from whence the larva is swallowed; (d) adult worms mature in the upper small-intestine (where they can live for 2–4 years) and large numbers of eggs are produced; (e) eggs are passed in faeces, and if deposited in warm, moist soil rhabditiform larvae emerge; (f) filariform larvae are produced and the cycle completed.

erythema and a vesicular or papular eruption) is unusual. Occasionally, but not often, a pulmonary reaction (with bronchospasm) is troublesome; minute haemorrhages are accompanied by eosinophilic and leucocytic infiltration. Abdominal discomfort (Maxwell et al. 1987), diarrhoea (rarely with blood and mucus) and an eosinophilia may be present. Serum IgE may be elevated. In the small-intestine, the adult worms attach to the mucosa and cause microscopic blood and serum protein loss but there is not significant enterocyte damage; therefore malabsorption is *not* a feature. Evidence that heavy infections produce growth impairment in children (Keymer and Bundy 1989) is poorly documented. Although there is some evidence for a duodenitis (Cook 1985a) further work is required. The clinical picture in advanced disease is dominated by an iron-deficient microcytic anaemia and hypoproteinaemia (World Health Organisation 1981). Rate of blood loss for *N americanus* and *A duodenale* is of the order of 0.03–0.05 and 0.16–0.34 ml per worm per day (World Health Organisation 1981) respectively; however, a good deal of iron is reabsorbed because the small-intestine possesses a substantial functional reserve. Clearly the degree of anaemia is dependent on dietary iron content, body iron reserves, and intensity and duration of infection; the chances of a heavy infection causing severe anaemia therefore vary in different geographical locations. A mixed anaemia (folate depletion being concurrently present, as in pregnancy) with megaloblastosis also occurs. The anaemia may be accompanied by systemic symptoms; cardiovascular decompensation can occur at a late stage although in Third World countries presentation with a haemoglobin concentration of 1.0 to 2.0 g/dl in the absence of signs of cardiac failure is not uncommon (Cook 1980). Although depigmentation is common, koilonychia is very unusual in tropical countries. Oedema is a further clinical manifestation, resulting from hypoalbuminaemia.

Diagnosis

Diagnosis is by identification of ova in faecal samples (preferably using a concentration technique) (Thienpont et al. 1986) or of adult worms in a duodenal-aspirate or jejunal-biopsy sample.

Management

Treatment is straightforward, provided financial constrictions allow the purchase of an effective anthelmintic. Whereas mebendazole and albendazole (which seems to be superior) (Cline et al. 1984; Cook 1988, 1989) are probably the most effective agents (both have broad-spectrum anthelmintic activity) they are too costly for many Third World countries where tetrachlorethylene has still to be used. Anaemia should be treated with an oral iron preparation, e.g. ferrous sulphate (rarely is an injectable iron preparation necessary and, even in severe anaemia, blood transfusion should be avoided for fear of precipitation of cardiac failure (Cook 1980)); if folate depletion is present concurrently, oral supplements are indicated.

Ascaris lumbricoides

The large roundworm, *Ascaris lumbricoides*, is one of man's most common parasites (Manni 1984; Editorial 1989). *A lumbricoides* (and *Trichuris trichiura*) eggs were detected in the intestine of Lindow man whose body was discovered after about 2000 years in a Cheshire bog in 1984 (Brothwell 1986). *A suum* is morphologically identical and can also mature in man. Although infection is most common in the developing Third World (Martin et al. 1983; Crompton et al. 1989), it occasionally occurs in European countries including the UK (Editorial 1985). Occasional cases have been reported in people who have not visited the tropics or subtropics, and the reasons for this have been summarized: (i) holiday travel abroad, (ii) infection acquired from immigrants, (iii) imported vegetables or fruit as a source, and (iv) acquisition of an *A suum* infection from contact with pigs (Lord and Bullock 1982). A recent estimate in a world context is 7800 million (Editorial 1985).

Parasitology and Pathogenesis

Ova (which are resistant to cold and disinfectants) are ingested by man from faecally contaminated soil and, after hatching in the small-intestine, minute

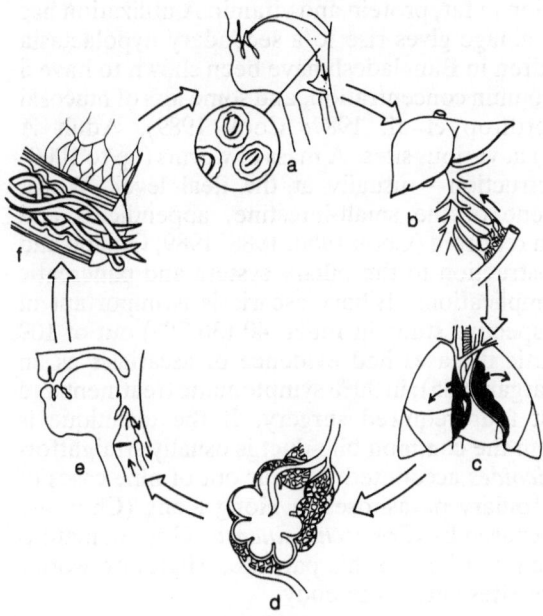

Fig. 3.3. Life-cycle of *Ascaris lumbricoides*. (a) An embryonated egg is ingested in contaminated food (or water) and swallowed; (b) in the small-intestine a larva is produced (following the action of the digestive enzymes on the egg-wall) which penetrates the mucosa and invades the portal-circulation; (c) haematogenous transmission to the heart and pulmonary circulation; (d) penetration of alveolar capillary into alveolar space takes place; (e) movement up the respiratory tract to the pharynx (this is similar to the hookworm), from whence the larva is swallowed; (f) the adult worm matures in the upper small-intestine where it can live for 2–5 years, and numerous eggs are produced which are excreted in faeces to complete the cycle.

larvae are liberated which penetrate blood and lymph vessels in the gut wall; some are carried to the liver via the portal circulation, whilst others pass through the thoracic duct. Figure 3.3 summarizes the life-cycle of *A lumbricoides*. Present understanding of host immunological mechanisms involved in ascariasis has been reviewed (World Health Organisation 1981). When they reach the lungs 4 to 16 days after infection, they perforate the alveolae and severe pulmonary symptoms (*Ascaris* pneumonia) may ensue; Löffler's syndrome consists of fever, productive cough, eosinophilia and radiographic evidence of pulmonary infiltration. At the end of this cycle. they reach the small-intestine, where maturation takes place.

Clinical Aspects

Children are frequently infected (Agugua 1983; El-Masry et al. 1983), and growth may be impaired (Nutrition Reviews 1981, 1983). However, as with hookworm infections, no conclusive evidence for interference with absorption has been demonstrated (Nutrition Reviews 1983). It seems likely, however, that *A lumbricoides* infection has a significant nutritional effect on children (Nesheim 1989); a reduction in fat, protein and vitamin A utilization has been documented, and mucosal damage gives rise to a secondary hypolactasia (Cook 1984a). Also, infected children in Bangladesh have been shown to have a significantly lower mean plasma albumin concentration, and some loss of mucosal integrity was demonstrated (Northrop et al. 1987; Cook 1989). Adult *A lumbricoides* can cause obstruction at various sites. A mass of worms (up to 1000) can produce small-intestinal obstruction – usually at the ileal level. Whilst volvulus, intussusception, gangrene of the small-intestine, appendicitis and intestinal perforation have all been reported (Cook 1980, 1988, 1989; Odaibo and Awogun 1988; Gordon 1989), obstruction to the biliary system and pancreatic duct are especially important complications. Biliary ascariasis is important in childhood (Lloyd 1981). In a prospective study in India, 40 (36.7%) out of 109 patients with biliary and pancreatic diseases had evidence of ascariasis as an aetiological factor (Khuroo and Zargar 1985); in 90% symptomatic treatment and anthelmintics led to cure, whilst four required surgery. If the technique is available, endoscopic removal from the common bile-duct is usually straightforward (Saul et al. 1984). *A lumbricoides* accounted for four out of nine cases of acute pancreatitis resulting from biliary parasitoses in Hong Kong (Choi and Wong 1984); the remainder were caused by *Clonorchis sinensis*. Granulomatous hepatitis and peritonitis have been ascribed to this parasite. Migrating worms have been located in various other sites within the body.

Diagnosis

Diagnosis, as with hookworm infections, depends on finding ova in faecal samples (preferably using a concentration technique) (Thienpont et al. 1986). Adult worms are sometimes passed in faeces or even vomited; alternatively they are occasionally 'hooked' with a jejunal-biopsy capsule or visualized during barium meal examination.

Management

Treatment is best carried out with mebendazole or albendazole (Bassily et al. 1984; Goldsmith 1988), although in developing Third World countries one of the piperazine salts is often used owing to low cost. Recently, a 100% cure rate has been claimed using ivermectin (Richard-Lenoble et al. 1988; Freedman et al. 1989; Naquira et al. 1989). Control of this parasitosis is an extremely difficult matter, but many countries have either developed or are developing national prevention programmes (Crompton et al. 1989).

Anisakis sp

Anisakis sp have been reported recently from several parts of the Western world including the UK (Lucas et al. 1985; Lewis and Shore 1985), USA (Kliks 1983; Brasitus 1984), France (Hubert et al. 1989) and Japan (Oshima 1987; Ishikura and Namiki 1989). Although not usually considered to be a common nematode in man, awareness of its existence is clinically important (Sakanari and McKerrow 1989). The adults (which belong to 24 genera of the family Anisakidae) inhabit the stomach of various species of fish (including mackerel and herring), amphibians, reptiles, mammals and birds. The larvae (which are difficult to classify) are occasionally pathogenic to man; these are therefore non-human nematodes of which the three main types are *Anisakis*, *Phocanema* and *Contracaecum*. Raw, undercooked, salted or pickled saltwater fish (sushi and sashimi (sliced raw fish fillet), or pickled herring) is the usual vehicle for transmission. In Japan, protection of marine mammals (including seals and porpoises) in the coastal waters has increased seawater contamination with *Anisakis* larvae, and this causes heavy infection in sea fish (Oshima 1987). Man is a dead-end host, i.e. larvae do not mature and ova are not found in faeces.

The site of human disease is usually the stomach or intestine; larvae attach to the mucosa which may ulcerate, and penetration through the muscle layer (with perforation) is possible. Following perforation, the mesentery, omentum and pancreas can be parasitized. Acute lesions develop within 12 hours – nausea, vomiting and epigastric pain (sometimes with haematemesis) – following ingestion of infected fish; with chronic lesions, symptoms and signs can resemble peptic ulcer disease. Disease of the small-intestine usually involves the ileocaecal region and presentation may be with appendicitis (Rushovich et al. 1983). Colonic infection is unusual.

Diagnosis is by finding larvae in vomit or gastrointestinal biopsies (usually surgical specimens taken at laparotomy). A peripheral eosinophilia and raised IgE are usual. No satisfactory serological tests are yet available (Ishikura and Namiki 1989). The disease is usually self-limiting and symptomatic treatment is the correct management if laparotomy can be avoided; no chemotherapy is effective (Ishikura and Namiki 1989).

Cestode Infections

Of the cestode infections the adult tapeworms *T solium* (pork) and *T saginata* (beef) – which mature in 5 to 12 weeks – do not usually produce significant human disease. Human infection is by ingesting viable cysticerci in measly pork or beef (Chap. 10). These infections are not strictly tropical and occur world-wide; one estimate is that 3 million and 45 million people are infected with the two species respectively. The scolex attaches to the mucosa of the small-intestine, usually the upper jejunum. Adults can reach 7 and 25 metres in length respectively.

Awareness of infection is usually apparent when segments are passed in the faeces; nausea and abdominal discomfort have been reported. Although other symptoms are documented it is difficult to evaluate their importance clinically. Occasionally, worms migrate to unusual sites, e.g. the appendix, and biliary and pancreatic ducts; intestinal obstruction and perforation have rarely been reported. Neurocysticercosis (Chap. 10) is undoubtedly the most important complication of taeniasis. Diagnosis is by identification of ova or proglottides in faecal samples. A mild eosinophilia and raised serum IgE may be present.

Treatment of uncomplicated taeniasis is straightforward: praziquantel and niclosamide both give good results (Richards and Schantz 1985; Cook 1989). In the case of *T solium* infections, some physicians recommend that an effective purge should be given 2 hours after the chemotherapeutic agent to eliminate all mature segments and thus avoid the remotely possible sequel of regurgitation of ova with the consequent development of cysticercosis.

Trematode Infections

These are dominated by *Heterophyes heterophyes* and *Fasciolopsis buski** (the largest fluke to infect man). *H heterophyes* is a small fluke found in South-east Asia and the Middle East, which attaches to the mucosa of the small-intestine and can penetrate, with a resultant granulomatous response. Abdominal pain, anorexia, nausea, and weight-loss can occur with heavy infections. Dogs, cats, foxes and other fish-eating mammals are reservoirs of infection. Raw or inadequately cooked fish is the usual source of infection. *F buski* is a parasite of South-east Asia, including Bangladesh (Gilman et al. 1982) and Indonesia (Hadidjaja et al. 1982), where one estimate is that 10 million people are infected annually, pigs forming the major reservoir. Adult worms attach to the duodenal and jejunal mucosa (and less commonly the pylorus, ileum and colon), having developed during the course of some three months, from metacercariae ingested on raw water plants – bamboo shoots, water chestnut and caltrop. There is localized inflammation, hypersecretion, ulceration and occasionally abscess formation. Diarrhoea and abdominal pain – similar to that of peptic ulcer disease – and anorexia, nausea and vomiting may ensue; intestinal stasis with partial obstruction has been documented. Oedema, involving the face in particular, occasionally occurs in heavy infections, especially in children; the mechanism for that is, however, unclear. Although impaired vitamin B_{12} absorption has been documented, there is no clear evidence of more generalized malabsorption or of protein-losing enteropathy (Jaroonvesama et al. 1986).

Diagnosis is by detection of faecal eggs; a peripheral eosinophilia may be present. The most effective treatment is probably praziquantel although it has not been extensively evaluated; niclosamide, tetrachlorethylene and hexylresorcinol are effective.

Relatively Unimportant Helminthic Infections

Although the list of such infections is a long one (Table 3.1) few are of interest from a clinical viewpoint. Of the nematodes, *Gnathostoma spinigerum*, reported mainly from Asian countries, can occasionally produce symptoms (including some involving the central nervous (Chap. 8) and urinary (Horohoe et al. 1984) systems) during the migratory stage in what is an abnormal host. Infection is by ingestion of poorly cooked freshwater fish, chicken, birds, frogs, snakes, etc. New evidence suggests that albendazole is effective (R. J. Horton, personal communication).

---

*This fluke was first visualized in 1843 by George Busk FRS (1807–1886) (Thomas 1970) during an operation on an Indian sailor, while on the second of the London hospital ships – *The Dreadnought* – which was anchored at Greenwich; this was one of the earliest venues of *clinical* tropical medicine in London (Cook 1990a). Busk, who later became President of the Royal College of Surgeons of England, Secretary of the Linnean Society of London and a prominent fellow of many learned societies, also made significant contributions to the study of Neanderthal man (Wood 1979; Reader 1988).

Angiostrongylus costaricensis, a filiform nematode (the female is 33 mm and the male 20 mm in length) which lives in the mesenteric arteries of the definitive host, can produce a granulomatous reaction with heavy eosinophilic infiltration of the intestinal wall – especially in the ileocaecal region – and occasionally at aberrant sites. Abdomen pain (appendicitis can be simulated), fever, anorexia and vomiting can occur, and a mass may be palpable on abdominal and rectal examination. Ova and adult worms can lodge in the liver. The infection occurs in Central and South America, from Mexico to Brazil. Rodents (especially the cotton rat) are the definitive, and a slug *Vaginulus plebeius* probably the main intermediate hosts; children can be infected when playing amongst infected grass. Diagnosis is usually made at laparotomy; an abnormal barium-meal and follow-through in the presence of an eosinophilia, and serology (using an ELISA), are of value. There is no effective treatment although albendazole might prove useful.

The remainder of the intestinal nematodes in this section – *Ternidens deminutus*, *Trichinella spiralis* and *Trichostrongylus orientalis* – are of limited clinical importance. *Ternidens deminutus*, a monkey parasite, is confined to Africa; the ileum is the region of the small-intestine most likely to be involved. Although adult *Trichinella spiralis* can sometimes be recovered from the intestinal mucosa in the early phase of infection, symptoms are usually mild, although severe diarrhoea has occasionally been reported in heavy infections. Trichiniasis (trichinosis) has a worldwide distribution, but is rarely responsible for human disease (Murrell and Nelson 1984); it has, however, produced significant morbidity and mortality in polar expeditions to the Arctic (Howell and Ford 1986), bears and walruses used as food being the source of infection. In other areas, pigs and wild carnivores harbour the parasite. Larval involvement of muscles, myocardium, and brain (Chap. 8) produce the major impact of this infection. (A high eosinophil count may make differentiation from other migratory intestinal nematodes and acute schistosomiasis (Chap. 7) important.) Treatment with high-dose mebendazole over a prolonged period (e.g. 20 mg/kg body-weight qds for $\geq$2 weeks) has been shown to be effective (Levin 1983). *Trichostrongylus orientalis* occurs in particular in Asia; adults lie with their heads embedded in the duodenal and jejunal mucosa. The ova found in faeces are similar to those of hookworm (Thienpont et al. 1986). Treatment is with levamisole.

The cestodes of lesser importance are: *Dipylidium caninum*, *Hymenolepis diminuta* and *H nana*. The first of these, the dog tapeworm, is nearly always asymptomatic. Proglottides can be found in faecal samples. Praziquantel and niclosamide are of value in treatment. The rodent tapeworm *H diminuta* occasionally produces mild gastrointestinal symptoms. Eggs are found in faecal samples; treatment is the same as for *D caninum*. *H nana* is usually transmitted directly from human to human. Very heavy infections in children can be associated with gastrointestinal symptoms: abdominal pain, diarrhoea, vomiting and pruritus ani. Diagnosis is by the detection of faecal ova (Thienpont et al. 1986). Treatment is with praziquantel (Farid et al. 1984) which kills both adult worms and larvae; nitrazoxamide (a nitrothiazole derivative) seems of value, and is also given as a single dose.

Of the trematodes, *Echinostoma* sp, primarily parasites of dogs, cats and other mammals, can occasionally produce human infections, largely in South-east Asia. Raw or inadequately cooked molluscs are the main source of infection. Adult worms attach to the mucosa of the small-intestine. Diarrhoea and abdominal pain can occur with heavy infections. Although praziquantel is probably effective, tetrachlorethylene and hexylresorcinol have been more widely used. *Gastrodiscoides hominis*, common in parts of India and South-east Asia, is occasionally responsible for diarrhoea; tetrachlorethylene is of value in treatment.

Infections for which Good Evidence of Interference with Absorption Exists

Table 3.2 summarizes those helminths for which there is good evidence of a causative role in malabsorption. The list is dominated by the nematodes *Strongyloides stercoralis* and *Capillaria philippinensis*. Strongyloidiasis (Cook 1986) (Chap. 5) is widespread throughout the tropics and subtropics, especially in South-east Asia. Epidemiology is very similar to that of the hookworm (see above). The related species *S fuelleborni* also causes severe malabsorption, especially in children (Cook 1980); most reports are from Zambia (Hira and Patel 1984) and Papua New Guinea (Ashford et al. 1978). As an experimental model of strongyloidiasis, *Nippostrongylus brasiliensis* infections in the rat have proved of considerable value (Carter et al. 1981). Treatment is usually with thiabendazole; however, other benzimidazoles, mebendazole (Mravak et al. 1983), albendazole (Cook 1990b), and cambendazole, have also been used (Bicalho et al. 1983) (Chap. 5).

Table 3.2. Helminths of small-intestine for which good evidence of an association with impaired absorption exists

Nematodes	*Strongyloides stercoralis* (Chap. 5)
	Capillaria philippinensis
Cestode	*Diphyllobothrium latum* (?)
Trematode	*Metagonimus yokogawai* (?)

Capillariasis has been considered in the past to be confined to the northern Philippines and Thailand (Singson et al. 1975); however, it has recently been identified in Egypt (Youssef et al. 1989). As with *S stercoralis* infections, autoinfection can occur and malabsorption, which may be gross, can lead to fatalities within a couple of months or so. The disease is contracted by consuming raw freshwater fish; a fish–bird cycle might be important epidemiologically (Cross and Basaca-Sevilla 1983). Men of 20 to 50 years of age are especially predisposed, and the disease can be epidemic and untreated carries a significant mortality. As with *S stercoralis* infections the adult worms can be demonstrated embedded in jejunal mucosa, but other sections of the gastrointestinal tract, e.g. oesophagus, stomach and colon are occasionally involved. Villus damage with infiltration of the lamina propria can be prominent. Gastrointestinal symptoms with large bulky 'malabsorption' stools are characteristic in heavy infections; absorption tests are grossly deranged. Diagnosis is by finding ova in faecal samples. Mebendazole seems to be the best therapeutic agent available, although thiabendazole is also effective; albendazole and flubendazole have also been used with good effect (Youssef et al. 1989).

Although *Diphyllobothrium latum*, the fish tapeworm, can occasionally induce vitamin B_{12} malabsorption (with resultant megaloblastic anaemia) this is an unusual event. Adult worms measure up to 10 metres in length. Although this infection, which is acquired through ingestion of raw fish, including salmon (Ruttenber et al. 1984), is often considered to be confined to cold areas, e.g. Finland, and in North American Eskimos, it is also widespread in tropical countries. The adult worms produce little in the way of small-intestinal mucosal damage; most carriers are asymptomatic, although gastrointestinal symptoms occasionally occur. Presentation can result from symptoms related to the anaemia. The vitamin B_{12} deficiency probably results from a competition between helminth and host, and is not therefore strictly an example of helminth-induced malabsorption. In severe disease, subacute combined degeneration of the spinal cord has been reported. Ova and proglottides are detected in faecal samples. Niclosamide and praziquantel are of value in treatment.

Metagonimus yokogawai infections closely resemble those caused by *Heterophyes heterophyes* (see above). There is, however, some evidence, albeit limited, that they can produce a malabsorptive state; further work is required.

Although suggestive evidence has been produced, there is little clear evidence of significant small-intestinal disease in *Schistosoma mansoni* infections (Fedail and Gadir 1985).

Summary of Helminth-Induced Symptoms and Signs, and Management

Tables 3.3 and 3.4 summarize some of the major gastrointestinal and systemic symptoms and signs produced by gastrointestinal helminths. Current treatment of intestinal helminthiases has been reviewed by Coulaud (1983), Most (1984) and Van den Bossche et al. (1985).

Table 3.3. Small-intestinal helminths: some associated gastrointestinal symptoms and signs

Epigastric pain (? duodenitis)
Malabsorptive state
Small-intestinal obstruction/intussusception
Right iliac fossa pain (+ mass)
Appendicitis-like syndrome
Intestinal perforation (?)
Biliary (large duct) obstruction
Pancreatic duct obstruction

Table 3.5 summarizes some chemotherapeutic agents which are currently in use for small-intestinal nematode infections with an indication of their relative efficacy (Gilles 1984); mebendazole, albendazole (Rossignol and Maisonneuve 1983), and flubendazole (Kan 1983) have revolutionized chemotherapy (Janssens

Table 3.4. Small-intestinal helminths: some associated systemic symptoms and signs

Anaemia: iron deficiency
Anaemia: B_{12} deficiency
Cardiac failure
Malabsorptive state
Hypoproteinaemia
Bronchospasm/pneumonitis
Overwhelming infection + septicaemia (Chap. 5)
Neurocysticercosis (Chap. 10)
Dermatological manifestations
(urticaria + 'larva currens') (Chap. 5)
Worm phobias

Table 3.5. Summary of some therapeutic agents currently used for small-intestinal nematode infections

Infection	Albendazole	Mebendazole	Pyrantel pamoate	Levamisole	Thiabendazole	Pyrvinium pamoate	Bephenium hydroxynaphthoate
Hookworm	+++	+++	++	++	++	–	++
Ascariasis	+++	+++	+++	+++	++	–	+
Strongyloidiasis (Chap. 5)	++	+	–	+	++	+	–
Trichostrongyliasis	?	++	++	+++	++	–	+

–, less than 30% cure; +, 30% to 60% cure; ++, 60% to 85% cure; +++, >85% cure.

1985; Cook 1990b). Mebendazole given as a single-dose is active against a wide range of nematode infections, including *A lumbricoides* and hookworm disease (Abadi 1985). Albendazole in particular has a wide range of activity and is given as a single-dose oral dose (400 mg); this has enormous potential in Third World populations (Ramalingam et al. 1983; Coulaud and Rossignol 1984). Treatment of trematode and cestode infections has been made much easier following the introduction of praziquantel (although niclosamide is still in use). At present, the least satisfactory gastrointestinal helminth to treat is *S stercoralis* (Chap. 5); thiabendazole, which has an incidence of side-effects of at least 50%, remains the best available chemotherapeutic agent but is by no means 100% effective (Grove 1982). Albendazole is still undergoing evaluation. That agent is also used for cutaneous larva migrans. Financial strictures remain a major problem regarding the use of most chemotherapeutic agents in Third World countries.

Whilst it is rarely possible to eliminate all worms from a definitive host on a large scale in a Third World setting (subsequent maintenance of a threshold level of worm 'burden' is usually the target), in a Western country elimination of every worm is or should be the major objective; most gastrointestinal helminths are potentially pathogenic.

Protozoa of the Small-Intestine

Table 3.6 summarizes the clinically important protozoan parasites of the small-intestine. In the immunointact individual *Giardia lamblia* dominates the list, whereas in the immunosuppressed (including AIDS patients) the coccidia (Chap. 4) assume a major pathogenic role.

Table 3.6. Protozoan infections of the small-intestine

	Immunointact	Immunosuppressed
Giardia lamblia	+	−
Cryptosporidium sp[a]	+	+
Isospora belli[a]	+	+
Sarcocystis hominis[a]	?	+
Microsporidium sp[a]	?	+
Blastocystis hominis[a]	?	+

[a]These organisms are reviewed in Chap. 4.
+, symptomatic infection.

Giardiasis

Apart from its widespread distribution in tropical countries, giardiasis is probably the most common human parasitic infection in the United Kingdom. Large outbreaks have also occurred in other European countries, the USA and Australia (Cook 1980; Farthing 1985). Seven per cent of the inhabitants of Holland who have not travelled abroad have *G lamblia* ova in a faecal sample; 21% of specimens from children between 5 and 9 years have been shown to be positive (Meuwissen et al. 1977). In Glasgow, 13.3% of Scottish, 10.2% of Asian, and 1.1% of Chinese and African children are infected with *G lamblia* (Goel et al. 1977).

In one study in India, 23% of 300 patients with non-dysenteric diarrhoea were found to be infected (Antia et al. 1966). Numerous epidemiological studies have now been recorded (Cook 1988, 1989). Giardiasis is largely a disease of travellers, however (Editorial 1977), and is frequently reported in them. In most outbreaks the organism has been isolated from water supplies including mountain-stream water (of interest in the context of hill-diarrhoea, see below). The infection does *not* seem to be unusually common in AIDS sufferers (Cook 1988).

G lamblia is frequently identified in the stool, duodenal aspirate, or jejunal biopsy of patients with post-infective tropical malabsorption (PIM) ('tropical sprue') (Wright et al. 1977). It seems possible that the epidemics of diarrhoeal disease described by Hillary (1766) in Barbados in the eighteenth century were associated with this parasite (Cook 1980). It is also possible that some epidemics of hill-diarrhoea in the nineteenth century (Grant 1854) resulted from a *G lamblia* infection; the descriptions of acute onset diarrhoea with excessive flatulence which started in the early hours of the morning, are consistent with giardiasis. An acute onset of diarrhoea with excessive flatulence and abdominal distension, reported in outbreaks of giardiasis in Colorado and Leningrad (Jokipii and

Jokipii 1977) is very similar to those nineteenth-century descriptions; significant malabsorption occurred in many. Faecal microscopy was widely used in the later nineteenth century, however, and it seems unlikely that this parasite would have been missed; awareness of its probable pathogenicity was not apparent, however, until the early twentieth century, and it could have been dismissed as being unimportant. Castellani (1905), working in Ceylon, was of the opinion that flagellates were important in producing diarrhoea if present in large numbers; he considered, however, that they also occurred in normal people, especially natives. *G lamblia* was associated with severe diarrhoea in soldiers during World War I (1914–1918) in both the Middle East and Indo-China (Vietnam) (Porter 1916; Fantham 1916).

Parasitology and Pathogenesis

G lamblia was first visualized by van Leeuwenhoek, in Delft, in 1681; he detected the trophozoite, using an early microscope, in his own stool (Dobell 1920). Many animal species in addition to man are infected, but whether they constitute a zoonotic reservoir for human infection remains debatable (Bemrick and Erlandson 1988; Faubert 1988). *G lamblia* is a flagellated protozoan which lives in close proximity to, and might actually invade, the jejunal mucosal cells (Saha and Ghosh 1977); evidence for this is, however, scanty (Sullam 1988). The trophozoite, which measures 12–18 μm in length, lives in the duodenum and jejunum; the highest concentration is present in the mucus which is adherent to the mucous membrane of the small-intestine. Figure 3.4 summarizes the life-cycle of *G*

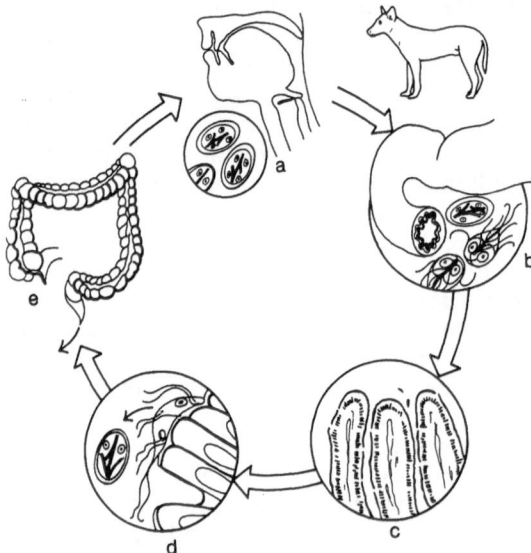

Fig. 3.4. Life-cycle of *Giardia lamblia*. (a) The cysts are ingested in contaminated water (or food) and swallowed (the importance of the domestic dog as a reservoir host is unclear, see Chap. 11); (b) each cyst gives rise to 2 trophozoites (10–20 μm × 7–10 μm) in the upper small-intestine; (c) and (d) the trophozoite adheres to the enterocyte by means of a 'sucker'; (e) encystment occurs in the lower intestinal lumen, and quadrinucleate cysts are produced; these are excreted in faeces and survive in moist soil for long periods of time.

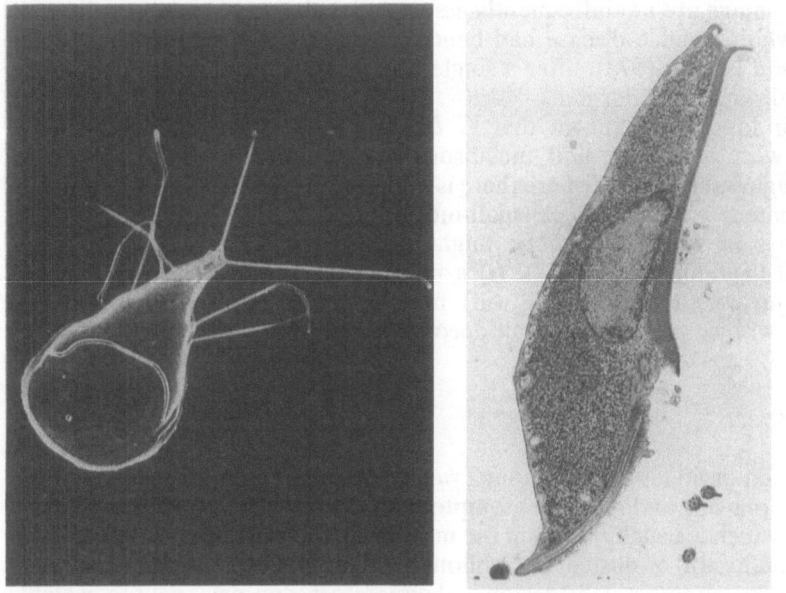

a b

Fig. 3.5. Scanning (a: × 2400) and transmission (b: × 6900) electron-micrographs of *G lamblia* trophozoites.

lamblia, and Figure 3.5 shows the mature trophozoite. *G lamblia* reproduces by binary fission. The cysts are oval and initially contain two nuclei and four after division in the mature cyst. As it descends the gastrointestinal tract it encysts, and it is in this form that it is most likely to be detected in a faecal specimen. It is possible to confuse degenerate cysts of *G lamblia* with isospora (Collins et al. 1978). Immunological aspects of a *G lamblia* infection have been reviewed (Farthing and Goka 1987; Sullam 1988). Humoral (*G lamblia*-specific IgG and secretory IgA) and cell-mediated immune mechanisms have been documented (Sullam 1988). Significant strain differences between surface antigens and excretory–secretory products have been documented (Nash 1988); infectivity and host response in gerbils and humans have also been shown to be different. Evidence for variability in strain pathogenicity is also emerging (Nash et al. 1987; Cook 1989); by using a DNA-probe, a great deal of genetic diversity has been demonstrated (Meloni et al. 1989) and this has important implications from taxonomic and epidemiological viewpoints. The organism can be cultivated in artificial media. The cyst form is resistant to the usual concentration of chlorine in domestic drinking water.

Although jejunal morphological changes have been associated with the organism, they are inconstant; villi may be shortened and stunted, and there may be an increase of mitoses in the enterocytes. Acute inflammatory lesions are often superimposed upon a non-specific chronic mucosal inflammatory exudate. Partial villous atrophy and an increase in the size and number of villus goblet cells have also been recorded.

The bile-ducts and gall-bladder are occasionally invaded. The degree of mucosal damage seems to bear little correlation with symptomatology; mild degrees of damage are not infrequently associated with severe malabsorption. A patient in whom coeliac disease had been excluded, had total villous atrophy (Levinson and Nastro 1978); after a single course of metronidazole, the biopsy became, and remained, normal.

It has for long been known that *G lamblia* infection in children can be associated with diarrhoea and malabsorption (Cortner 1959). Similarly in hypogammaglobulinaemia – where there is impaired immunity, this organism has been associated with abnormal small-intestinal structure and function. The possible ways in which *G lamblia* might produce malabsorption have been summarized (Tandon et al. 1977): (i) a mechanical barrier to absorption, (ii) mucosal injury without invasion, (iii) mucosal invasion, and (iv) bacterial overgrowth with subsequent bile-salt deconjugation.

Clinical Aspects

The incubation period is usually about 2 weeks, but may be up to several months. Many infections are undoubtedly asymptomatic (Kaezmersky and Jones 1989). Diarrhoea, which is usually worst in the mornings, and is watery, explosive, and sometimes bulky and offensive, but without blood or pus, is, however, characteristic. Weakness, abdominal distension and discomfort, anorexia, nausea, weight-loss, flatulence, vomiting, belching, depression, and failure to thrive in children (Cook 1988), are important symptoms. The brush-border damage often gives rise to secondary hypolactasia (Cook 1984a; Belosevic et al. 1989). The acute stage may last from a few days to several months. Wright et al. (1977) reported 40 patients with clinical giardiasis; symptoms had been present for up to 5 years, and 23 had evidence of malabsorption. The reason why some infections are asymptomatic is unknown; this is not related to parasite load. Differences in host susceptibility may be important. Clinical features in homosexual men are similar to those in heterosexuals (Sullam 1988); neither the frequency of infection, nor complication-rate seems to differ. Diagnosis of giardiasis is made from a history of diarrhoea, often alternating with constipation, colic, and typical malabsorption stools with excessive flatus; it often starts with an acute onset, and is frequently epidemic. The overall clinical presentation is often identical to that of PIM (Cook 1984b; 1990c), and any grade of severity may be encountered; the presence and severity of malabsorption can be demonstrated with appropriate biochemical investigations. However, many people harbour this parasite for many years without experiencing any symptoms, or suffer at most mild abdominal discomfort and occasional morning diarrhoea. Very rarely death has been attributed to giardiasis; acute ulceration of the jejunum was present (McGrath et al. 1940).

Diagnosis

The trophozoites can frequently be demonstrated in jejunal fluid; plugs or threads of mucus should be stained on a microscope-slide with Giemsa, without centrifugation. Alternatively, they can be demonstrated in jejunal biopsy samples. The 'Enterotest' (string) test (in which a nylon thread containing a gelatin capsule at its distal end is swallowed and positioned in the jejunum, and to which trophozoites of *G lamblia* adhere, and are identified microscopically) is often of value (Beal et al. 1970). Cysts can be identified in faecal specimens. Presence of *G lamblia* cysts or trophozoites in a faecal specimen is erratic, and the patient may be symptomatic for several weeks before parasites are detectable (Jokipii and Jokipii 1977); identification of cysts in a wet faecal-film (without concentration) is probably an underused diagnostic technique (Gibb 1989). Detection of parasites in duodenal or jejunal fluid is usually a more satisfactory, but time-consuming, method of diagnosis.

Circulating antibody to *G lamblia* (Ridley and Ridley 1976) is detectable, and probably indicates increased jejunal mucosal permeability with absorption of parasite antigen. An IIF has been shown to be useful diagnostically in infected children (Rojas et al. 1989). Recently, an ELISA has been reported to possess 70% sensitivity and 50% specificity (Cook 1989).

Amini (1963) demonstrated steatorrhoea in 3 out of 8 adults with a *G lamblia* infection, and that resolved after treatment. Ament and Rubin (1972) demonstrated both steatorrhoea and mucosal lesions in 4 out of 7 patients; they also tended to recover after treatment. Petersen (1972), in a review of giardiasis, concluded that malabsorption occasionally, but by no means always, occurs in infected adults. However, although the association is common, the causal role of *G lamblia per se* in the pathogenesis of malabsorption is still unclear and many patients with giardiasis are completely asymptomatic. Although there is now limited evidence that the organism invades the duodenal and jejunal mucosa (see above), it is by no means easy to comprehend how a flagellated protozoan can actively penetrate tissue. The presence of *G lamblia* trophozoites in the ileal region is difficult to assess; in practice, attempts to isolate the organism are usually directed at detection of trophozoites in the upper jejunum, and the cysts in a faecal sample. Some patients with giardiasis have a significant overgrowth of enterobacteria in the small-intestinal lumen (Tomkins et al. 1976) with free bile-acids in the duodenal aspirate (Tandon et al. 1977). Giardia, and/or closely associated enterobacteria might cause bile-salt deconjugation, and subsequent malabsorption (Cook 1980). *G lamblia* infections are common in Africa; however, PIM is very unusual on that continent (Cook 1984b; 1990c). Those observations are consistent with the probability that the parasite merely alters the luminal internal milieu, which is subsequently colonized by bacteria. Malabsorption is usually cured with metronidazole (see below); however, that compound also eradicates anaerobic bacteria, which can themselves deconjugate bile-salts and cause diarrhoea. The role of *G lamblia per se* in the production of malabsorption is therefore unclear. The mechanism might very well be similar to that in PIM (see above).

The role of dogs and other pets as reservoir hosts remains unclear (Chap. 11). Other members of the household should certainly be tested for infection.

Management

Detection of *G lamblia* in an asymptomatic patient is not in itself an indication for chemotherapy (Kaczmarski and Jones 1989). Standard chemotherapy for giardiasis is with either metronidazole ('Flagyl'), tinidazole, or mepacrine (Bassily et al. 1970; Cook 1988, 1989a). Metronidazole should be given either as a 10-day course at a dose of 200 mg bd, or preferably a 3-day course of 2 g daily; the latter regime probably gives a slightly higher cure rate. Furazolidone has given good results in infected children, but has produced a less impressive result in adults (Sullam 1988). Alcohol should be strictly avoided during treatment with metronidazole due to the possibility of a confusional state. The benzoyl ester of metronidazole has been shown to produce longer sustained plasma concentrations than metronidazole (Homeida et al. 1986); this might have a practical importance. An alternative agent is tinidazole, either at a dose of 150 mg bd for 7 days, or as a single 2.0 g dose given orally; in a report from Sudan (Salih and Abdalla 1977) that agent eradicated the parasite in 32 of 33 symptomatic patients; the only failure was in a patient given the single dose regimen. Nausea, skin-rash, and worsening of abdominal pain and diarrhoea were reported in some patients on the 7-day course. In a report from Egypt (El Masry et al. 1978), a single 2.0 g dose cured 53 of 55 patients with a heavy *G lamblia* infection. A single 2.0 g dose was also used in a study in Iran (Farahmandian et al. 1978); a reduction of 94.5% in positive faecal tests was claimed. Forty-five patients with symptomatic giardiasis were treated with tinidazole by Jokipii and Jokipii (1978); 150 mg bd for 7 days, cured 14 of 19 (74%), and a single dose of 2.0 g, 24 out of 26 (92%). Mild side-effects were noted after the higher dose. Most treatment failures were detected a few weeks after therapy, and that stresses the importance of a long follow-up. Mepacrine can be given as 100 mg tds for 10 days; acute haemolysis may be produced in the presence of glucose-6-phosphate dehydrogenase deficiency. In one study, mepacrine (300 mg daily for 10 days) cured 63%, and metronidazole (2 g daily for three days) 91% of infections (Wright et al. 1977). A synergistic (or additive) effect has been claimed when metronidazole and mepacrine are used in combination (Taylor et al. 1987). Twelve 5-nitroimidazole and 10 other compounds have been compared for their activity against *G intestinalis* in a suckling mouse model (Boreham et al. 1986); ronidazole, satranidazole and fexinidazole were 2.8, 2.0 and 2.0 times more active than tinidazole. In another recent study, 23 chemotherapeutic agents were assessed using an in vitro assay (Crouch et al. 1986); tinidazole, metronidazole and furazolidone had a powerful effect on both growth and adherence whilst mepacrine only affected growth; these authors also considered that mefloquine, doxycycline and rifampicin warranted further study.

Parasites of the Biliary Tract

Three unrelated trematodes are involved: *Clonorchis* sp, *Opisthorchis* sp, and *Fasciola* sp (Cook 1980). The first two are largely confined to South-east Asia (Cook 1980); examples are therefore uncommon in the UK and are usually discovered incidentally by the identification of eggs in a faecal specimen. They are usually asymptomatic, although heavy infections can give rise to fever, diarrhoea, epigastric pain, anorexia, tender hepatomegaly and/or jaundice. Biliary tract obstruction accompanied by stone-formation, cholangitis, and multiple small liver-abscesses are the major complications.

Snails constitute the intermediate host; these are infected by ingestion of eggs ($27\text{--}35 \times 12\text{--}19$ μm for *C sinensis*, and $26 \times 13\text{--}15$ μm for *O viverrini*) which have been released in bile and excreted in human faeces; cercariae develop within the snail, and attach to fish in which they encyst as metacercariae. Human infection occurs when infected raw or undercooked fish is ingested; smoking, pickling, and drying do not necessarily kill the metacercariae. Following ingestion, the flukes (1.0–2.5 cm long × 3–5 mm wide) ascend the biliary tree from the duodenum and lodge in medium and large bile-ducts – especially in the left lobe. Many animal species (including dogs and cats) act as reservoir hosts. Human infection can continue for at least 30 years. Excessive mucin formation with desquamation and adenomatous hyperplasia of duct epithelium progresses to bile-duct thickening, dilatation, tortuosity, and ductal and periductal fibrosis. Biliary stasis results in pericholangitis, cholangiohepatitis, pyelophlebitis and multiple abscesses; biliary cirrhosis is a rare sequel. Entry to the pancreatic duct, causing dilatation and fibrosis, is a relatively common event. Cholangiocarcinoma is a late result in both *C sinensis* and *O viverrini* infections. Although suggested, an increase in gallstones in *C sinensis* infection has not been confirmed by ultrasonography (Hou et al. 1989).

Diagnosis is by detection of eggs in a faecal specimen or duodenal fluid. Ultrasonography and CT-scanning often outline the adult worms in the biliary tree; strictures alternating with dilatation may be present. There may be an associated leucocytosis and eosinophilia.

Praziquantel (3 oral doses of 25 mg/kg given on a single day) is the best available chemotherapeutic agent (Bunnag and Harinasuta 1980; Liu et al. 1982; Lin and Chapman 1987; Goldsmith 1988); an alternative is niclofolan (Eckhardt and Heckers 1981).

Fascioliasis results from infection with the sheep liver-fluke *Fasciola hepatica* (3 cm in length × 1.5 cm wide). It is distributed world-wide and infection is often traced to infected watercress (which contains metacercariae). Snails act as the intermediate host, and a wide range of mammals may be affected. Metacercariae excyst in the duodenum, penetrate the intestinal wall, enter the peritoneal cavity, and penetrate the liver capsule; they migrate to the biliary system from the hepatic parenchyma. Eggs, which are passed in faeces, measure 130–150 μm × 63–90 μm.

Clinically, acute, chronic latent, and chronic obstructive syndromes are described. In the former, there may be systemic symptoms, an enlarged tender liver, a leucocytosis, and eosinophilia. Liver function tests are deranged. Presentation as a pyrexia of undetermined origin has been described (Salama et al. 1988).

Diagnosis is by detection of eggs in a faecal specimen (they do not normally appear until 3–4 months after the initial infection), duodenal fluid, or by needle liver-biopsy or laparotomy. Ultrasonography may also give valuable additional information (Salama et al. 1988; Bassily et al. 1989). Serology may be useful and an indirect haemagglutination test gives high sensitivity but there is considerable cross-reaction with other helminths.

Treatment is with oral bithionol (30–50 mg/kg on alternative days for 10–15 doses); the daily doses should be divided into two or three equal parts. A recent report from France has described encouraging preliminary results using triclabendazole (Loutan et al. 1989). An alternative agent is dehydroemetine (Farid et al. 1986). Praziquantel is less effective (Farag et al. 1986; Farid et al. 1986).

Conclusions

Gastrointestinal and biliary helminths (nematodes, trematodes and cestodes) constitute some of the most common and important infective agents of mankind, and are responsible for much morbidity and some mortality. Whereas many symptoms and signs are confined to the small-intestine and less often the associated digestive organs, systemic manifestations are also numerous; this applies especially to indigenous populations of developing Third World countries. A minority of small-intestinal helminths has been causally related to intestinal malabsorption. Clearly, however, not all gastrointestinal helminths are associated with disease and it is important to separate these two groups; when present at high concentration (and especially in infants and children) some of the least pathogenic are not, however, entirely asymptomatic. Numerically, the most important biliary helminths are: *Clonorchis sinensis* and *Opisthorchis viverrini*; however, *Ascaris lumbricoides* is an underdiagnosed cause of large-duct biliary obstruction. Maintenance of a high 'index of suspicion' is necessary and this applies especially to Western populations, in whom rapid and extensive travel to areas of the world with substandard sanitation and contaminated food and water supplies is now common; first evidence of infection in them may result from a serious clinical complication. Recent advances have focused on treatment, and especially the introduction of the benzimidazole compounds (especially albendazole) (Goldsmith 1988) for nematode, and praziquantel for cestode and trematode, infections. Mass elimination of gastrointestinal helminths in developing Third World countries remains a major challenge.

Of the protozoan infections, *Giardia lamblia* is without doubt the most important in the immunointact individual; whereas most infections are asymptomatic, severe malabsorption may co-exist, but the mechanism of its production remains unclear.

References

Abadi K (1985) Single dose mebendazole therapy for soil-transmitted nematodes. Am J Trop Med Hyg 34:129–133

Agugua NEN (1983) Intestinal ascariasis in Nigerian children. J Trop Paediatr 29:237–239

Akogun OB (1989) Some social aspects of helminthiasis among the people of Gumau District, Bauchi State, Nigeria. J Trop Med Hyg 92:193–196

Allardyce RA, Bienenstock J (1984) The mucosal immune system in health and disease, with an emphasis on parasitic infection. Bull WHO 62:7–25

Ament ME, Rubin CE (1972) Relation of giardiasis to abnormal intestinal structure and function in gastrointestinal immunodeficiency syndromes. Gastroenterology 62: 216–226

Amini F (1963) Giardiasis and steatorrhoea. J Trop Med Hyg 66:190–192

Antia FP, Desai HG, Jeejeebhoy KN (1966) Giardiasis in adults: incidence, symptomatology and absorption studies. Ind J Med Sci 20:471–477

Ashford RW, Vince JD, Gratten MJ, Miles WE (1978) Strongyloides infection associated with acute infantile disease in Papua New Guinea. Trans R Soc Trop Med Hyg 72:554

Bassily S, Farid Z, Mikhail JW, Kent DC, Lehman JS (1970) The treatment of *Giardia lamblia* infection with mepacrine, metronidazole and furazolidone. J Trop Med Hyg 73: 15–18

Bassily S, El-Masry NA, Trabolsi B, Farid Z (1984) Treatment of ancylostomiasis and ascariasis with albendazole. Ann Trop Med Parasitol 78:81–82

Bassily S, Iskander M, Youssef FG, El-Masry N, Bawden M (1989) Sonography in diagnosis of fascioliasis. Lancet i:1270–1271

Beal CB, Viens P, Grant RGL, Hughes JM (1970) A new technique for sampling duodenal contents: demonstation of upper small-bowel pathogens. Am J Trop Med Hyg 19:349–352

Beaver PC (1988) Light, long-lasting *Necator* infection in a volunteer. Am J Trop Med Hyg 39:369–372

Belosevic M, Faubert GM, MacLean JD (1989) Disaccharidase activity in the small intestine of gerbils (*Meriones unguiculatus*) during primary and challenge infections with *Giardia lamblia*. Gut 30:1213–1219

Bemrick WJ, Erlandsen SL (1988) Giardiasis – is it really a zoonosis? Parasitol Today 4:69–71

Bicalho SA, Leão OJ, Pena Q (1983) Cambendazole in the treatment of human strongyloidiasis. Am J Trop Med Hyg 32:1181–1183

Boreham PFL, Phillips RE, Shepherd RW (1986) The activity of drugs against *Giardia intestinalis* in neonatal mice. J Antimicrob Chemother 18:393–398

Brasitus TA (1984) 'Sushi' anyone? Gastroenterology 86:368–369

Brothwell D (1986) The bogman and the archeology of people. British Museum Publications, London, pp 73–76

Bundy DAP (1989) Ascariasis. Lancet i:1336

Bunnag D, Harinasuta T (1980) Studies on the chemotherapy of human opisthorchiasis in Thailand. I. Clinical trial of praziquantel. Southeast Asian J Trop Med Publ Health 11:528–531

Carter EA, Bloch KJ, Cohen S, Isselbacher KJ, Walker WA (1981) Use of hydrogen gas (H_2) analysis to assess intestinal absorption. Studies in normal rats and in rats infected with the nematode, *Nippostrongylus brasiliensis*. Gastroenterology 81:1091–1097

Castellani A (1905) Diarrhoea from flagellates. Br Med J ii:1285–1287

Choi TK, Wong J (1984) Severe acute pancreatitis caused by parasites in the common bile duct. J Trop Med Hyg 87:211–214

Cline BL, Little MD, Bartholomew RK, Halsey NA (1984) Larvicidal activity of albendazole against *Necator americanus* in human volunteers. Am J Trop Med Hyg 33:387–394

Collins JP, Keller KF, Brown L (1978) 'Ghost' forms of *Giardia lamblia* cysts initially misdiagnosed as *Isospora*. Am J Trop Med Hyg 27:835–836

Cook GC (1980) Tropical gastroenterology. Oxford University Press, Oxford, p 484

Cook GC (1981) Specific infective conditions – including diseases of the tropics. In: Thomson JPS, Nicholls RJ, Williams CB (eds) Colorectal disease; an introduction for surgeons and physicians. Heinemann, London, pp 187–199

Cook GC (1984a) Hypolactasia: geographical distribution, diagnosis, and practical significance. In: Chandra RK (ed) Critical reviews in tropical medicine, vol 2. Plenum Press, New York, pp 117–139

Cook GC (1984b) Aetiology and pathogenesis of postinfective tropical malabsorption (tropical sprue) Lancet i:721–723

Cook GC (1985a) Parasitic infection. In: Booth CC, Neale G (eds) Disorders of the small intestine. Blackwell Scientific Publications, Oxford, pp 283–298

Cook GC (1985b) Infective gastroenteritis and its relationship to reduced gastric acidity. Scand J Gastroenterol 20[Suppl 111]:17–23

Cook GC (1985c) Intestinal parasitic infection. In: Jewell DP, Chapman R (eds) Topics in gastroenterology 13. Blackwell Scientific Publications, Oxford, pp 71–96

Cook GC (1986) The clinical significance of gastrointestinal helminths – a review. Trans R Soc Trop Med Hyg 80:675–685

Cook GC (1987) *Strongyloides stercoralis* hyperinfection syndrome: how often is it missed? Q J Med 64;625–629

Cook GC (1988) Intestinal parasitic infections. Current Opin Gastroenterol 4:113–123

Cook (1989) Parasitic infections of the gastrointestinal tract: a worldwide clinical problem. Current Opin Gastroenterol 5:126–139

Cook GC (1990a) Early history of clinical tropical medicine in London. J R Soc Med 83:38–41

Cook GC (1990b) Use of benzimidazole chemotherapy in human helminthiases: indications and efficacy. Parasitol Today (in press)

Cook GC (1990c) The small-intestine and its role in chronic diarrhoeal disease in the tropics. In: Gracey M (ed) Diarrhea. Telford Press, New Jersey (in press)

Cortner JA (1959) Giardiasis, a cause of celiac syndrome. Am J Dis Child 98:311–316

Coulaud JP (1983) Traitement des nematodoses intestinales. Ann Soc Belg Med Trop 63:5–20

Coulaud JP, Rossignol JF (1984) Albendazole: a new single dose anthelmintic. Acta Trop 41:87–90

Crompton DWT, Nesheim MC, Pawlowski ZS (eds) (1989) Ascariasis and its prevention and control. Taylor and Francis, London and New York, p 406

Cross JH, Basaca-Sevilla V (1983) Experimental transmission of *Capillaria philippinensis* to birds. Trans R Soc Trop Med Hyg 77:511–514

Crouch AA, Seow WK, Thong HY (1986) Effect of twenty-three chemotherapeutic agents on the adherence and growth of *Giardia lamblia* in vitro. Trans R Soc Trop Med Hyg 80:893–896

Dobell C (1920) The discovery of the intestinal protozoa of man. Proc R Soc Med 13[section of the history of medicine]:1–15

Eckhardt T and Heckers H (1981) Treatment of human fascioliasis with niclofolan. Gastroenterology 81:795–798
Editorial (1977) Giardiasis. Br Med J ii:538–539
Editorial (1985) Ascaris infections: Lancet ii:1284
Editorial (1989) Ascariasis. Lancet i:997–998
Elkins DB (1984) A survey of intestinal helminths among children of different social communities in Madras, India. Trans R Soc Trop Med Hyg 78:132–133
El-Masry NA, Farid Z, Miner WF (1978) Treatment of giardiasis with tinidazole. Am J Trop Med Hyg 27:201–202
El-Masry NA, Trabolsi B, Bassily S, Farid Z (1983) Albendazole in the treatment of *Ancylostoma duodenale* and *Ascaris lumbricoides* infections. Trans R Soc Trop Med Hyg 77:160–161
Fantham HB (1916) Remarks on the nature and distribution of the parasites observed in the stools of 1305 dysenteric patients. Lancet i:1165–1166
Farag HF (1985) Intestinal parasitosis in the population of the Yemen Arab Republic. Trop Geogr Med 37:29–31
Farag HF, Ragab M, Salem A, Sadek N (1986) A short note on praziquantel in human fascioliasis. J Trop Med Hyg 89:79–80
Farahmandian I, Sheiban F, Sanati A (1978) Evaluation of the effect of a single dose of tinidazole (Fasigyn) in giardiasis. J Trop Med Hyg 81:139–140
Farid Z, El-Masry MA, Wallace CK (1984) Treatment of *Hymenolepis nana* with a single dose of praziquantel. Trans R Soc Trop Med Hyg 78:280
Farid Z, Trabolsi B, Boctor F, Hafez A (1986) Unsuccessful use of praziquantel to treat acute fascioliasis in children. J Infect Dis 154:920–921
Farthring MJG (1985) Giardiasis. In: Jewell DP, Chapman RW (eds) Topics in Gastroenterology 13. Blackwell, Scientific Publications, Oxford, pp 97–118
Farthing MG, Goka AKJ (1987) Immunology of giardiasis. Baillière Clin Gastroenterol 1:589–604
Fashuyi SA (1988) An observation of the dynamics of intestinal helminth infections in two isolated communities of south-western Nigeria. Trop Geogr Med 40:226–232
Faubert GM (1988) Evidence that giardiasis is a zoonosis. Parasitol Today 4:66–68
Feachem RG, Guy MW, Harrison S, Iwago KO, Marshall T, Mbere N, Muller R, Wright AM (1983) Excreta disposal facilities and intestinal parasitism in urban Africa: preliminary studies in Botswana, Ghana and Zambia. Trans R Soc Trop Med Hyg 77:515–521
Fedail SS, Gadir AFMA (1985) The pathology of the small intestine in human schistosomiasis mansoni in the Sudan. Trop Med Parasitol 36:94–96
Freedman DO, Zierdt WS, Lujan A, Nutman TB (1989) The efficacy of ivermectin in the chemotherapy of gastrointestinal helminthiasis in humans. J Infect Dis 159:1151–1153
Gibb AP (1989) Identification of unsuspected cases of giardiasis by wet-film microscopy. Lancet ii:216–217
Gilles HM (1984) Intestinal namatode infections. In: Strickland GT (ed) Hunter's tropical medicine, 6th edn. Saunders, Philadelphia, pp 620–647
Gilles HM (1985) Selective health care: strategies for control of disease in the developing world. XVII. Hookworm infection and anaemia. Rev Inf Dis 7:111–118
Gilman RH, Mondal G, Maksud M, Alam K, Rutherford E, Gilman JB, Khan MU (1982) Endemic focus of *Fasciolopsis buski* infection in Bangladesh. Am J Trop Med Hyg 31:796–802
Goel KM, Shanks RA, McAllister TA, Follett EAC (1977) Prevalence of intestinal parasitic infestation, salmonellosis, brucellosis, tuberculosis, and hepatitis B among immigrant children in Glasgow. Br Med J i:676–679
Goldsmith RS (1988) Recent advances in the treatment of helminthic infections: ivermectin, albendazole, and praziquantel. In: Leech JH, Sande MA, Root RK (eds) Parasitic infections. Churchill Livingstone, Edinburgh and New York, pp 327–347
Goldsmith R, Markell EK (1984) Cestode infections. In: Strickland GT (ed) Hunter's tropical medicine, 6th edn. Saunders, Philadelphia, pp 758–771
Gordon ME, (1989) Ascariasis. Lancet i:1336
Grant A (1854) Remarks on hill diarrhoea and dysentery, with brief notices of some of the Himalayan sanitaria. Ind Ann Med Sci[2nd Edn]:311–348
Greenwood BM, Whittle HC (1981) Immunology of medicine in the tropics. Edward Arnold, London, pp 178–210
Grove DI (1982) Treatment of strongyloidiasis with thiabendazole: an analysis of toxicity and effectiveness. Trans R Soc Trop Med Hyg 76:114–118
Hadidjaja P, Dahri HM, Roesin R, Margono SS, Djalins J, Hanafiah M (1982) First autochthonous case of *Fasciolopsis buski* infection in Indonesia. Am J Trop Med Hyg 31:1065

Hall A, Latham MC, Crompton DWT, Stephenson LS, Wolgemuth JC (1982) Intestinal parasitic infections of men in four regions of rural Kenya. Trans R Soc Trop Med Hyg 76:728–733

Hillary W (1766) Observations on the changes of the air and the concomitant epidemical diseases, in the island of Barbadoes, 2nd edn. Hawes Clarke and Collins, London, pp 276–297

Hira PR, Patel BG (1984) Hookworms and the species infecting man in Zambia. J Trop Med Hyg 87:7–10

Homeida MA, Daneshmend TK, Ali HM, Kaye CM (1986) Metronidazole metabolism following oral benzoylmetronidazole suspension in children with giardiasis. J Antimicrob Chemother 18:213–220

Horohoe JJ, Ritterson AL, Chessin LN (1984) Urinary gnathostomiasis. JAMA 251:255–256

Hou M-F, Ker C-G, Sheen P-C, Chen E-R (1989) The ultrasound survey of gallstone diseases of patients infected with Clonorchis sinensis in Southern Taiwan. J Trop Med Hyg 92:108–111

Howell M, Ford P (1986) The ghost disease and twelve other stories of detective work in the medical field. Penguin Books, Harmondsworth, pp 17–52

Hubert B, Bacou J, Belveze H (1989) Epidemiology of human anisakiasis: incidence and sources in France. Am J Trop Med Hyg 40:301–303

Ishikura H, Namiki M (eds) (1989) Gastric anisakiasis in Japan: epidemiology, diagnosis, treatment. Springer, Berlin Heidelberg New York

Janssens PG (1985) Chemotherapy of gastrointestinal nematodiasis in man. In: Van den Bossche H, Thienpont D, Janssens PG (eds) Chemotherapy of gastrointestinal helminths. Springer-Verlag, Berlin Heidelberg New York, pp 183–406

Jaroonvesama N, Charoenlarp K, Areekul S (1986) Intestinal absorption studies in Fasciolopsis buski infection. Southeast Asian J Trop Med Publ Health 17:582–586

Jokipii AMM, Jokipii L (1977) Prepatency of giardiasis. Lancet i:1095–1097

Jokipii AMM, Jokipii L (1978) Comparative evaluation of two dosages of tinidazole in the treatment of giardiasis. Am J Trop Med Hyg 27:758–761

Kaczmarski EB, Jones DM (1989) Let sleeping Giardia lie. Lancet ii:872

Kan SP (1983) The anthelmintic effects of flubendazole on Trichuris trichiura and Ascaris lumbricoides. Trans R Soc Trop Med Hyg 77:668–670

Keymer A, Bundy D (1989) Seventy-five years of solicitude. Nature 337:114

Khuroo MS, Zargar SA (1985) Biliary ascariasis: a common cause of biliary and pancreatic disease in an endemic area. Gastroenterology 88:418–423

Kliks MM (1983) Anisakiasis in the western United States: four new case reports from California. Am J Trop Med and Hyg 32:526–532

Latham MC (1989) Ascariasis. Lancet i:1270

Latham MC, Stephenson LS, Hall A, Wolgemuth JC, Elliott TC, Crompton DWT (1982) A comparative study of the nutritional status, parasitic infections and health of male roadworkers in four areas of Kenya. Trans R Soc Trop Med Hyg 76:734–740

Levin ML (1983) Treatment of trichinosis with mebendazole. Am J Trop Med Hyg 32:980–983

Levinson JD, Nastro LJ (1978) Giardiasis with total villous atrophy. Gastroenterology 74:271–275

Lewis R, Shore JH (1985) Anisakiasis in the United Kingdom. Lancet ii:1019

Lin AC, Chapman SW (1987) Praziquantel and clonorchiasis. Antimicrob Agents Chemother 31:1291

Liu Y-H, Qiu Z-D, Wang X-G, Wang Q-N, Qu Z-Q, Chen R-X, Liu J-B, Zhang C-D, Qin S-A (1982) Praziquantel in clonorchiasis sinensis: a further evaluation of 100 cases. China Med J 95:89–94

Lloyd DA (1981) Massive hepatobiliary ascariasis in childhood. Br J Surg 68:468–473

Lord WD, Bullock WL (1982) Swine ascaris in humans. New Engl J Med 306:1113

Loutan L, Bouvier M, Rojanawisut B, Stalder H, Rouan MC, Buescher G, Poltera AA (1989). Single treatment of invasive fascioliasis with triclabendazole. Lancet ii:383

Lucas SB, Cruse JP, Lewis AAM (1985) Anisakiasis in the United Kingdom. Lancet ii:843–844

Manni JJ (1984) Ascariasis: effect of treating a single case upon the local population. Trop Doctor 14:142

Martin J, Keymer A, Isherwood RJ, Wainwright SM (1983) The prevalence and intensity of Ascaris lumbricoides infections in Moslem children from northern Bangladesh. Trans R Soc Trop Med Hyg 77:702–706

Maxwell C, Hussain R, Nutman TB, Poindexter RW, Little MD, Schad GA, Ottesen EA (1987) The clinical and immunologic responses of normal human volunteers to low dose hookworm (Necator americanus) infection. Am J Trop Med Hyg 37:126–134

McGrath J, O'Farrell PT, Boland SJ (1940) Giardial steatorrhoea: a fatal case with organic lesions. Irish J Med Sci 6:802–816

Meloni BP, Lymbery AJ, Thompson RCA (1989) Characterization of Giardia isolates using a non-radiolabeled DNA probe, and correlation with the results of isoenzyme analysis. Am J Trop Med Hyg 40:629–637

Meuwissen JHET, Tongeren JHM, Werkman HPT (1977) Giardiasis. Lancet ii:32–33

Most H (1984) Treatment of parasitic infections of travelers and immigrants. N Engl J Med 310:298–304

Mravak S, Schopp W, Bienzle U (1983) Treatment of strongyloidiasis with mebendazole. Acta Trop 40:93–94

Murrell KD, Nelson GS (1984) Trichinosis. In: Strickland GT (ed) Hunter's tropical medicine, 6th edn. Saunders, Philadelphia, pp 689–695

Naquird C, Jimenez G, Guerra JG, Bernal R, Naliu DR, Neu D, Aziz M (1989) Ivermectin for human Strongyloidiasis and other intestinal helminths. Am J Trop Med Hyg 40:304–309

Nash TE (1988) Biologic differences among isolates of *Giardia lamblia*. In: Leech JH, Sande MA, Root RK (eds) Parasitic infections. Churchill Livingstone, Edinburgh and New York, pp 133–145

Nash TE, Herrington DA, Losonsky GA, Levine MM (1987) Experimental human infections with *Giardia lamblia*. J Infect Dis 156:974–984

Nesheim MC (1989) Ascariasis and human nutrition. In: Crompton DWT, Nesheim MC, Pawlowski ZS (eds) Ascariasis and its prevention and control. Taylor and Francis, London and New York, pp 87–100

Northrop CA, Lunn PG, Wainwright M, Evans J (1987) Plasma albumin concentrations and intestinal permeability in Bangladeshi children infected with *Ascaris lumbricoides*. Trans R Soc Trop Med Hyg 81:811–815

Nutrition Reviews (1981) Infections as deterrents of child growth. Nutr Rev 39:328–330

Nutrition Reviews (1983) Ascariasis, giardiasis and growth. Nutr Rev 41:149–151

Odaibo SK, Awogun IA (1988) Small intestinal perforation by *Ascaris lumbricoides*. Trans R Soc Trop Med Hyg 82:154

Oshima T (1987) Anisakiasis – is the sushi bar guilty? Parasitol Today 3:44–48

Petersen H (1972) Giardiasis (Lambliasis) Scand J Gastroenterol 7[Supp 14]:1–44

Porter A (1916) An enumerative study of the cysts of *Giardia* (*lamblia*) *intestinalis* in human dysenteric faeces. Lancet i:1166–1169

Ramalingam S, Sinniah B, Krishnan U (1983) Albendazole, an effective single dose, broad spectrum anthelmintic drug. Am J Trop Med Hyg 32:984–989

Reader J (1988) Missing links: the hunt for earliest man. Penguin Books, Harmondsworth, pp 11–12

Richard-Lenoble D, Kombila M, Rupp EA, Pappayliou ES, Gaxotte P, Nguiri C, Aziz MA (1988) Ivermectin in loiasis and concomitant *O. volvulus* and *M. perstans* infections. Am J Trop Med Parasitol 39:480–483

Richards F, Schantz PM (1985) Treatment of *Taenia solium* infections. Lancet i:1264–1265

Ridley MJ, Ridley DS (1976). Serum antibodies and jejunal histology in giardiasis associated with malabsorption. J Clin Pathol 29:30–34

Rojas L, Torres DR, Mediola BJ, Finlay CM (1989) Detection of specific anti-giardia serum antibody by an immunofluorescence test in children with clinical giardiasis. Am J Trop Med Hyg 40:477–479

Rossignol JF, Maisonneuve H (1983) Albendazole: placebo-controlled study in 870 patients with intestinal heminthiasis. Trans R Soc Trop Med Hyg 77:707–711

Rushovich AM, Randall EL, Caprini JA, Westenfelder GO (1983) Omental anisakiasis: a rare mimic of appendicitis. Am J Clin Pathol 80:517–520

Ruttenber AJ, Weniger BG, Sorvillo F, Murray RA, Ford SL (1984) Diphyllobothriasis associated with salmon consumption in Pacific coast states. Am J Trop Med Hyg 33:455–459

Saha TK, Ghosh TK (1977) Invasion of small intestinal mucosa by *Giardia lamblia* in man. Gastroenterology 72:402–405

Sakanari JA, McKerrow JH (1989) Anisakiasis. Clin Microbiol Rev 2:278–284

Salama HM, Abdel-Wahab MF, Farid Z (1988) Hepatobiliary disorders presenting as fever of unknown origin in Cairo, Egypt: the role of diagnostic ultrasonography. J Trop Med Hyg 91:147–149

Salih SY, Abdalla RE (1977) Symptomatic giardiasis in Sudanese adults and its treatment with tinidazole. J Trop Med Hyg 80:11–13

Saul C, Pias VM, Jannke HA, Braga NHM (1984) Endoscopic removal of *Ascaris lumbricoides* from the common bile duct. Am J Gastroenterol 79:725–727

Singson CN, Banzon TC, Cross JH (1975) Mebendazole in the treatment of intestinal capillariasis. Am J Trop Med Hyg 24:932–934

Sullam PM (1988) Amebiasis and giardiasis in homosexual men. In: Leech JH, Sande MA, Root RK (eds) Parasitic infections. Churchill Livingstone, Edinburgh and New York, pp 147–175

Tandon BN, Tandon RK, Satpathy BK, Shriniwas (1977) Mechanism of malabsorption in giardiasis: a study of bacterial flora and bile salt deconjugation in upper jejunum. Gut 18:176–181

Taylor GD, Wenman WM, Tyrrell DLJ (1987) Combined metronidazole and quinacrine hydrochloride therapy for chronic giardiasis. Can Med Assoc J 136:1179–1182

Thienpont D, Rochette F, Vanparijs OFJ (1986) Diagnosing helminthiasis by coprological examination, 2nd edn. Janssen Research Foundation, Beerse, Belgium, p 205

Thomas KB (1970) George Busk. In: Dictionary of scientific biography. Scribner, New York, pp 616–618

Tomkins AM, Wright SG, Drasar BS, James WPT (1976) Colonization of jejunum by enterobacteria and malabsorption in patients with giardiasis. Gut 17:397

Udonsi JK (1983) *Necator americanus* infection: a longitudinal study of an urban area in Nigeria. Ann Trop Med Parasitol 77:305–310

Van den Bossche H, Thienpont D, Janssens PG (eds) (1985) Chemotherapy of gastrointestinal helminths. Springer-Verlag, Berlin Heidelberg New York, p 719

Variyam EP, Banwell JG (1984) Worm infections. In: Bouchier IAD, Allan RN, Hodgson HJF, Keighley MRB (eds) Textbook of gastroenterology. Baillière Tindall, London, pp 1074–1091

Walker WA (1984) Immunoregulation of small intestinal function. Gastroenterology 86:577–579

Warren KS (1988) Hookworm control. Lancet ii:897–898

Wong B (1984) Parasitic diseases in immunocompromised hosts. Am J Med 76:479–486

Wood BA (1979) The 'Neanderthals' of the College of Surgeons. Ann R Coll Surg Engl 61:385–389

World Health Organization (1981) Intestinal protozoan and helminthic infections. Technical Report Series No. 666. WHO, Geneva, p 152

Wright SG, Tomkins AM, Ridley DS (1977). Giardiasis: clinical and therapeutic aspects. Gut 18:343–350

Youssef FG, Mikhail EM, Mansour NS (1989) Intestinal capillariasis in Egypt: a case report. Am J Trop Med Hyg 40:195–196

Chapter 4

Small-Intestinal Coccidiosis: The Cause of Diverse Symptomatology, and a Major Problem in AIDS

In the last stages of this illness a diarrhoea helps to waste the little remainder of flesh and strength.

William Heberden (1710–1801),
Commentaries on the history and cure of diseases

Introduction

Several human protozoan infections have recently assumed prominence in the context of severe immunosuppressive states (including the acquired immune deficiency syndrome (AIDS)), in which they occur as 'opportunists'. *Pneumocystis carinii* (Blaser and Cohn 1986; Cook 1987a), *Toxoplasma gondii* (Navia et al. 1986; Cook 1987a), and *Leishmania donovani* (Badaró et al. 1986; Montalban et al. 1987) (the causative agent of visceral leishmaniasis or Kala-azar) are protozoa which can parasitize the respiratory, central nervous, and reticulo-endothelial systems respectively (Chaps. 2, 9 and 12). Gastrointestinal defence mechanisms, as well as systematic ones, are, however, compromised in AIDS sufferers (Rodgers et al. 1986; Siegal et al. 1986) and here too various protozoa (coccidia) are, as a consequence, allowed to run riot! Numerically, *Cryptosporidium* sp is the most important of the human coccidial infections (Whiteside et al. 1984; Casemore et al. 1985; Fayer and Ungar 1986; Cook 1987b; 1988a,b; 1990; Current 1988; Soave and Johnson 1988; Tzipori 1988; Casemore 1989). This organism was first demonstrated by Tyzzer in 1907 to parasitize the stomach and small-intestine of mice (Casemore et al. 1985; Fayer and Ungar 1986); its causative role in diarrhoea in turkeys and calves was elucidated in 1955 and 1971 respectively (Cook 1990). *Isospora belli* (Whiteside et al. 1984; Forthal and Guest 1984; DeHovitz et al. 1986; Gelb and Miller 1986; Cook 1987b; Soave and Johnson 1988) and *Sarcocystis hominis* (Greve 1985; Cook 1987a; Dubey et al.

1989) are also important in the immunosuppressed. The precise pathological roles of *Microsporidium* sp (clearly associated with AIDS) (Desportes et al. 1985; Cook 1987a; Rijpstra et al. 1988; Shadduck 1989); and *Blastocystis hominis** (Garcia et al. 1984; Vannatta et al. 1985; Markell and Udkow 1986; Masry et al. 1988; Miller and Minshew 1988; Kain and Noble 1989; Llibre et al. 1989; Rolston et al. 1989) are so far poorly delineated, despite the fact that the latter has been known since 1912 to be an inhabitant of the human small-intestine (Garcia et al. 1984). There seems to be no doubt that the clinical significance of all these organisms depends upon the magnitude of the infection, and that this correlates inversely with underlying immune competence.

Recent interest in human coccidia is by no means confined to the immunosuppressed and those with AIDS, however. It has recently become clear that some, at least, are causatively important in self-limiting diarrhoea in infants and children (Wolfson et al. 1985; Hira et al. 1989), and in travellers' diarrhoea, in immunocompetent individuals (see below); simultaneous infection with *Giardia lamblia* has also been reported from several countries. The clinical importance of the coccidia varies geographically (like some systemic protozoan parasites, including *L donovani*); these intestinal protozoa are more prevalent in many Third World countries (e.g. Haiti, Uganda, Zambia and India) compared with most industrialized ones (Quinn et al. 1986; Cook 1987b, 1989; Sewankambo et al. 1987; Pal et al. 1989).

Until recently, cryptosporidiosis was considered to be a zoonotic disease; indeed, the first recorded human case involved a 3-year-old girl who lived on a farm (Nime et al. 1976). However, within the past few years, person-to-person transmission (Cook 1987b) and infection from contaminated water supplies (probably by cattle faeces) (D'Antonio et al. 1985; Isaac-Renton et al. 1987) have become increasingly apparent. The exact size of the problem in contamination of domestic water supplies (by animal and human sewage) is not yet entirely clear. It seems clear, however, that whereas farm animals are more important in rural areas, person-to-person and water-borne transmission are particularly relevant in an urban setting (Editorial 1989; Cook 1990). Food-borne transmission has been poorly documented. Airborne (Højlyng et al. 1987) and perinatal (Låhdevirta et al. 1987) routes of infection have recently been suggested in addition. Recently an outbreak caused by infected swimming-pool water, which had been polluted with sewage, was reported in England (Galbraith 1989). The potential reservoir for human infection must be vast; it is widely spread in the animal kingdom, and oocysts, which are stable in excreta, are resistant to many chemical agents (Fayer and Ungar 1986). Whilst *I belli* infections also result largely from ingested oocysts in contaminated food and water (Cook 1987a), a *Sarcocystis hominis* infection usually originates from ingestion of bradyzoites in raw beef or pork (especially cardiac and oesophageal muscle) (Cook 1987a; Dubey et al. 1989); person-to-person transmission is probably unusual.

---

*The correct taxonomic position of *B hominis* remains unclear; however, recent evidence indicates that it was incorrectly classified with the Sporozoa and should be transferred to a new suborder (Blastocystina) of the subphyllum Sarcodina (Zierdt 1988).

Parasitology and Pathogenesis

The small-intestinal coccidia have a history dating back several million years. It is from them that the haematogenous protozoa, *Plasmodium* sp (the causative agents of malaria), originated (Chap. 1) (Bruce-Chwatt 1985; Casemore et al. 1985). They belong to the class Sporozoa of the phylum Apicomplexa (Cook 1990); Cryptosporidiidae (to which *Cryptosporidium* sp belongs), Eimeriidae, and Sarcocystidae are families which belong to the suborder Eimeria of the order Eucoccidiia. Although 18 species were named following the initial description, the most recent classification has reduced this to four: *C nasorum* (fish), *C crotali* (reptiles), *C meleagradis* (birds) and *C parvum* [or *C muris*] (mammals) (Current 1988); some investigators consider this to be a single-species genus, however. Their life-cycles, which are complex and involve six stages, have still not been satisfactorily unravelled; they vary from species to species (Forthal and Guest 1984; Casemore et al. 1985; Desportes et al. 1985; Fayer and Ungar 1986;

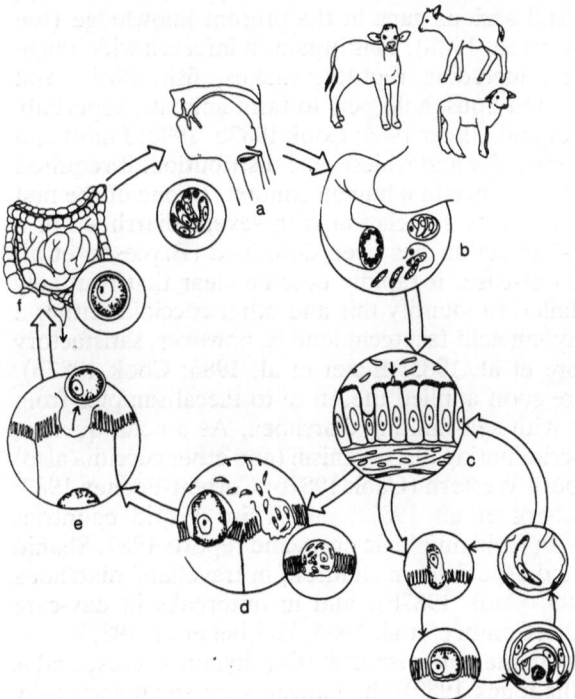

Fig. 4.1. Life-cycle of *Cryptosporidium* sp. (a) Oocysts (3–5 μm) are ingested in contaminated food or water (many animal species, most importantly calves, can act as a reservoir for infection) and swallowed; (b) sporozoites are released in the upper small-intestine (following the action of digestive enzymes); (c) each sporozoite is capable of entering an enterocyte, in which the asexual cycle takes place (the intracellular, extracytoplasmic trophozoite emerges and transforms into a schizont which produces 8 merozoites and they can in turn infect other enterocytes); (d) microgametes (♂) are formed which burst out of the infected cell and are able to fuse with an intracellular macrogamete (♀); (e) the resultant zygote (oocyst) secretes an outer wall and enters the small-intestinal lumen; (f) the oocyst is excreted in faeces, sporulates, and is infective; the unsporulated oocyst is also potentially infective, sporulation occurring *after* ingestion.

Cavalier-Smith 1987; Casemore 1989). In some instances light- and electron-microscopy are currently open to different interpretations (Casemore et al. 1985). Figure 4.1 summarizes the major features of the life-cycle of *Cryptosporidium* sp. Excystation (infective sporozoites are released from the oocysts), merogony (asexual replication), gametogony (gamete formation), fertilization, oocyst-wall formation, and sporogony (sporozoite formation) can all be demonstrated (Cook 1987b, 1988b). *Cryptosporidium* sp has an apical complex but possesses neither cilia nor flagella. Figure 4.2 shows electron-micrographic appearances of *Cryptosporidium* sp. It now seems clear that it is an intracellular, but extracytoplasmic organism. Absence of mitochondria in *Cryptosporidium* sp brings it perhaps into line with the intraluminal protozoa (including *Giardia lamblia*) (Cavalier-Smith 1987); *I belli*, which does possess these organelles, has points in common with other intracytoplasmic enterocytic parasites (Forthal and Guest 1984). Development of *Cryptosporidium* sp in cell culture (at 35, 37 and 41 °C) has been described, and much will doubtless be learned using this technique (Current and Haynes 1984; Cook 1987b; Lumb et al. 1988).

Overall, most known facts about coccidia relate to *Cryptosporidium* sp, although even here there are still serious gaps in the present knowledge (see above) (Casemore et al. 1985; Current 1988). This organism infects a wide range of animal species (see above), including reptiles, snakes, fish, birds, and mammals ranging from rodents and household pets to farm animals, especially calves (O'Donoghue 1985; Fayer and Ungar 1986; Cook 1987b, 1990; Janoff and Reller 1987). Despite its great antiquity and widespread distribution, it required AIDS to bring it (in 1982) to prominence in a human context. In one of the first cases of AIDS in the UK, in 1978, its association with severe diarrhoea in a Portuguese man with an HIV-2 infection has been described (Bryceson et al. 1988). After recognition in this disease, it rapidly became clear that routinely used faecal staining-methods failed to identify this and other coccidia; either a modified Ziehl–Neelsen or Kinyoun acid-fast technique is, however, satisfactory (Ma and Soave 1983; Casemore et al. 1985; Elsser et al. 1986; Cook 1987b). These laboratory methods were soon applied therefore to faecal-samples from immunocompetent individuals with self-limiting diarrhoea. As a consequence, there are now extensive data incriminating this organism (and other coccidia also) in acute diarrhoeal disease in both Western (Cook 1987b; Corbett-Feeney 1987; Thomson et al. 1987; Wittenberg et al. 1987), and Third World countries (Højlyng et al. 1986; Cook 1987b; Epidemiologic notes and reports 1987; Shahid et al. 1987). It has been reported especially in children, in travellers' diarrhoea ('turista') (Soave and Ma 1985; Cook 1987b), and in outbreaks in day-care centres in the USA and Canada (Combee et al. 1986; Heijbel et al. 1987).

There are several reasons why human microsporidiosis (phylum Microspora) is a relatively obscure disease (Shadduck 1989); the parasites are small and easily overlooked, stain poorly, evoke little or no tissue response, often require electron-microscopy for recognition, and cannot be detected serologically.

It is possible that both humoral and cell-mediated immunity (CMI) are involved in limiting the length of disease in the immuno-intact individual (Cook 1990). Most immunocompetent individuals possess *C parvum*-specific serum antibodies for several months (up to 2 years) after recovery from a *Cryptosporidium* sp infection; this fact is difficult to comprehend considering that the organism is confined to the microvillous region of the enterocyte. Normal T-cell function has been recorded in hypogammaglobulinaemic patients with a severe

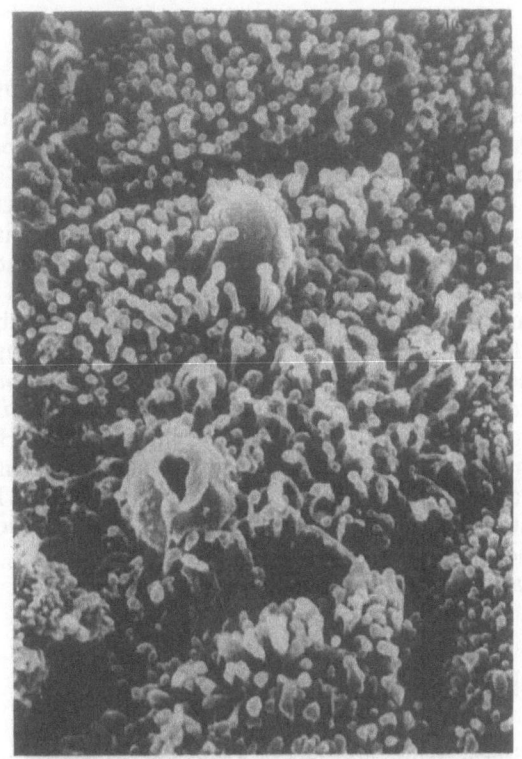

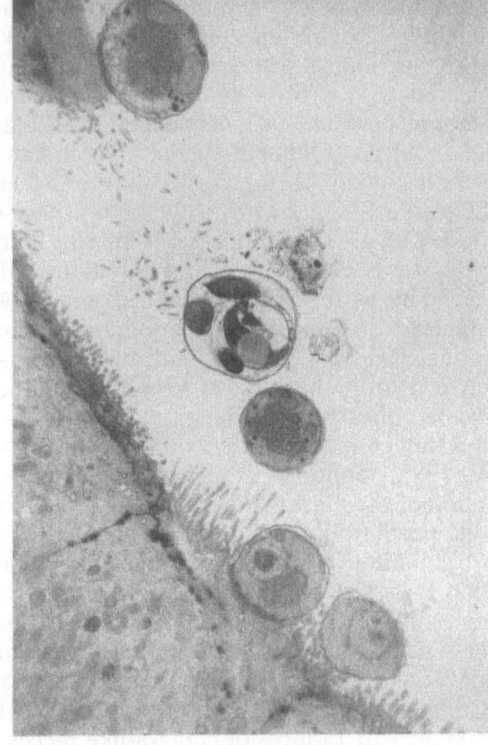

Fig. 4.2a,b. a Scanning electron-micrograph of *Cryptosporidium* sp oocysts situated at the brush-border of an enterocyte (× 6000) in an HIV-2 positive patient (Cook 1987a); b transmission electron-micrograph of oocysts, some of which are lying within (but in an extracytoplasmic position) an enterocyte (× 3600).

infection, and in T-cell deficient nude white mice, diarrhoea (with persisting oocyst excretion) continues for much longer than in immunocompetent litter-mates. Measles (which impairs CMI) is a probable predisposing factor in the Third World. Also, a high *Cryptosporidium* sp antibody titre has been demon-strated in some AIDS patients with a severe infection. Suckling rodents develop a heavy infection, whilst adults merely get a trivial one after an oral inoculation with a calf or human *Cryptosporidium* isolate. It seems likely that silent *Microsporidium* sp infections are not unusual in man; impairment of T-cell function produces, as in mice, clinically detectable disease.

In many AIDS sufferers, other intestinal opportunistic infections are fre-quently present in association with coccidia: *Salmonella* sp, *Shigella* sp, *Campylo-bacter jejuni*, *Mycobacterium tuberculosis*, *M. avium-intracellulare*, cytomegalovirus (CMV), herpes simplex virus (HSV) and *Candida albicans*, etc.; small-intestinal Kaposi's sarcoma and lymphoma may be present in addition (Page et al. 1983). The precise role of HIV-1 and HIV-2 in the pathogenesis of the enterocyte and colonocyte damage, and diarrhoea and malabsorption remains unclear (Miller et al. 1988; Ullrich et al. 1989), although there seems no doubt that they do impart a significant effect.

Clinical Aspects

Clinical manifestations of a coccidial infection usually vary greatly between the immune intact and the immunocompromised individual. The size of the infecting dose required to produce human disease is unknown; infant macaques develop a self-limiting illness after inoculation with 10 oocysts. Heavy infections are associated with protracted diarrhoea, severe malabsorption and weight-loss (Malebranche et al. 1983; Modigliani et al. 1985), and are an especial problem in AIDS in Africa (Quinn et al. 1986; Sewankambo et al. 1987); similar symptoms have occasionally been recorded in the presence of intact immunity (Edelman and Oldfield 1988). However, in the presence of intact immunity, a cryptospori-dial infection usually produces self-limiting diarrhoea of 2–14 days' duration (with 2 to 10 stools daily) after an incubation period of 4 to 14 days; this may be preceded by an 'influenza-like' illness and a low-grade fever (Current et al. 1983; Jokipii and Jokipii 1986). Abdominal discomfort (colic), anorexia, nausea, vomiting, headache, cough, and mild weight-loss are additional symptoms. A reactive arthropathy has also been documented (Hay et al. 1987). In travellers in particular, the clinical syndrome resembles very closely that caused by a *G. lamblia* infection (both infections may in fact be present simultaneously) (Jokipii et al. 1985), although flatulence and 'bloating' tend to be less common and duration of the illness shorter. Up to 13% of acute diarrhoeal episodes in Third World paediatric practice have been attributed to cryptosporidiosis (Cook 1987b); limited evidence indicates that breast-feeding provides relative pro-tection (Mata et al. 1984). *Cryptosporidium* sp is also important in immuno-compromised states apart from AIDS; these include lymphomas, leukaemias and those resulting from cytotoxic therapy (Casemore et al. 1985; Fayer and Ungar 1986; Cook 1987b). In the immune-compromised host, the resultant small-intestinal diarrhoea (the pathophysiology of which is poorly understood) may be torrential: 1 to 15 litres of cholera-like faeces daily for many weeks or months, and this is frequently accompanied by malabsorption with grossly deranged absorption tests (Malebranche et al. 1983; Modigliani et al. 1985). Fever may also be a feature, and death an almost certain sequel. However, there are also rare reports of mild and self-limiting cryptosporidial enteritis in AIDS (Berkowitz and Seidel 1985; Scaglia et al. 1986).

Disease caused by *Isospora belli* is in most respects similar and clinically indistinguishable (Soave and Johnson 1988); the incubation period in the immunointact is approximately 1 week, and oocysts can be recovered from faecal samples for 9 to 15 days after infection (Cook 1987a). One estimate is that 15% of AIDS sufferers in Haiti are infected with *I belli* (DeHovitz et al. 1986). In a *Sarcocystis hominis* infection, diarrhoea and abdominal pain usually begin 14 to 18 days after infection (Cook 1987a; Dubey et al. 1989). Rarely, parasites can be demonstrated in other organs; a recent case-report from France, documented *Sarcocystis* sp schizonts in a sputum specimen (Lancastre et al. 1989).

In AIDS although the jejunum is usually most severely affected, *Cryptosporidium* sp may involve any part of the gastrointestinal tract, from mouth to anus; in a heavy infection the colon can be severely affected. Histological changes include: villous atrophy, an increase in crypt length, and mild to moderate infiltration (consisting mostly of mononuclear cells) in the lamina propria. The gall-bladder and biliary system may also be severely involved (acute and gangrenous cholecystitis have been recorded) (Cockerill et al. 1986; Margulis et al. 1986; Kahn et al. 1987; Soave and Johnson 1988), sometimes simultaneously with a CMV infection; histological appearances closely resemble those of idiopathic sclerosing cholangitis (Margulis et al. 1986; Cook 1987a,b). Respiratory tract involvement presenting with chronic cough, dyspepsia, bronchiolitis and pneumonitis has been reported in the immunocompromised individual. Multisystem involvement has been recorded (Gross et al. 1986), possibly as a result of haematogenous spread (Gentile et al. 1987). Disseminated infection with *I belli* has also been documented; a chronic granulomatous response has been recorded in the mesenteric and tracheobronchial lymph glands (Restrepo et al. 1987). In severe *Sarcocystis hominis* infection, intestinal obstruction has been reported in Thailand (Cook 1987a).

Diagnosis

Diagnosis of the coccidial infections is by detection of oocysts in faecal samples using appropriate staining techniques (see above) (Casemore 1989); concentration and formalin–ether sedimentation methods are of value (Current 1988; Soave and Johnson 1988). The fact that human infection was first documented in AIDS patients was due to the fact that faecal oocysts are present in far greater numbers in this condition. The concentration of oocysts is significantly higher in fluid compared with a formed faecal sample. Recently, atypical oocysts in faecal smears have been reported (Baxby et al. 1987); they may fail to stain by standard techniques. Detection of faecal oocysts by an indirect fluorescent antibody procedure (Stibbs and Ongerth 1986), and a fluorescein-labelled IgG monoclonal antibody technique (McLauchlin et al. 1987; Soave and Johnson 1988), have given encouraging results. Oocysts should be distinguished from yeasts by using an iodine wet-mount or acid-fast staining technique. All diagnostic laboratories should now possess at least one technician who has had considerable experience of *Cryptosporidium* sp identification; a test-sample can easily be maintained for 12 months if stored at 4 °C in either 2.5% potassium dichromate or 10% formalin. Methods for detection of oocysts in contaminated water have also been described (Musial et al. 1987; Ongerth and Stibbs 1987). Coccidial oocysts can also be detected in a jejunal-biopsy specimen, in some of which 'villous atrophy with blunting' has been recorded (Whiteside et al. 1984; Modigliani et al. 1985; Cook 1987a); the actual mechanism(s) of malabsorption in all of the human coccidial infections is far from clear. In AIDS, *Cryptosporidium* sp oocysts can sometimes be visualized in sputum and lung-biopsy material (Ma et al. 1984; Miller et al. 1984).

Serum antibody to *Cryptosporidium* sp has been detected using an indirect immunofluorescent technique (IIFT) (Campbell and Current 1983; Casemore 1987). An ELISA for IgG and IgM detection has been developed using calf-derived oocysts as the antigen source (Ungar et al. 1986); this is of value in both people with AIDS and those who are immunocompetent (Soave and Johnson 1988). This test is not yet available commercially.

Management

Chemotherapy for coccidiosis is not indicated in those whose immune response is intact (Current et al. 1983); infection is self-limiting, but oral rehydration may be required in the acute phase of the illness. Shedding of oocysts continues for 8 to 50 (mean 12–14) days (Jokipii and Jokipii 1986; Stehr-Green et al. 1987); a carrier-state and relapse seem to be very unusual. When the immune response is diminished, or virtually absent, as in AIDS, chemotherapy is badly needed but relatively ineffective (Hart and Baxby 1985). Table 4.1 summarizes some of the

Table 4.1. Some therapeutic regimens which have been used against the major small-intestinal coccidial infections in immunocompromised (including AIDS) patients (Cook 1987a)

Infection (Fayer and Ungar 1986; Cook 1987b)	Chemotherapeutic agent	Suggested dose regimen (often continued indefinitely)	Side-effects
Cryptosporidium sp.	Spiramycin	1 g qds; oral, daily for 2–4 weeks	Gastrointestinal, epigastric pain, acute colitis, dermatitis

(Amongst many other agents used, with almost complete failure are the following: 'co-trimoxazole', erythromycin, furazolidone + tetracycline, diloxanide furoate, amprolium, polyamines, quinine + clindamycin, amphotericin B + flucytosine, α-difluoromethylornithine, α-interferon, interleukin-2)

| *Isospora belli* | Pyrimethamine + sulphadiazine | 75 mg⎱ oral daily for 4–8 g ⎰ 7 days | (as for sulphonamides) |
| | Trimethoprim + sulphamethoxazole ('co-trimoxazole') | 160 mg ⎱ tab 2 qds, oral 800 mg ⎰ daily for 10 days, then 2 bd for 3 weeks | (see text) |

(Metronidazole and furazolidone (100 mg qds for 100 days) have also proved of value; however, tetracycline, ampicillin, spiramycin, nitrofurantoin and chloroquine have proved relatively ineffective) (Whiteside et al. 1984; DeHovitz et al. 1986)

chemotherapeutic agents (with suggested dose regimens) which have been used (Cook 1987a). In cryptosporidiosis, the macrolide antibiotic spiramycin (1–3 g daily for 2 or more weeks) (Portnoy et al. 1984; Casemore et al. 1985; Fayer and Ungar 1986; Cook 1987a,b; Tuazon and Labriola 1987) is the only chemotherapeutic agent presently known to be of any value, although much of the evidence for its efficacy is anecdotal (about 70 others have been tested); even when temporarily successful, recurrence is usual, however, in those with AIDS. Amongst the compounds so far tested are: 'co-trimoxazole', erythromycin, furazolidone + tetracycline, diloxanide furoate, amprolium, polyamines, quinine + clindamycin, amphotericin B + flucytosine, α-difluoromethylornithine, α-interferon, and interleukin-2. Many other lines of treatment have been used but with very limited success (Current 1988). The value of zidovudine (AZT) is so far unclear (Chandrasekar 1987; Cook 1989). Delay in initiating immunosuppressive chemotherapy until a mild or subclinical *Cryptosporidium* sp infection has been eliminated may prevent a life-threatening illness. Recently, hyperimmune bovine colostrum (which contains IgG antibodies) has been given orally, but results are to date contradictory (Tzipori et al. 1986; Saxon and Weinstein 1987; Tzipori et al. 1987). Cows' milk globulin has also been used. Bovine transfer factor has been reported to be of value in AIDS-associated *Cryptosporidium* sp infection; immunomodulation, or passive transfer of antibodies or lymphocytes might also have a place in management. Codeine phosphate, diphenoxylate or loperamide may be necessary to control severe diarrhoea; rehydration is obviously important, and in a severe infection must be carried out intravenously.

Treatment of an *I belli* infection in the immunosuppressed is more satisfactory (Table 4.1): trimethoprim (0.64 g) + sulphamethoxazole (3.20 g) daily for 10 days followed by 0.32 g + 1.60 g daily for 3 weeks, or furazolidone (400 mg daily for 10 days) have both proved effective (DeHovitz et al. 1986; Cook 1987a,b; Tuazon and Labriola 1987). Pyrimethamine + sulphadiazine, nitrofurantoin, and metronidazole have also been considered to be of value (Cook 1987a,b; Soave and Johnson 1988; Cook 1989). *Sarcocystis hominis* infections in the immunosuppressed individual respond to metronidazole (500 mg tds for 7 days) (Vannatta et al. 1985; Siegal et al. 1986); iodoquinol, paromomycin and several other agents are also reported to be effective (Dubey et al. 1989). *B hominis* infection in the immunointact individual apparently responds to metronidazole (Guirges and Al-Waili 1987) but only poorly to tinidazole (Masry et al. 1988); in association with HIV infection it has been shown to respond to di-iodohydroxyquinoline (650 mg three times daily for 21 days) (Llibre et al. 1989). There is no known effective chemotherapy for microsporidiosis, although successes have been claimed after sulfisoxazole, and trimethoprim-sulphamethoxazole followed by sulphadiazine (Shadduck 1989); fumagillin has proved effective in vitro.

Prevention

Oocysts (which can remain viable for 9–12 months in vitro) are excreted in faeces for 2 weeks (and rarely up to 3 months) after diarrhoea has ceased; this fact is obviously important in infection control. Rodents, puppies and kittens are other reservoir hosts which are probably important. Disease in farm animals must be recognized and treated. In prophylaxis, the pasteurization of raw milk renders it non-infective (Anderson 1985). Most disinfectants are, however, of very limited value against oocysts of *Cryptosporidium* sp (Cook 1987b). They are destroyed by heat (>65°C for 30 minutes) and freezing at −20°C; 5% ammonia, commercial bleach (sodium hypochlorite) and 10% formol saline are also effective. Routine chlorination of drinking water has no effect on oocyst infectivity. Filtration of domestic water supplies is of limited value because the small size of *Cryptosporidium* sp oocysts (3–5 μm) allows them to pass through all but the finest filters. Special precautions should be used to prevent infection in immunosuppressed people including those with AIDS; also, the risk of contracting an infection from an AIDS patient should be appreciated, especially by nursing staff and other medical personnel.

Conclusions

A vast amount of evidence has recently accumulated that this intriguing group of small-intestine pathogens, recognized by veterinarians for nearly a century, is important in several human situations. Microsporidiosis is likely to become increasingly recognized in AIDS. The saga still contains serious gaps, however, and results of further collaboration with protozoologists, immunologists, pharmacologists and, by no means least, veterinarians, will be keenly awaited. Hopefully, diagnostic methods, especially serological ones, will improve. Current chemotherapy is unsatisfactory and advances here will be awaited with particular interest. Will effective vaccines be forthcoming in the future? Much also still remains to be elucidated as to why the small-intestinal coccidia (together with other protozoa) so readily 'run riot' with fatal consequences in the immunosuppressed individual.

References

Anderson BC (1985) Moist heat inactivation of *Cryptosporidium* sp. Am J Publ Health 75:1433–1434
Badaró R, Carvalho EM, Rocha H, Queiroz AC, Jones TC (1986) *Leishmania donovani*: an opportunistic microbe associated with progressive disease in three immunocompromised patients. Lancet i:647–649
Baxby D, Blundell N, Hart CA (1987) Excretion of atypical oocysts by patients with cryptosporidiosis. Lancet i:974
Berkowitz CD, Seidel JS (1985) Spontaneous resolution of cryptosporidiosis in a child with acquired immunodeficiency syndrome. Am J Dis Child 139:967
Blaser MJ, Cohn DL (1986) Opportunistic infections in patients with AIDS: clues to the epidemiology of AIDS and the relative virulence of pathogens. Rev Infect Dis 8:21–30
Bruce-Chwatt LJ (1985) Essential malariology, 2nd edn. Heinemann, London, pp 1–11
Bryceson A, Tomkins A, Ridley D, Warhurst D, Goldstone A, Bayliss G, Toswill J, Parry J (1988) HIV-2-associated AIDS in the 1970s. Lancet ii:221
Campbell PN, Current WL (1983) Demonstration of serum antibodies to *Cryptosporidium* sp. in normal and immunodeficient humans with confirmed infections. J Clin Microbiol 18:165–169

Casemore DP (1987) The antibody response to cryptosporidium: development of a serological test and its use in a study of immunologically normal persons. J Infect 14:125–134

Casemore DP (1989) Human cryptosporidiosis. In: Reeves DS, Geddes AM (eds) Recent advances in infection. Churchill Livingstone, Edinburgh, pp 209–236

Casemore DP, Sands RL, Curry A (1985) Cryptosporidium species a 'new' human pathogen. J Clin Pathol 38:1321–1336

Cavalier-Smith T (1987) Eukaryotes with no mitochondria. Nature 326:332–333

Chandrasekar PH (1987) 'Cure' of chronic cryptosporidiosis during treatment with azidothymidine in a patient with the acquired immune deficiency syndrome. Am J Med 83:187

Cockerill FR, Hurley DV, Malagelada J-R, LaRusso NF, Edson RS, Katzmann JA, Banks PM, Wiltsie JC, Davis JP, Lack EE, Ishak KG, Scoy RE van (1986) Polymicrobial cholangitis and Kaposi's sarcoma in blood product transfusion-related acquired immune deficiency syndrome. Am J Med 80:1237–1241

Combee CL, Collinge ML, Britt EM (1986) Cryptosporidiosis in a hospital-associated day care center. Pediatr Infect Dis 5:528–532

Cook GC (1987a) Opportunistic parasitic infections associated with the acquired immune deficiency syndrome (AIDS): parasitology, clinical presentation, diagnosis and management. Q J Med 65:967–983

Cook GC (1987b) Cryptosporidium sp. and other intestinal coccidia: a bibliography. Bureau of Hygiene and Tropical Diseases, London, pp V-XIV

Cook GC (1988a) Small-intestinal coccidiosis: an emergent clinical problem. J Infect 16:213–219

Cook GC (1988b) Intestinal parasitic infections. Curr Opin Gastroenterol 4:113–123

Cook GC (1989) Parasitic infections of the gastrointestinal tract: a worldwide clinical problem. Curr Opin Gastroenterol 5:126–139

Cook GC (1990) Cryptosporidiosis. In: Strickland GT (ed) Hunter's tropical medicine, 7th edn. Saunders, Philadelphia (in press)

Corbett-Feeney G (1987) Cryptosporidium among children with acute diarrhoea in the west of Ireland. J Infect 14:79–84

Current WL (1988) The biology of Cryptosporidium. In: Leech JH, Sande ML, Root RK (eds) Parasitic infections. Churchill Livingstone, New York and Edinburgh, pp 109–132

Current WL, Haynes TB (1984) Complete development of Cryptosporidium in cell culture. Science 224:603–605

Current WL, Reese NC, Ernst JV, Bailey WS, Heyman MB, Weinstein WM (1983) Human cryptosporidiosis in immunocompetent and immunodeficient persons: studies of an outbreak and experimental transmission. N Engl J med 308:1252–1257

D'Antonio RG, Winn RE, Taylor JO (1985) A waterborne outbreak of cryptosporidiosis in normal hosts. Ann Intern Med 103:886–888

DeHovitz JA, Pape JW, Boncy M, Johnson WD (1986) Clinical manifestations and therapy of Isospora belli infection in patients with the acquired immunodeficiency syndrome. N Engl J Med 315:87–90

Desportes I, Charpentier Y le, Galian A, Bernard F, Cochand-Priollet B, Lavergne A, Ravisse P, Modigliani R (1985) Occurrence of a new microsporidan: Enterocytozoon bieneusi n.g., n. sp., in the enterocytes of a human patient with AIDS. J Protozool 32:250–254

Dubey JP, Speer CA, Fayer R (1989) Sarcocystosis of animals and man. CRC Press, Boca Rafon, p 215

Edelman MJ, Oldfield EC (1988) Severe cryptosporidiosis in an immunocompetent host. Arch Intern Med 148:1873–1874

Editorial (1989) Troubled waters. Lancet ii:251–252

Elsser KA, Moricz M, Proctor EM (1986) Cryptosporidium infections: a laboratory survey. Can Med Assoc J 135:211–213

Epidemiologic notes and reports (1987) Cryptosporidiosis: New Mexico 1986. MMWR 36:561–563

Fayer R, Ungar BLP (1986) Cryptosporidium spp. and cryptosporidiosis. Microbiol Rev 50:458–483

Forthal DN, Guest SS (1984) Isospora belli enteritis in three homosexual men. Am J Trop Med Hyg 33:1060–1064

Galbraith NS (1989) Cryptosporidiosis: another source. Br Med J 298:276–277

Garcia LS, Bruckner DA, Clancy MN (1984) Clinical relevance of Blastocystis hominis. Lancet i:1233–1234

Gelb A, Miller S (1986) AIDS and gastroenterology. Am J Gastroenterol 81:619–622

Gentile G, Baldassarri L, Caprioli A, Donelli G, Venditti M, Avvisati G, Martino P (1987) Colonic vascular invasion as a possible route of extraintestinal cryptosporidiosis. Am J Med 82:574–575

Greve E (1985) Sarcosporidiosis – an overlooked zoonosis: man as intermediate and final host. Dan Med Bull 32:228–230

Gross TL, Wheat J, Bartlett M, O'Connor KW (1986) AIDS and multiple system involvement with *Cryptosporidium*. Am J Gastroenterol 81:456–458

Guirges SY, Al-Waili NS (1987) *Blastocystis hominis*: evidence for human pathogenicity and effectiveness of metronidazole therapy. Clin Exp Pharmacol Physiol 14:333–335

Hart A, Baxby D (1985) Management of cryptosporidiosis. J Antimicrob Chemother 15:3–4

Hay EM, Winfield J, McKendrick MW (1987) Reactive arthritis associated with cryptosporidium enteritis. Br Med J 295:248

Heijbel H, Slaine K, Seigel B, Wall P, McNabb SJN, Gibbons W, Istre GR (1987) Outbreak of diarrhea in a day care center with spread to household members: the role of *Cryptosporidium*. Pediatr Infect Dis J 6:532–535

Hira PR, Al-Ali F, Zaki M, Saleh Q, Sharda D, Behbehani K (1989) Human cryptosporidiosis in the Arabian Gulf: first report of infections in children in Kuwait. J Trop Med Hyg 92:249–252

Højlyng N, Holten-Andersen W, Jepsen S (1987) Cryptosporidiosis: a case of airborne transmission. Lancet ii:271–272

Højlyng N, Mølbak K, Jepsen S (1986) *Cryptosporidium* spp., a frequent cause of diarrhea in Liberian children. J Clin Microbiol 23:1109–1113

Isaac-Renton JL, Fogel D, Stibbs HH, Ongerth JE (1987) *Giardia* and *Cryptosporidium* in drinking water. Lancet i:973–974

Janoff EN, Reller LB (1987) *Cryptosporidium* species, a protean protozoan. J Clin Microbiol 25:967–975

Jokipii L, Jokipii AMM (1986) Timing of symptoms and oocyst excretion in human cryptosporidiosis. N Engl J Med 315:1643–1647

Jokipii L, Pohjola S, Jokipii AMM (1985) Cryptosporidiosis associated with traveling and giardiasis. Gastroenterology 89:838–842

Kahn DG, Garfinkle JM, Klonoff DC, Pembrook LJ, Morrow DJ (1987) Cryptosporidial and cytomegaloviral hepatitis and cholecystitis. Arch Pathol Lab Med 111:879–881

Kain K, Noble M (1989) *Blastocystis hominis* infection in humans. Rev Infect Dis 11:508–509

Lähdevirta J, Jokipii AMM, Sammalkorpi K, Jokipii L (1987) Perinatal infection with *Cryptosporidium* and failure to thrive. Lancet i:48–49

Lancastre F, Delalande A, Deluol A-M, Matrat C, Georges E, Roux P (1989) Sarcosporidiosis revealed in sputum. Lancet i:791

Llibre JM, Tor J, Manterola JM, Carbonell C, Foz M (1989) *Blastocystis hominis* chronic diarrhoea in AIDS patients. Lancet i:221

Lumb R, Smith K, O'Donoghue PJ, Lauser JA (1988) Ultrastructure of *Cryptosporidium* sporozoites to tissue culture cells. Parasitol Res 74:531–536

Ma P, Soave R (1983) Three-step stool examination for cryptosporidiosis in 10 homosexual men with protracted watery diarrhoea. J Infect Dis 147:824–828

Ma P, Villanueva TG, Kaufman D, Gillooley JF (1984) Respiratory cryptosporidiosis in the acquired immune deficiency syndrome: use of modified cold Kinyoun and Hemacolor stains for rapid diagnoses. JAMA 252:1298–1301

Malebranche R, Arnoux E, Guérin JM, Pierre GD, Laroche AC, Péan-Guichard C, Elis R, Morisset PH, Spira T, Mandeville R, Drotman P, Seemayer T, Dupay J-M (1983) Acquired immunodeficiency syndrome with severe gastrointestinal manifestations in Haiti. Lancet ii:873–878

Margulis SJ, Honig CL, Soave R, Govoni AF, Mouradian JA, Jacobson IM (1986) Biliary tract obstruction in the acquired immunodeficiency syndrome. Ann Intern Med 105:207–210

Markell EK, Udkow MP (1986) *Blastocystis hominis*: pathogen or fellow traveler? Am J Trop Med Hyg 35:1023–1026

Masry NA El, Bassily S, Farid Z (1988) *Blastocystis hominis*: clinical and therapeutic aspects. Trans R Soc Trop Med Hyg 82:173

Mata L, Bolaños H, Pizarro D, Vives M (1984) Cryptosporidiosis in children from some highland Costa Rican rural and urban areas. Am J Trop Med Hyg 33:24–29

McLauchlin J, Casemore DP, Harrison TG, Gerson PJ, Samuel D, Taylor AG (1987) Identification of *Cryptosporidium* oocysts by monoclonal antibody. Lancet i:51

Miller ARO, Griffin GE, Batman P, Farquar C, Forster SM, Pinching AJ, Harris JRW (1988) Jejunal mucosal architecture and fat absorption in male homosexuals infected with human immunodeficiency virus. Q J Med 69:1009–1019

Miller RA, Minshew BH (1988) *Blastocystis hominis*: an organism in search of a disease. Rev Infect Dis 10:930–938

Miller RA, Wasserheit JN, Kirihara J, Coyle MB (1984) Detection of *Cryptosporidium* oocysts in sputum during screening for mycobacteria. J Clin Microbiol 20:1192–1193

Modigliani R, Bories C, Charpentier Y le, Salmeron M, Messing B, Galian A, Rambaud JC, Lavergne A, Cochand-Priollet B, Desportes I (1985) Diarrhoea and malabsorption in acquired immune deficiency syndrome: a study of four cases with special emphasis on opportunistic protozoan infestations. Gut 26:179–187

Montalban C, Sevilla F, Moreno A, Nash R, Celma ML, Muñoz RF (1987) Visceral leishmaniasis as an opportunistic infection in the acquired immunodeficiency syndrome. J Infect 15:247–250

Musial CE, Arrowood MJ, Sterling CR, Gerba CP (1987) Detection of *Cryptosporidium* in water by using polypropylene cartridge filters. Appl Environ Microbiol 53: 687–692

Navia BA, Petito CK, Gold JW, Cho ES, Jordan BD, Price RW (1986) Cerebral toxoplasmosis complicating the acquired immune deficiency syndrome: clinical and neuropathological findings in 27 patients. Ann Neurol 19:224–238

Nime FA, Burek JD, Page DL, Holscher MA, Yardley JH (1976) Acute enterocolitis in a human being infected with the protozoan *Cryptosporidium*. Gastroentology 70:592–598

O'Donoghue PJ (1985) *Cryptosporidium* infections in man, animals, birds and fish. Aust Vet J 62:253–258

Ongerth JE, Stibbs HH (1987) Identification of *Cryptosporidium* oocysts in river water. Appl Environ Microbiol 53:672–676

Pal S, Bhattacharya SK, Das P, Chaudhuri P, Dutta P, De SP, Sen D, Saha MR, Nair GB, Pal SC (1989) Occurrence and significance of *Cryptosporidium* infection in Calcutta. Trans R Soc Trop Med Hyg 83:520–521

Pape JW, Liautaud B, Thomas F, Mathurin J-R, Amand M-M A St, Boncy M, Pean V, Pamphile M, Laroche AC, Johnson WD (1983) Characteristics of the acquired immunodeficiency syndrome (AIDS) in Haiti. New Engl J Med 309:945–950

Portnoy D, Whiteside ME, Buckley E, MacLeod CL (1984) Treatment of intestinal cryptosporidiosis with spiramycin. Ann Intern Med 101:202–204

Quinn TC, Mann JM, Curran JW, Piot P (1986) AIDS in Africa: an epidemiologic paradigm. Science 234:955–963

Restrepo C, Macher AM, Radany EH (1987) Disseminated extraintestinal isosporiasis in a patient with acquired immune deficiency syndrome. Am J Clin Pathol 87:536–542

Rijpstra AC, Canning EU, Ketel RJ van, Schattenkerk JKME, Laarman JJ (1988) Use of light microscopy to diagnose small-intestinal microsporidiosis in patients with AIDS. J Infect Dis 157:827–831

Rodgers VD, Fassett R, Kagnoff MF (1986) Abnormalities in intestinal mucosal T cells in homosexual populations including those with the lymphadenopathy syndrome and acquired immunodeficiency syndrome. Gastroentology 90:552–558

Rolston KVI, Winans R, Rodriguez S (1989) *Blastocystis hominis*: pathogen or not? Rev Infect Dis 11:661–662

Saxon A, Weinstein W (1987) Oral administration of bovine colostrum anti-cryptosporidia antibody fails to alter the course of human cryptosporidiosis. J Parasitol 73:413–415

Scaglia M, Senaldi G, Di Perri G, Minoli L (1986) Unusual low-grade cryptosporidial enteritis in AIDS: a case report. Infection 14:87–88

Sewankambo N, Mugerwa RD, Goodgame R, Carswell JW, Moody A, Lloyd G, Lucas SB (1987) Enteropathic AIDS in Uganda: an endoscopic, histological and microbiological study. AIDS 1:9–13

Shadduck JA (1989) Human microsporidiosis and AIDS. Rev Infect Dis 11:203–207

Shahid NS, Rahman ASMH, Sanyal SC (1987) *Cryptosporidium* as a pathogen for diarrhoea in Bangladesh. Trop Geogr Med 39:265–270

Siegal FP, Lopez C, Fitzgerald PA, Shah K, Baron P, Leiderman IZ, Imperato D, Landesman S (1986) Opportunistic infections in acquired immune deficiency syndrome result from synergistic defects of both the natural and adaptive components of cellular immunity. J Clin Invest 78:115–123

Soave R, Johnson WD (1988) *Cryptosporidium* and *Isospora belli* infections. J Infect Dis 157:225–229

Soave R, Ma P (1985) Cryptosporidiosis: traveler's diarrhea in two families. Arch Intern Med 145:70–72

Stehr-Green JK, McCaig L, Remsen HM, Rains CS, Fox M, Juranek DD (1987) Shedding of oocysts in immunocompetent individuals infected with *Cryptosporidium*. Am J Trop Med Hyg 36:338–342

Stibbs HH, Ongerth JE (1986) Immunofluorescence detection of *Cryptosporidium* oocysts in fecal smears. J Clin Micobiol 24:517–521

Thomson MA, Benson JWT, Wright PA (1987) Two-year study of *Cryptosporidium* infection. Arch Dis Child 62:559–563

Tuazon CU, Labriola AM (1987) Management of infectious and immunological complications of
    acquired immunodeficiency syndrome (AIDS): current and future prospects. Drugs 33:66–84
Tzipori S (1988) Cryptosporidiosis in perspective. Adv Parasitol 27:63–129
Tzipori S, Roberton D, Chapman C (1986) Remission of diarrhoea due to cryptosporidiosis in an
    immunodeficient child treated with hyperimmune bovine colostrum. Br Med J 293:1276–1277
Tzipori S, Roberton D, Cooper DA, White L (1987) Chronic cryptosporidial diarrhoea and
    hyperimmune cow colostrum. Lancet ii:344–345
Ullrich R, Zeitz M, Heise W, L'age M, Höffken G, Riecken EO (1989) Small intestinal structure and
    function in patients infected with human immunodeficiency virus (HIV): evidence for HIV-induced
    enteropathy. Ann Intern Med 111:15–21
Ungar BLP, Soave R, Fayer R, Nash TE (1986) Enzyme immunoassay detection of immunoglobulin
    M and G antibodies to *Cryptosporidium* in immunocompetent and immunocompromised persons. J
    Infect Dis 153:570–578
Vannatta JB, Adamson D, Mullican K (1985) *Blastocystis hominis* infection presenting as recurrent
    diarrhea. Ann Intern Med 102:495–496
Whiteside ME, Barkin JS, May RG, Weiss SD, Fischl MA, MacLeod CL (1984) Enteric coccidiosis
    among patients with the acquired immunodeficiency syndrome. Am J Trop Med Hyg 33:1065–1072
Wittenberg DF, Smith EG, Ende J van den, Becker PJ (1987) *Cryptosporidium*-associated diarrhoea
    in children. Ann Trop Paediatr 7:113–117
Wolfson JS, Richter JM, Waldron MA, Weber DJ, McCarthy DM, Hopkins CC (1985) Cryptospor-
    idiosis in immunocompetent patients. New Engl J Med 312:1278–1282
Zierdt CH (1988) *Blastocystis hominis*, a long misunderstood intestinal parasite. Parasitol Today
    4:15–17

Chapter 5

Strongyloides stercoralis and Its Hyperinfection Syndrome: The Index of Suspicion Is Still Far Too Low

> And he was eaten of worms, and gave up the ghost.
>
> *Acts of the Apostles*, chapter 12, verse 23

Introduction

There has recently been an increase in awareness that infection with the intestinal helminth *Strongyloides stercoralis* can continue for very long periods of time (Cook 1987). Several reports have recorded infection lasting for 40 years or more in men who were formerly prisoners of war in South-east Asia during World War II (ex-FEPOWs) (Gill and Bell 1979; Pelletier 1984; Proctor et al. 1985; Hill 1988; Pelletier et al. 1988). Many of them worked on the Burma–Siam railway (Hardie 1983); whether malnutrition, impaired immunity, or other factors accounted for the very high rate of infection in this group is undetermined. A high rate of persisting infection (but lower than in the prisoners) has been recorded in Burma Star veterans who were not captured (Gill and Bell 1987). In many members of this group, the infection is still present.

S stercoralis is a small nematode which occurs primarily in tropical and subtropical locations (especially West Africa, the Caribbean and South-east Asia); however, it is also widely distributed in eastern Europe, including Hungary, Romania, and southern areas of Poland and the USSR. A high prevalence has also been reported in northern Italy (Genta et al. 1988). A recent report of infection in a young woman at Nottingham, England, strongly suggests that the parasite was acquired in a local recreational park (Sprott et al. 1987). There is increasing evidence that *S stercoralis* infection is a major problem in some chronic care institutions (Proctor et al. 1987).

Parasitology and Pathogenesis

Human infection with *S stercoralis* is usually acquired through penetration of intact skin by the filariform larvae which can survive for many weeks in moist soil contaminated with human faeces; this mode of transmission is exactly comparable with that of the hookworms *Ancylostoma duodenale* and *Necator americanus* (Cook 1980, 1986) (Chap. 3). Infection by the faecal–oral route is also possible. Many animals including dogs and some subhuman primates, can act as reservoir hosts. Normond (1876) working in Cochin China (southern Vietnam) is credited with the first description of the causative organism, which he detected in human faecal samples. It was initially considered to consist of two species: *Anguillula stercoralis* (in the faeces) and *A intestinalis* (in the bowel) (Castellani and Chalmers 1919). That they were one and the same organism was however clear to Manson in 1898; this author gave little credence, though, to a pathological role of this parasite. Following a complex life-cycle (also similar to that of the hookworms) (Fig. 5.1) in which the larvae migrate successively from the circulation to the lungs, trachea and pharynx, they are swallowed and thence enter the small-intestine where maturation to adult worms takes place whilst they are embedded in the duodenal and jejunal mucosa. Most of the evidence for these migratory routes has been derived from experimental animal studies (Tindall and Wilson 1988; Dawkins 1989; Genta and Grove 1989) and further work is required (Schad 1989). The egg-laying female is approximately 2 mm, and the male 0.7 mm in length. After hatching, the eggs (still within the small-intestine) produce rhabditiform larvae, which can sometimes be detected in faecal samples (Fig. 5.1); this stage differs from that of the hookworm, and underlies the mechanism for extreme chronicity of this infection. These larvae, which can transform prematurely into filariform larvae, have the potential of invading the mucosa of the ileum, colon, appendix and rectum, and the perianal skin (the internal and external '*autoinfection cycles*'). Thereafter, by recurrent migratory cycles, infection can be maintained for the remainder of the individual's life whether he/she lives in a tropical or temperate area. The cycle can continue for at least 40–50 years. It is probable that there are significant strain variations with increased virulence in some geographical locations (Genta et al. 1988) and that autoinfection occurs more commonly with strains of the parasite acquired in some of them, e.g. South-east Asia. There is a possibility that passage from host to host might diminish the ability of *S stercoralis* to disseminate (Genta 1989b); evidence for this has been produced in an experimental model using corticosteroid-treated beagle dogs.

Animal models have been used to study the *S stercoralis* hyperinfection syndrome with widespread dissemination (see below) (Grove et al. 1983; Schad et al. 1984; Genta et al. 1986); the dog is particularly susceptible and understanding of the syndrome has been increased by such studies. It is clear that the syndrome is dependent on intensity and duration of infection; more information on host–parasite interactions, and the precise value of various chemotherapeutic agents, might be forthcoming from these studies. The patus monkey *Erythrocebus patus* can be used as a further experimental model, and has been studied from both pathological and immunological viewpoints (Genta et al. 1984; Harper et al. 1984). Corticosteroid administration did not alter the immune response significantly – as assessed by an effect on anti-larval surface IgG and

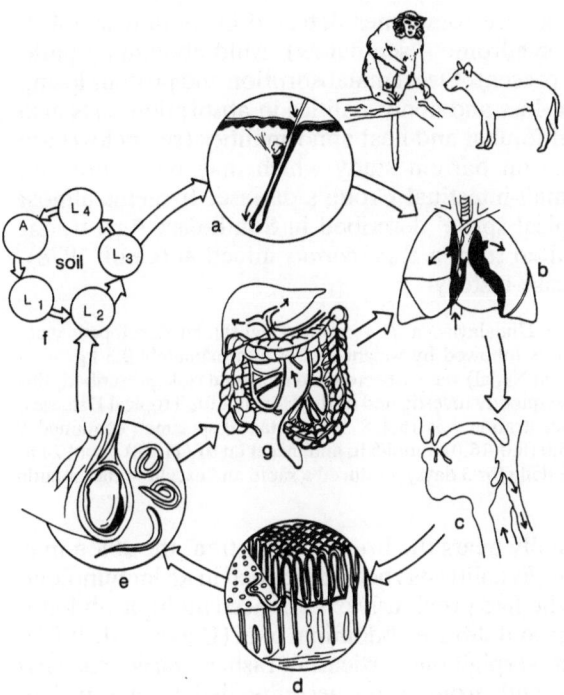

Fig. 5.1. Life-cycle of *Strongyloides stercoralis*. (a) Filariform (third-stage) larva enters the cutaneous circulation (infection can also occur after ingestion) (many animals including subhuman primates and dogs can act as reservoir hosts); (b) haematogenous transmission to the heart and pulmonary circulation, where penetration of an alveolar capillary into an alveolar space takes place; (c) movement up respiratory tree to the pharynx, from whence the larva is swallowed; (d) *S stercoralis* larva develops into an adult female (which is a protanderous hermaphrodite, measuring 2 mm in length and 0.04 mm wide) in the upper small-intestinal mucosa and submucosa; (e) embryonated eggs are shed into the surrounding tissues where second-stage larva hatches and migrates into the small-intestinal lumen; (f) larvae are excreted in faeces, and if deposited in moist soil develop into free-living adult males and females (the free-living cycle takes several weeks for completion); (g) unlike most intestinal nematodes, internal (colorectal) and external (perianal) *autoinfection cycles* can occur; this allows repeated re-infection to continue for at least 40–50 years (in the absence of the external cycle).

specific IgE antibody responses to *S stercoralis* antigens: local intestinal immune and non-immune mechanisms were considered to be more important protective mechanisms against disseminated strongyloidiasis (Genta et al. 1986a; Genta 1989b).

Clinical Aspects

Clinical sequelae of a *S stercoralis* infection are numerous. At the site of larval penetration there may be a transient itchy erythematous rash; this is followed by various diverse systemic manifestations as the invasive cycle gets under way (Cook 1980; Gilles 1984). Pulmonary symptoms, including bronchospasm, of varying severity may occur (larvae are sometimes detected in sputum samples, especially in the hyperinfection syndrome – see below). Mild abdominal pain, diarrhoea and blood loss may be present. Overt malabsorption and protein-losing enteropathy with marked weight-loss and abnormalities in absorption tests also occur; concurrent morphological jejunal and ileal abnormalities (see below) are reflected in radiological changes on barium study which may be severe and difficult to differentiate from small-intestinal Crohn's disease. It seems almost certain that some cases of 'tropical sprue' described in South-east Asia by Sir Patrick Manson and others resulted from a *S stercoralis* infection (Cook 1978). The following is an illustrative case-history:

Whilst on a climbing expedition in the Himalayas, a 71-year-old Englishman developed acute diarrhoea (up to 12 stools daily); this was followed by weight-loss of approximately 9.5 kg. A *G lamblia* infection (which is very common in Nepal) was suspected and metronidazole prescribed; this had no effect, however, and he was subsequently investigated at the Hospital for Tropical Diseases, London. His peripheral eosinophil concentration was $16.4 \times 10^9/l$, a faecal specimen contained *S stercoralis* larvae, xylose excretion was 5.0 (8.0–16.0) mmol/5 h, and faecal fat 91 (11–18) mmol/24 h. A thiabendazole course (25 mg/kg twice daily for 3 days) produced a rapid and excellent therapeutic response.

Although the small-intestine usually bears the brunt of infection, the colon may also be affected; chronic *S stercoralis* colitis has been described in an immunologically competent young woman who had previously experienced multiple abdominal operations for haematochezia and diffuse abdominal pain (Berry et al. 1983). In chronic infection, recurrent serpiginous urticarial rashes (*larva currens*) located on the trunk, buttocks and groins (and accompanied by a transient eosinophilia) may persist for many years; in one study carried out on ex-FEPOWs (see above), 92% had had such rashes (Pelletier 1984). Figure 5.2 gives an example of the 'larva currens' rash. This should be distinguished from *larva migrans* (Chap. 11) which is usually caused by the dog hookworm *Ancylostoma braziliense* and is usually present on the feet; infection is usually acquired by walking bare-foot on beaches contaminated with dog faeces.

The *hyperinfection syndrome* occurs usually, but not always (Seymour and Finucane 1989), in the presence of immunosuppression. It may be associated with corticosteroid (not infrequently given for chronic asthma, which in some probably resulted from strongyloidiasis) or other immunosuppressive drug administration, HTLV-I infection, reticuloses, systemic lupus erythematosus, lepromatous leprosy, malnutrition and other debilitating illnesses. The syndrome is characterized by widespread dissemination of larvae throughout the body, and has been recognized for at least six decades (Scowden et al. 1978; Cook 1980; Igra-Siegman et al. 1981; Cook 1985; Case Records of the Massachusetts General Hospital 1987). It is frequently accompanied by a Gram-negative septicaemia (usually caused by *Escherichia coli* and other enterobacteriaceae), pneumonia and meningitis (see below); fatal paralytic ileus is a frequent sequel in the untreated. Filariform larvae can be visualized in most organs (albeit often at post-mortem examination) (Igra-Siegman et al. 1981; Genta and Gomes 1989); lungs, liver, spleen, kidneys (larvae may rarely be detected in a urine specimen), myocardium, meninges, and the lymphatics of the gall bladder, pancreas, adrenals, thyroid and parathyroid glands may all be affected. Cerebrospinal fluid and pleural and pericardial effusions occasionally contain larvae. Secondary bacterial infection occurs in up to 45% of cases, producing bacteraemia, meningitis, peritonitis and endocarditis. Whereas dissemination of organisms

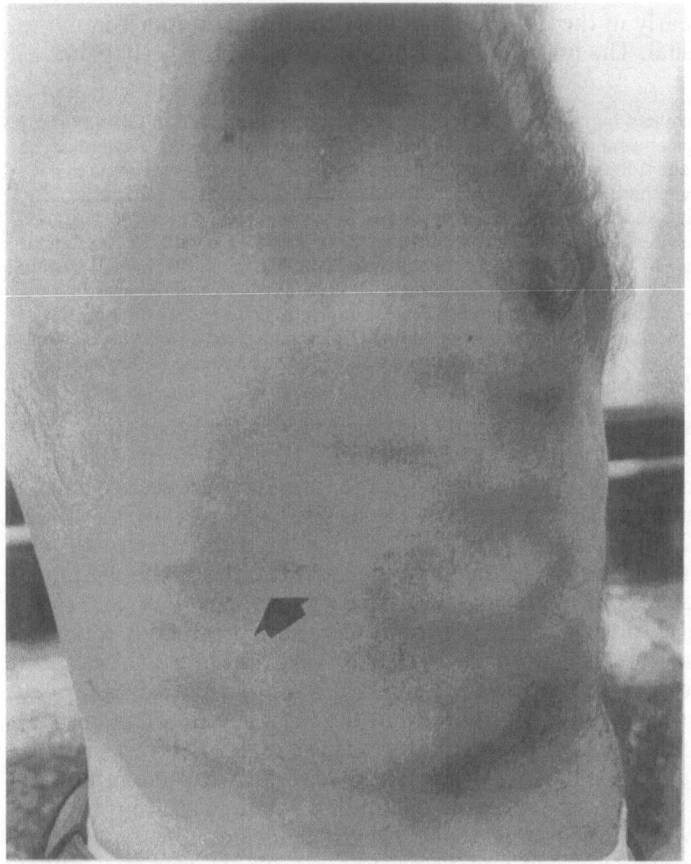

Fig. 5.2. 'Larva currens' in a 64-year-old former Far-east prisoner of war 37 years after the end of World War II (1939–1945). Transient itchy eruptions had for many years recurred intermittently over the trunk and buttocks; he had consulted numerous medical practitioners. *Strongyloides stercoralis* could not be detected in either faecal samples or by the 'Enterotest'. He was, however, successfully treated with thiabendazole (see text).

from mucosal ulcerations in the small-intestine is probably important in some cases, active transmission of enteric bacteria across the small-intestinal and colonic mucosa by invading filariform larvae seems more probable.

Clinically this syndrome, which is more common in men than women, usually begins insidiously. Severe anorexia, abdominal pain and constipation may simulate small-intestinal obstruction; the consequences of a laparotomy can be disastrous. Alternatively, it may masquerade as a malabsorption disorder (sometimes identical with post-infective malabsorption – 'tropical sprue' (Cook 1978; 1980)) with or without clinical evidence of obstruction. Acute presentation is also possible. The fatality rate is high and a figure of 77% has been recorded (Igra-Siegman et al. 1981), but the syndrome is often superimposed upon a serious underlying condition, often of malignant origin. A serious delay in diagnosis is common and the condition is first recognized at post-mortem in at least 50% of cases. Prognosis depends upon the time at which chemotherapy is started; when given early in the disease to an individual with an intact immune system, recovery is usual. The following is an illustrative case-history (Pagliuca et al. 1988):

A 27-year-old Ghanian man had lived in the UK for 5 years; he had not returned to Ghana or any other tropical or subtropical country during that time. An HTLV-I associated T-lymphocytic lymphoma was diagnosed and treated with corticosteroids and cytotoxic agents. He was found to have *S stercoralis* larvae in a faecal specimen and was given mebendazole (an agent which is not particularly effective in strongyloidiasis). Shortly afterwards, he developed abdominal pain, a paralytic ileus, and meningitis. On examination he was thin, had marked hepatomegaly (associated with the lymphoma) and was severely dyspnoeic. At this time *S stercoralis* larvae were detected in both faecal and sputum specimens. In addition peripheral blood, and later cerebrospinal fluid (Chap. 8), was shown to contain faecal organisms. A chest-radiograph showed extensive dense infiltrates throughout both lung fields, an abdominal-radiograph evidence of paralytic ileus, and his bones contained several lucent areas compatible with the underlying lymphoma. He was treated with a prolonged course of thiabendazole and the strongyloidiasis was cured.

The hyperinfection syndrome has recently received increasing recognition in a variety of situations: acute lymphoblastic leukaemia (Bezares et al. 1983), in association with renal transplant (usually in the presence of corticosteroid administration) (Boram et al. 1981; Hoy et al. 1981; Fowler et al. 1982; Lijovetsky et al. 1982; Bush and Gabriel 1983), during the course of corticosteroid treatment of the nephrotic syndrome (Vattana and Prasarnsarakit 1983), and in children, most of whom were malnourished (Panyathanya et al. 1983; Thisyakorn and Dithisawad 1983). The syndrome has also recently been reported in an ex-FEPOW (see above) (Stewart and Heap 1985) and in an American Vietnamese war veteran (Hakim and Genta 1986); both of these cases proved fatal. The suggestion has been made that use of the H_2 receptor antagonists in immunosuppressed individuals might predispose to the condition by reducing the gastric acid concentration (Ainley et al. 1986); a 56-year-old West Indian woman with the syndrome who was receiving cimetidine while suffering from a lymphoma was shown at endoscopy to be heavily infected. Larvae may be demonstrable in sputum (Vattana and Prasarnsarakit 1983), bronchial smear (Lijovetzky et al. 1982), or ascitic fluid (Vattana and Prasarnsarakit 1983). Other reports describe co-existent meningitis associated with Gram-negative bacteraemia – usually caused by *E coli* (Vishwanath et al. 1982; Smallman et al. 1986); while bacteria may be demonstrable, the meningitis may sometimes be 'aseptic' with only larvae demonstrable in CSF (Thisyakorn and Dithisawad 1983) (Chap. 8). Clinically, the syndrome can masquerade as cerebral vasculitis (Wachter et al. 1984). Periumbilical purpura, resulting from widespread skin involvement has also been reported (Kalb and Grossman 1986).

It has been suggested that the presence of a *S stercoralis* infection might actively predispose to human T-cell leukaemia virus (HTLV) infection (Nakada et al. 1984); however, it seems far more likely that this infection results from a general impairment of immunity in infected individuals (see above) (Gill and Bell 1984).

Diagnosis

Diagnosis in both immune-intact and immunosuppressed individuals is usually by detection of larvae (and much less commonly eggs) in faecal samples (Cook 1980;

Gilles 1984; Grove 1989a; Speare 1989); however, in at least 50% of cases they will not be demonstrable. The formalin–ether concentration technique gives the highest diagnostic yield (Pelletier 1984; Proctor et al. 1985). Faecal culture is also possible and adult *S stercoralis* can be identified (Speare 1989). Duodenal fluid may be examined for larvae and embryonated eggs (and occasionally adult worms), and is more often positive. The 'Enterotest' (string test) is of value; a nylon thread containing a gelatin capsule at its distal end is swallowed, and when withdrawn 4 or 5 hours later contains attached larvae which can be detected by microscopy. In the hyperinfection syndrome, larvae can also be visualized in other body fluids (see above). Shortened, blunted villi can be demonstrated in a jejunal biopsy specimen; infiltration of the lamina propria, with adult worms, larvae and/or eggs in the mucosa or crypts is diagnostic (Cook 1980). Peripheral eosinophilia (which may be gross) is present intermittently; in the hyperinfection syndrome, especially when corticosteroids are being administered, this is usually absent. In ex-FEPOWs the presence of an eosinophilia can be considered to be strong presumptive evidence of a persisting *S stercoralis* infection (Gill and Bailey 1989).

Small-intestinal radiological changes (see above) are rarely diagnostic, but paralytic ileus with small-intestinal obstruction should put this diagnosis to the fore. Specific serological tests are not readily available; however, an IgG ELISA has recently given high sensitivity and specificity (Genta 1988; Genta et al. 1988; Pelletier et al. 1988; Bailey 1989). *S stercoralis* antibodies cross-react with several of the filariases (including *Wuchereria bancrofti* and *Loa loa* (Case records of the Massachusetts General Hospital 1987; Genta 1988)), and serological examination for filariasis may thus give a positive result. It seems likely that serology will prove to be of value in diagnosing disseminated disease (Genta 1988). Total IgE concentration might be of greater value however, in predicting a chemotherapeutic cure (Pelletier et al. 1988).

Management

Treatment is unsatisfactory at present and newer chemotherapeutic agents are required (Cook 1986, 1987; Pelletier et al. 1988; Grove 1989b). Thiabendazole (25 mg/kg bd on three consecutive days (maximum 3 g daily)) produces a cure in 60%–70% of immune-competent individuals (Hill 1988); clinical cure of up to 93% has been claimed in one study (Pelletier 1984). However, side-effects (anorexia, nausea, vomiting, diarrhoea and dizziness) are common (Hill 1988). Pruritus, xanthopsia, neurotoxicity, leucopenia, bradycardia and hypotension are rare side-effects. In the hyperinfection syndrome, high success rates of up to 60% have also been claimed (Scowden et al. 1978). However, this syndrome has been reported after renal transplantation despite standard courses of thiabendazole (Fowler et al. 1982); an initial 10–15-day course, followed by standard 3-day courses (25 mg/kg on 3 consecutive days) monthly for 6 months has been recommended (Bush and Gabriel 1983). Courses of up to 15 days have been used (Igra-Siegman et al. 1981). Low-dose, long-term interrupted courses have also been recommended in immunosuppressed individuals (Shelhamer et al. 1982).

Albendazole has produced encouraging results in experimental (Grove et al. 1988) and human (Pungpak et al. 1987) studies. An acceptable result has been achieved with 400 mg albendazole daily for 3 days, and repeated after one week (Cook 1989). Further evaluation is required, however, and there is a strong suggestion that it will not be effective in the hyperinfection syndrome. Cure rates of up to 100% have recently been recorded using oral ivermectin (Freedman et al. 1989; Naquira et al. 1989). Less satisfactory agents include mebendazole (100 mg twice daily for 4 days), levamisole and pyrantel embonate. In an experimental study using normal and immunosuppressed dogs infected with a human strain of *S stercoralis*, cambendazole gave a superior result when compared with thiabendazole and mebendazole (Grove and Northern 1988); none of them, however, eliminated infection in those which were immunosuppressed. It has been suggested that cyclosporin A might diminish the likelihood of the hyperinfection syndrome in immunosuppressed patients by virtue of its parasitocidal activity (Schad 1986).

Conclusions

In the immunointact individual, a *Strongyloides stercoralis* infection may be completely asymptomatic; however, with a heavy infection, malabsorption with weight-loss sometimes occurs. The migratory cycle can give rise to an intensely irritant skin eruption (larva currens) and bronchospasm. A peripheral-blood eosinophilia is a frequent, but by no means constant, accompaniment.

S stercoralis hyperinfection syndrome is a frequently fatal but potentially treatable condition. Therefore individuals with a history of tropical exposure, even many decades previously, and immigrants to the United Kingdom (especially those from the Caribbean (Dacre 1988) and West Africa) should be screened for this parasite; alternatively a course of thiabendazole should be given to members of these groups before immunosuppressive treatment is commenced. During immunosuppressive therapy a repeated search for the parasite should be mandatory. A case can be made for giving prophylactic thiabendazole to all immunosuppressed patients if doubt exists that this infection has been eliminated (Vishwanath et al. 1982). A high 'index of suspicion' is also required in everyone with a compromised immune response for any reason, especially those with a lymphoma. It is also important to appreciate that immunity need not necessarily be compromised for this condition to be present (Igra-Siegman et al. 1981; Smallman et al. 1986). Presentation may be with unexplained gastrointestinal symptoms, an 'atypical' pneumonia, bacteraemia or meningitis. The recent literature on the hyperinfection syndrome suggests that it is being diagnosed too late and not infrequently at post-mortem; this state of affairs is clearly extremely unsatisfactory.

Surprisingly, perhaps, the hyperinfection syndrome does not seem to be a common sequel in AIDS (Chap. 2); although a handful of cases have been recorded (Maayan et al. 1987), there is no good evidence from any geographical location (including Africa) for an increased prevalence. The reason(s) for this is unclear.

References

Ainley CC, Clarke DG, Timothy AR, Thompson RPH (1986) *Strongyloides stercoralis* hyperinfection associated with cimetidine in an immunosuppressed patient: diagnosis by endoscopic biopsy. Gut 27:337–338

Bailey JW (1989) A serological test for the diagnosis of *Strongyloides* antibodies in ex Far East prisoners of war. Ann Trop Med Parasitol 83:241–247

Berry AJ, Long EG, Smith JH, Gourley WK, Fine DP (1983) Chronic relapsing colitis due to *Strongyloides stercoralis*. Am J Trop Med Hyg 32:1289–1293

Bezares RF, Carreras LO, Marin CA, Fuchs CAR, Pinto M de T, Nuñez EN (1983) Fatal *Strongyloides stercoralis* hyperinfection in acute leukaemia. Lancet i:481

Boram LH, Keller KF, Justus DE, Collins JP (1981) Strongyloidiasis in immunosuppressed patients. Am J Clin Pathol 76:778–781

Bush A, Gabriel R (1983) Recurrent hyperinfestation with *Strongyloides stercoralis* in a renal allograft recipient. Br Med J 286:52

Case records of the Massachusetts General Hospital (1987) Case 47–1987: *Strongyloides stercoralis* hyperinfection syndrome. N Engl J Med 317:1332–1342

Castellani A, Chalmers AJ (1919) Manual of tropical medicine, 3rd edn. London: Baillière, Tindall and Cox, London, pp 628–629

Cook GC (1978) Tropical sprue: implications of Manson's concept. J R Coll Phys Lond 12:329–349

Cook GC (1980) Tropical gastroenterology. Oxford University Press, Oxford, pp 309–314

Cook GC (1985) Parasitic infection. In: Booth CC, Neale G (eds) Disorders of the small intestine. Blackwell Scientific Publications, Oxford, pp 283–298

Cook GC (1986) The clinical significance of gastrointestinal helminths – a review. Trans R Soc Trop Med Hyg 80:675–685

Cook GC (1987) *Strongyloides stercoralis* hyperinfection syndrome: how often is it missed? Q J Med 64:625–629

Cook GC (1989) Parasitic infections of the gastrointestinal tract: a worldwide clinical problem. Curr Opin Gastroenterol 5:126–139

Dacre J (1988) Strongyloidiasis. Br Med J 296:1328

Dawkins HJS (1989) *Strongyloides ratti* infections in rodents: value and limitations as a model for human strongyloidiasis. In: Grove DI (ed) Strongyloidiasis: a major roundworm infection of man. Taylor and Francis, London, pp 287–332

Fowler CG, Lindsay I, Lewin J, Sweny P, Fernando ON, Moorhead JF (1982) Recurrent hyperinfestation with *Strongyloides stercoralis* in a renal allograft recipient. Br Med J 285:1394

Freedman DO, Zierdt WS, Lujan A, Nutman TB (1989) The efficacy of ivermectin in chemotherapy of gastrointestinal helminthiasis in humans. J Infect Dis 159:1151–1153

Genta RM (1988) Predictive value of an enzyme-linked immunosorbent assay (ELISA) for the serodiagnosis of strongyloidiasis. Am J Clin Pathol 89:391–394

Genta RM (1989a) *Strongyloides stercoralis*: loss of ability to disseminate after repeated passage in laboratory beagles. Trans R Soc Trop Med Hyg 83:539–541

Genta RM (1989b) Immunology. In: Grove DI (ed) Strongyloidiasis: a major roundworm infection of man. Taylor and Francis, London, pp 133–153

Genta RM, Gomes MC (1989) Pathology. In: Grove DI (ed) Strongyloidiasis: a major roundworm infection of man. Taylor and Francis, London, pp 105–132

Genta RM, Grove DI (1989) *Strongyloides stercoralis* infections in animals. In: Grove DI (ed) Strongyloidiasis: a major roundworm infection of man. Taylor and Francis, London, pp 251–269

Genta RM, Harper JS, Gam AA, London WT, Neva FA (1984) Experimental disseminated strongyloidiasis in *Erythrocebus patas*. II. Immunology. Am J Trop Med Hyg 33:444–450

Genta RM, Schad GA, Hellman ME (1986) *Strongyloides stercoralis*: parasitological, immunological and pathological observations in immunosuppressed dogs. Trans R Soc Trop Med Hyg 80:34–41

Genta RM, Gatti S, Linke MJ, Cevini C, Scaglia M (1988) Endemic strongyloidiasis in northern Italy: clinical and immunological aspects. Q J Med 68:679–690

Gill GV, Bailey JW (1989) Eosinophilia as a marker for chronic strongyloidiasis – use of a serum ELISA test to detect asymptomatic cases. Ann Trop Med Parasitol 83:249–252

Gill GV, Bell DR (1979) *Strongyloides stercoralis* infection in former Far East prisoners of war. Br Med J ii:572–574

Gill GV, Bell DR (1984) Strongyloidiasis and impaired immunity. Lancet i:858

Gill GV, Bell DR (1987) *Strongyloides stercoralis* infection in Burma Star veterans. Br Med J 294:1003–1004
Gilles HM (1984) Strongyloidiasis. In: Strickland GT (ed) Hunter's tropical medicine, 6th edn. Saunders, Philadelphia, pp 641–645
Grove DI (1989a) Diagnosis. In: Grove DI (ed) Strongyloidiasis: a major roundworm infection of man. Taylor and Francis, London, pp 175–197
Grove DI (1989b) Treatment. In: Grove DI (ed) Strongyloidiasis: a major roundworm infection of man. Taylor and Francis, London, pp 199–231
Grove DI, Northern C (1988) The effects of thiabendazole, mebendazole and cambendazole in normal and immunosuppressed dogs infected with a human strain of *Strongyloides stercoralis*. Trans R Soc Trop Med Hyg 82:146–149
Grove DI, Heenan PJ, Northern C (1983) Persistent and disseminated infections with *Strongyloides stercoralis* in immunosuppressed dogs. Int J Parasitol 13:483–490
Grove DI, Lumsden J, Northern C (1988) Efficacy of albendazole against *Strongyloides ratti* and *S stercoralis in vitro*, in mice, and in normal and immunosuppressed dogs. J Antimicrob Chemother 21:75–84
Hakim SZ, Genta RM (1986) Fatal disseminated strongyloidiasis in a Vietnam war veteran. Arch Pathol Lab Med 110:809–812
Hardie R (1983) The Burma–Siam railway: the secret diary of Dr Robert Hardie 1942–45. Imperial War Museum, London, p 178
Harper JS, Genta RM, Gam A, London WT, Neva FA (1984) Experimental disseminated strongyloidiasis in *Erythrocebus patas*. I Pathology. Am J Trop Med Hyg 33:431–443
Hill JA (1988) Strongyloidiasis in ex-Far East prisoners of war. Br Med J 296:753
Hoy WE, Roberts NJ, Bryson MF, Bowles C, Lee JCK, Rivero AJ, Ritterson AL (1981) Transmission of strongyloidiasis by kidney transplant? Disseminated strongyloidiasis in both recipients of kidney allografts from a single cadaver donor. JAMA 246:1937–1939
Igra-Siegman Y, Kapila R, Sen P, Kaminski ZC, Louria DB (1981) Syndrome of hyperinfection with *Strongyloides stercoralis*. Rev Infect Dis 3:397–407
Kalb RE, Grossman ME (1986) Periumbilical purpura in disseminated strongyloidiasis. JAMA 256:1170–1171
Lijovetzky G, Reinhartz T, Rivkind A, Rubinger D (1982) Fatal case of strongyloidiasis in an immunosuppressed patient. Israel J Med Sci 18:1048–1050
Maayan S, Wormser GP, Widerhorn J, Sy ER, Kim YE, Ernst JA (1987) *Strongyloides stercoralis* hyperinfection in a patient with the acquired immune deficiency syndrome. Am J Med 83:945–948
Manson P (1898) Tropical diseases: a manual of the diseases of warm climates. Cassell, London, pp 550–553
Nakada K, Kohakura M, Komoda H, Hinuma Y (1984) High incidence of HTLV antibody in carriers of *Strongyloides stercoralis*. Lancet i:633
Naquira C, Jiminez G, Guerra JG, Bernal R, Nalin DR, Neu D, Aziz M (1989) Ivermectin for human strongyloidiasis and other intestinal helminths. Am J Trop Med Hyg 40:304–309
Normond LA (1876) Sur la maladie dite diarrhée de Cochinchine. CR Acad Sci (Paris) 83:316–318
Pagliuca A, Layton DM, Allen S, Mufti GJ (1988) Hyperinfection with *strongyloides* after treatment for adult T cell leukaemia–lymphoma in an African immigrant. Br Med J 297:1456–1457
Panyathanya R, Sriumpai S, Tantranond R (1983) Fatal strongyloidiasis in Siriraj Hospital, Bangkok, Thailand. Southeast Asian J Trop Med Publ Health 14:294–297
Pelletier LL (1984) Chronic strongyloidiasis in World War II Far East ex-prisoners of war. Am J Trop Med Hyg 33:55–61
Pelletier LL, Baker CB, Gam AA, Nutman TB, Neva FA (1988) Diagnosis and evaluation of treatment of chronic strongyloidiasis in ex-prisoners of war. J Infect Dis 157:573–576
Proctor EM, Isaac-Renton JL, Robertson WB, Black WA (1985) Strongyloidiasis in Canadian Far East war veterans. Can Med Ass J 133:876–878
Proctor EM, Muth HAV, Proudfoot DL, Allen AB, Fisk R, Isaac-Renton J, Black WA (1987) Endemic institutional strongyloidiasis in British Columbia. Can Med Ass J 136:1173–1176
Pungpak S, Bunnag D, Chindanond D, Radmoyos B (1987) Albendazole in the treatment of strongyloidiasis. Southeast Asian J Trop Med Publ Health 18:207–210
Schad GA (1986) Cyclosporin may eliminate the threat of overwhelming strongyloidiasis in immunosuppressed patients. J Infect Dis 153:178
Schad GA (1989) Morphology and life history of *Strongyloides stercoralis*. In: Grove DI (ed) Strongyloidiasis: a major roundworm infection of man. Taylor and Francis, London, pp 85–104
Schad GA, Hellman ME, Muncey DW (1984) *Strongyloides stercoralis*: hyperinfection in immuno-suppressed dogs. Exp Parasitol 57:287–296

Scowden EB, Schaffner W, Stone WJ (1978) Overwhelming strongyloidiasis: an unappreciated opportunistic infection. Medicine (Baltimore) 57:527–544

Seymour R, Finucane P (1989) Hyperinfection with *Strongyloides*. Br Med J 298:386

Shelhamer JH, Neva FA, Finn DR (1982) Persistent strongyloidiasis in an immunodeficient patient. Am J Trop Med Hyg 31:746–751

Smallman LA, Young JA, Shortland-Webb WR, Carey MP, Michael J (1986) *Strongyloides stercoralis* hyperinfestation syndrome with *Escherichia coli* meningitis: report of two cases. J Clin Pathol 39:366–370

Speare R (1989) Identification of species of *Strongyloides*. In: Grove DI (ed) Strongyloidiasis: a major roundworm infection of man. Taylor and Francis, London, pp 11–83

Sprott V, Selby CD, Ispahani P, Toghill PJ (1987) Indigenous strongyloidiasis in Nottingham. Br Med J 294:741–742

Stewart JB, Heap BJ (1985) Fatal disseminated strongyloidiasis in an immunocompromised former war prisoner of the Japanese. J R Army Med Corps 131:47–49

Thisyakorn U, Dithisawad J (1983) Disseminated strongyloidiasis in children: a case report. J Med Assoc Thailand 66:410–411

Tindall NR, Wilson PAG (1988) Criteria for a proof of migration routes of immature parasites inside hosts exemplified by studies of *Strongyloides ratti* in the rat. Parasitology 96:551–563

Vattana SS, Prasarnsarakit N (1983) Disseminated strongyloidiasis: a case report. J Med Assoc Thailand 66:61–64

Vishwanath S, Baker RA, Mansheim BJ (1982) *Strongyloides* infection and meningitis in an immunocompromised host. Am J Trop Med Hyg 31:857–858

Wachter RM, Burke AM, MacGregor RR (1984) *Strongyloides stercoralis* hyperinfection masquerading as cerebral vasculitis. Arch Neurol 41:1213–1216

Chapter 6

Colorectal Parasitic Infections: Invasive *Entamoeba histolytica* and Its Role in Colonic and Hepatic Disease

Recall from Time's abysmal chasm
That piece of primal protoplasm
The First Amoeba, strangely splendid,
From whom we're all of us descended.

Arthur Guiterman (1871–1943),
Ode to the Amoeba

Introduction

In all developing Third World countries – both tropical and subtropical – socioeconomic conditions and standards of hygiene and sanitation are less than perfect. In consequence human infection with a large range of colorectal parasites is common (Cook 1980, 1986a,b, 1988, 1989). Travellers and tourists are also frequently infected and a 'high index of suspicion' is required if this group of diseases is to be diagnosed (Walker and Williams 1985). Recently, intestinal parasitic infections have received considerable prominence in relation to immunosuppression (Chaps. 2 and 4) (Cook 1980, 1986b), and this is especially so in patients with HIV infections and in particular those with the end-stage AIDS syndrome (Casemore et al. 1985); active male homosexuals who are HIV-negative are also at a significantly greater risk from some of these infections (Weller 1985).

In the tropics and subtropics, underlying malnutrition and impaired immunity, which are often closely intertwined, are important predisposing factors; they are probably more important, however, in the context of protozoan rather than helminthic infections of the lower gastrointestinal tract (Greenwood and Wittle 1981). The role of hypochlorhydria in predisposing individuals to these infections

remains unclear; for many years this condition has been recognized as predisposing to certain bacterial infections (Hurst 1934), and several studies also suggest
that parasitic infections are also more common (Cook 1985a). Now that H_2-
receptor-antagonists are widely prescribed even in developing countries, the
importance of hypochlorhydria and, more importantly, achlorhydria requires re-
evaluation in this context (Cook 1985a).

Protozoan Infections

Table 6.1 summarizes the more important colorectal protozoan parasites. These
are dominated by *Entamoeba histolytica* (Cook 1980; Martínez-Palomo 1987;
Ravdin 1988).

Table 6.1. Colorectal protozoa

Luminal	
Pathogenic	*Entamoeba histolytica*
	E polecki
	Balantidium coli
	Giardia lamblia (?)[a]
	Cryptosporidium sp (?)[b]
	Blastocystis hominis (?)[b]
Non-pathogenic[c]	*Dientamoeba fragilis*(?)
	E coli
	Iodamoeba bütschlii
	Endolimax nana
	Chilomastix mesnili
	Trichomonas hominis
	Retortamonas intestinalis
Mural (non-luminal)	*Enteromonas hominis*
	Trypanosoma cruzi (Chagas' disease)
	megacolon (Chap. 12)

[a]See Chap. 3.
[b]See Chap. 4.
[c]The possibility cannot be ruled out that some, or all of these can
produce symptoms when present at high concentration, or in
immunosuppressed (including AIDS) patients.

Entamoeba histolytica

The history of this infection has been reviewed (Kean 1988). The overall
prevalence of amoebiasis is difficult to assess; one estimate is that in one year, 480
million people were infected with *E histolytica* and of these 36 million developed a
disabling colitis or extraintestinal 'abscesses', and there were 40 000 deaths
(Walsh 1986); in numerical terms this would make it the third most important
human parasitic infection, following malaria (Chap. 1) and schistosomiasis

(Chap. 7). The prevalence of this infection in industrialized countries has declined with urbanization and better standards of hygiene and sanitation; however, it remains extremely common in developing countries (Ravdin 1989) and in tourists (Lalla et al. 1988; Cook 1989).

Parasitology and Pathogenesis

E histolytica is a member of the family Entamoebidae, and belongs to the subphylum Sarcodina, class Lobosea, order Amoebida. It is distinguished from other species (e.g. *E coli*) by several morphological features. Figure 6.1 summarizes the life-cycle of *E histolytica*. The motile trophozoite has an average diameter of 25 μm (range 10–60 μm) and contains a single 3–5 μm nucleus with a distinct central nucleolus; the cytoplasm is finely granular and may contain ingested red blood cells. Figure 6.2 shows several trophozoites of *E histolytica* in culture. The cysts are smaller (averaging 12 μm in diameter) and have one to four nuclei; the cytoplasm may contain visible chromatoidal bars and on occasion, glycogen granules. While trophozoites can only survive for a few hours outside the human host, cysts (the cause of human infection) remain viable in a moist environment for several weeks or months. After passage through the stomach, excystation occurs and the trophozoites either remain in the colonic lumen or

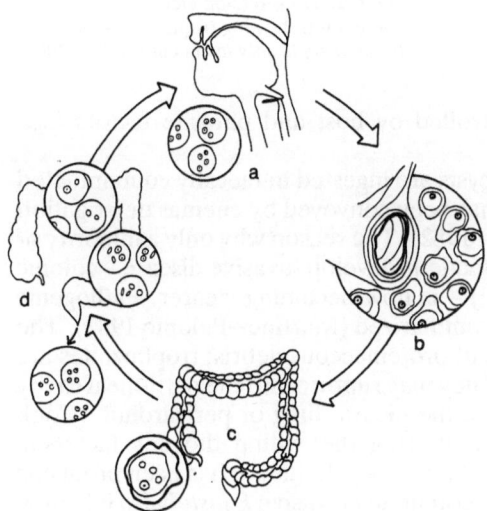

Fig. 6.1. Life-cycle of *Entamoeba histolytica*. (a) Cyst (9–15 μm) which contains four nuclei and a central karyosome, is ingested in contaminated food or water and swallowed; (b) excystation occurs (following the action of digestive enzymes) in the small-intestine, and eight motile trophozoites are liberated; (c) trophozoite (20–30 μm diameter) which possesses a single nucleus with a central karyosome surrounded by chromatin; if it belongs to an 'invasive' zymodeme it ingests red blood cells which are present in its cytoplasm (and invasion of other organs – most importantly the liver – may take place; by taking this course it departs from the life-cycle and is 'committing suicide'); (d) encystment occurs in the colonic lumen; this is complete when all four nuclei are present and the chromatoidal bars (ordered arrays of ribosomes) have disappeared. Cysts passed in a faecal sample can remain viable for up to one month in favourable conditions.

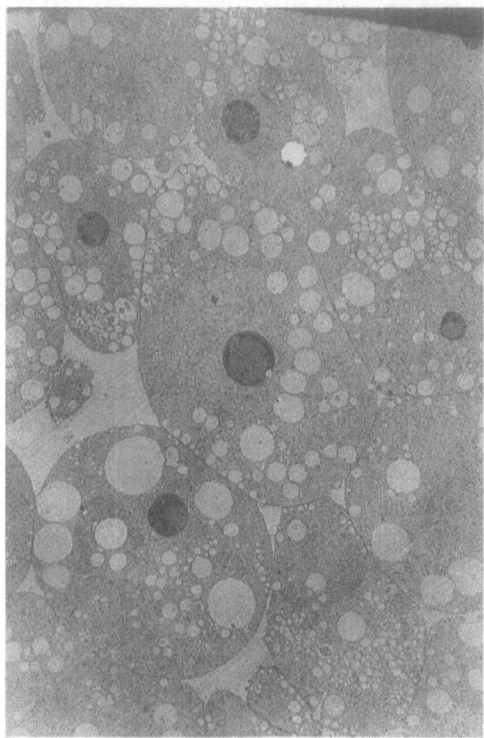

Fig. 6.2. Transmission electron-micrograph showing trophozoites of *Entamoeba histolytica* in culture (× 1200).

produce invasive disease; this is controlled by host and parasite factors (see below).

The usual route of infection is oral; cysts are ingested in faecally contaminated food or water. Occasionally infection has been conveyed by enemas or irrigation fluid used for colonic lavage (Istre et al. 1982). The reason why only a minority of individuals harbouring *E histolytica* infections develop invasive disease – colonic and sometimes hepatic (liver 'abscess') – is now becoming clearer. Pathogenic features of invasive disease have been summarized (Martínez-Palomo 1987). The 'abscess' cavity does not contain pus, but proteinaceous debris; trophozoites are present at the periphery of the cavity. They may rupture into the peritoneal cavity or spread by direct extension to involve the pleura, lung or pericardium (Cook 1980). Host factors involved in the response (together with pathogenic factors in human disease) have been reviewed (Sullam 1988). Evidence has been produced which indicates a greater resistance to a potentially invasive *E histolytica* infection in Old compared with New World subhuman primates (Beaver et al. 1988). In a hamster model, invasive hepatic disease is modulated by host immune-responses to the plasma-membrane protein of *E histolytica* (Vinayak and Sharma 1989). Invasive *E histolytica* which actually produces invasive hepatic disease have 'opted out' of the parasite's life-cycle, and although causing serious disease in the human host have pursued a potentially suicidal course!

Sargeaunt and his colleagues in London have demonstrated that *E histolytica* can be divided into benign and 'aggressive' strains (zymodemes) by an analysis of their isoenzyme patterns (Sargeaunt et al. 1978; Sargeaunt 1987, 1988); at present nine zymodemes have been positively associated with *clinical* disease, whereas 13 seem to be non-invasive (Editorial 1985). Genomic DNA differences have recently been demonstrated between pathogenic and non-pathogenic strains (Tannich et al. 1989). This work is consistent with an hypothesis formulated by Brumpt in 1925 that *E histolytica* can be divided into pathogenic (*E dysenteriae*) and non-pathogenic (*E dispar*) strains (Brumpt 1925). The crucial question, however, is whether these two zymodeme (and DNA) groupings represent completely separate entities or whether under certain circumstances they can switch from one type to the other (Martínez-Palomo 1987). Environmental factors, including nutrition, have been suggested to be important factors in the determination of the invasiveness of *E histolytica* (Barker et al. 1976). The stability of the two separate isoenzyme groupings has been challenged by Mirelman et al. (1986a,b; Mirelman 1987, 1988); these workers have demonstrated that the axenization of a strain with a non-pathogenic isoenzyme pattern resulted in reversion to a pathogenic zymodeme pattern with acquisition of virulence, as measured in a hamster model. These observations suggest that culture conditions and bacterial associates can modify isoenzyme patterns; they did not seem to be caused by the induction of selective pressure on heterogeneous populations because the results were obtained with the use of cloned cultures. Does *E histolytica* therefore consist of only one species which can change its expression of virulence? Is gene-switching in fact occurring?

A further interesting and enigmatic fact has recently emerged: although *E histolytica* infection is common in homosexual men (Weber 1985; Sullam 1988), pathogenic zymodemes seem to occur only rarely in this group and, consequently, invasive disease is rare; most are therefore asymptomatic. This is difficult to comprehend because some male homosexuals must be infected with pathogenic strains. These findings would presumably be more consistent with a factor(s) in the colorectum of male homosexuals which rendered all *E histolytica* non-pathogenic in that environment. [A recent report from Japan has in fact documented *E histolytica* isolates from four practising homosexual men (all of whom had invasive disease) which belonged to invasive zymodemes (Nozaki et al. 1989).]

However, these observations do not solve the problem as to *how* this protozoan invades human tissue (Sullam 1988). Recently, evidence has been presented for enterotoxigenicity (Feingold et al. 1985) and proteolytic properties (Lushbaugh et al. 1984) in some amoebae; adherence lectins have also been studied (Ravdin et al. 1985; Ravdin 1988, 1989). The galactose lectin mediates attachment of trophozoites to colonic mucins; an understanding of this would presumably be important in vaccine development. However, to date, these factors have not been correlated with the various zymodemes (Cook 1989).

Clinical Aspects

Infection may be asymptomatic (which is the case in 90%–99% of infected individuals) or result in acute or chronic invasive colitis, or hepatic disease resulting in an 'abscess' or 'abscesses' (Cook 1980; Martínez-Palomo 1987). Invasive colonic disease usually presents with bloody diarrhoea, abdominal pain and frequently fever also. Ulcerations are characteristically flask-shaped and extend into the submucosa. A fulminant (necrotizing) form of colitis with total colonic involvement, and frequently perforation, is characteristically associated with corticosteroid administration; this serious complication carries a high mortality rate (Ellyson et al. 1986; Shukla et al. 1986). Chronic lesions (amoebomas) can mimic colorectal carcinomas.

Amoebic colitis, which carries a significant mortality rate, is most common in infants and children (2–3 years) and those >40 years; this differs from a group of patients with diarrhoeal disease of other aetiologies who were studied in Bangladesh, and in whom a unimodal age-distribution curve was demonstrated (Wanke et al. 1988). These authors also found a significant association between amoebic colitis and a prior measles rash, malnutrition, hyponatraemia, hypokalaemia and hypoproteinaemia. Invasive amoebiasis has repeatedly been shown to be more common in males than females (Cook 1980; Walsh 1986); however, a higher prevalence exists during pregnancy (Wanke et al. 1988). Differentiation from shigella-colitis on clinical grounds has received attention in Bangladesh (Speelman et al. 1987); those with amoebic colitis were older, had a longer pre-hospital illness, lower body-weight, were less often febrile, and in addition had a lower haematocrit, higher leucocyte count and fewer faecal leucocytes. It is extremely important to differentiate this entity from inflammatory bowel disease (IBD); clinical presentation is often identical. Furthermore, IBD is not uncommonly unmasked by tropical exposure. At the Hospital for Tropical Diseases, London, a recent retrospective study demonstrated that 32 out of 129 previously asymptomatic UK residents who presented with bloody diarrhoea during or immediately after tropical exposure, had underlying IBD, usually ulcerative colitis (Harries et al. 1985); only 27 of them had amoebic colitis. The mechanism for this precipitation of overt disease is unclear but is presumably associated with an alteration of the luminal flora; bacteria or viruses, or both, might be important (Gorbach 1982).

The association of 'tropical liver abscess' with *E histolytica* was first demonstrated by Councilman and Lafleur (1891) and later by Rogers (1922). While recognizing an association between 'abscess of the liver' and dysentery, Manson (1898) speculated that *Amoeba coli* might play a pathogenic role; other possibilities noted were that (i) this organism might be a carrier of pus-forming bacteria, and (ii) it was merely a harmless epiphenomenon. Amoebic liver 'abscess', which occurs in about 2% of adults infected with *E histolytica* (Martínez-Palomo 1987), usually presents with right upper abdominal pain and/or a febrile illness. Figure 6.3 shows an example of invasive hepatic amoebiasis. Right shoulder-tip pain and right-sided chest pathology are other common presentations of this disease. Tender hepatomegaly and fever are usually present. Chemotherapy (see below) should be instituted as soon as the diagnosis has been established.

Diagnosis

Diagnostically, trophozoites in a *fresh* faecal sample or rectal scraping or biopsy is the surest means of diagnosis; ingestion of the host's erythrocytes is characteristic. *E histolytica* trophozoites can occasionally be detected in liver 'pus', and an indirect fluorescent antibody technique has been applied (Yang 1989). Although

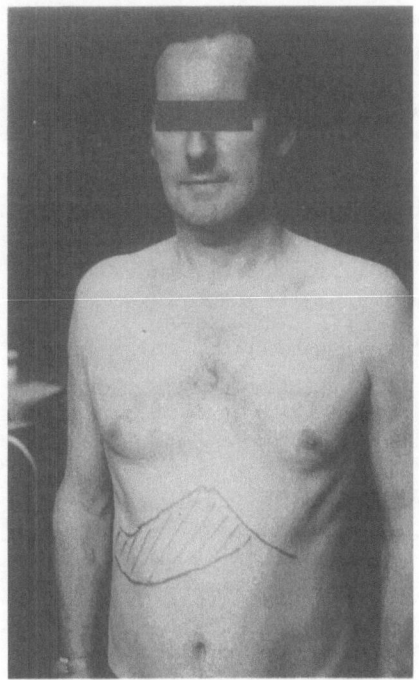

Fig. 6.3. A 45-year-old man who had travelled extensively in tropical countries, mostly in South-east Asia. Presentation was with a febrile illness and a tender enlarged liver. Serological tests for invasive amoebiasis were strongly positive (IFAT 1:640), and ultrasonography showed a single 'abscess' of approximately 10 cm diameter. Response to metronidazole followed by diloxanide furoate (see text) was rapid, and complete.

first developed in 1925, in vitro faecal culture remains primarily an investigative technique. Immunological tests for *E histolytica* infection have been reviewed and their value in epidemiological surveys assessed (Healy 1986). The immuno-fluorescent antibody test (IFAT), is of considerable value in severe *invasive* amoebiasis (Ambroise-Thomas 1980); however, even in this situation, some 5% of results are negative in the early, acute stage of an hepatic '*abscess*'. In amoebic *colitis*, although up to 75% of cases give positive results, the titre is usually much lower than it is in invasive disease involving the liver. A rapidly performed indirect haemagglutination test for serodiagnosis has been documented (Parija et al. 1989). An ELISA designed to detect circulating immune complexes of *E histolytica* proteins as a diagnostic test in hepatic amoebiasis has been reported (Gandhi et al. 1988). It is important to recognize that immunosuppression can give rise to false-negative results. Detection of *E histolytica* antigen in faecal material using an ELISA has been reported (Grundy et al. 1987; Joyce and Ravdin 1988). A technique utilizing immunofluorescence with monoclonal antibodies to separate pathogenic from non-pathogenic *E histolytica* might prove useful in clinical management (Strachan et al. 1988). Unfortunately the isoen-zyme technique used to identify the subspecies takes several days to perform and is of little or no value in clinical medicine; it will, however, continue to be valuable in epidemiological work (Cook 1989). Ultrasonography and CT-scanning are extremely valuable techniques for localizing an hepatic 'abscess(es)' and for differentiating it from other intrahepatic space-occupying lesions (Table 6.2); when aspiration is carried out (see below), it can be performed under ultrasonographic control. Figure 6.4 shows an ultrasound scan of an amoebic liver 'abscess' in an adult before and after chemotherapy.

Table 6.2. Ultrasonographic features of an amoebic liver 'abscess' compared with other space-occupying hepatic lesions

Amoebic 'abscess'	Well defined
	Usually high; often sub-diaphragmatic
	Hyperreflective
	(Usually enlarges after chemotherapy is initiated)
Pyogenic abscess	Poorly defined (usually)
	'Ragged' loculated appearance
	Change from diffuse to transonic in days or weeks
Hydatid cyst	Septate
	Germinal layer and daughter cysts may be visible
	Transonic

Management

Mortality rate from invasive amoebiasis fell from >80% during the nineteenth century to around 10%–20% in the early 1970s, and to 2% after the introduction of metronidazole (Martínez-Palomo 1987). Rogers (1912) first successfully administered emetine, although ipecac bark had been used in Peru since the seventeenth century (Kean 1988). Treatment of amoebic colitis is now usually straightforward: 800 mg metronidazole ('Flagyl') tds is given orally for 5–10 days. Recently tinidazole, 2 g daily for 3 days, has also been used, but evidence of cure, using controlled trials, is far less extensive. Ornidazole is also effective (Cook 1989); in one study a 94% cure rate was achieved (Bassily et al. 1987). Other agents which have been used are: paromomycin (an aminoglycoside) (25–30 mg/kg daily, in 3 divided doses, for 7 days), iodoquinol, tetracycline and quinfamide (Sullam 1988). Aspiration of a liver 'abscess' is indicated only when (i) a large 'abscess(es)' is present in a sick patient, or (ii) the abscess(es) impinges upon a vital organ such as the pericardium. A recent controlled trial in India has clearly demonstrated that in an uncomplicated case routine aspiration is not indicated (Sharma et al. 1989). Resolution of an amoebic 'abscess' can be assessed by ultrasonography or CT-scanning; it is very slow but this is entirely consistent with successful chemotheraphy (Sheen et al. 1989). During the first few days of treatment it is usual for the 'abscess' to *increase* slightly in diameter.

When available, diloxanide furoate ('Furamide'), 500 mg tds for 10 days, should always follow the 5-nitroimidazole compound. Diloxanide is an excellent luminal amoebicide, whereas both metronidazole and tinidazole have relatively weak activity on the cyst-stage. Numerous examples exist of second amoebic liver abscesses arising when a full course of metronidazole has not been followed by diloxanide. Should all *E histolytica* cyst-carriers be treated? This is a difficult question but in a Western country where this compound is readily available the

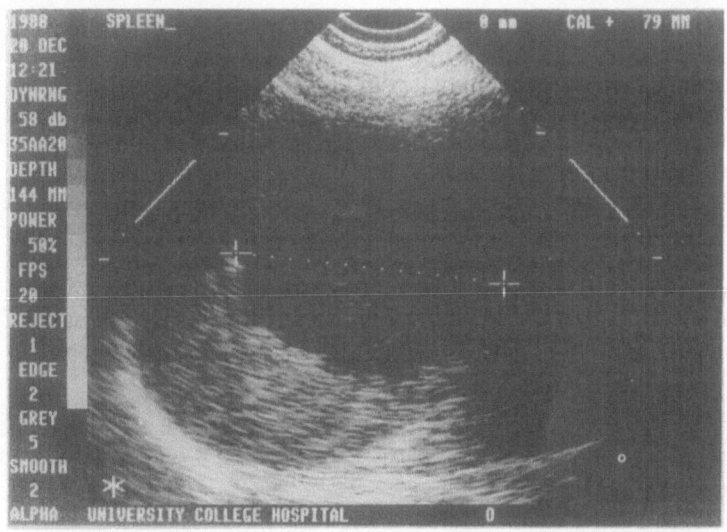

a

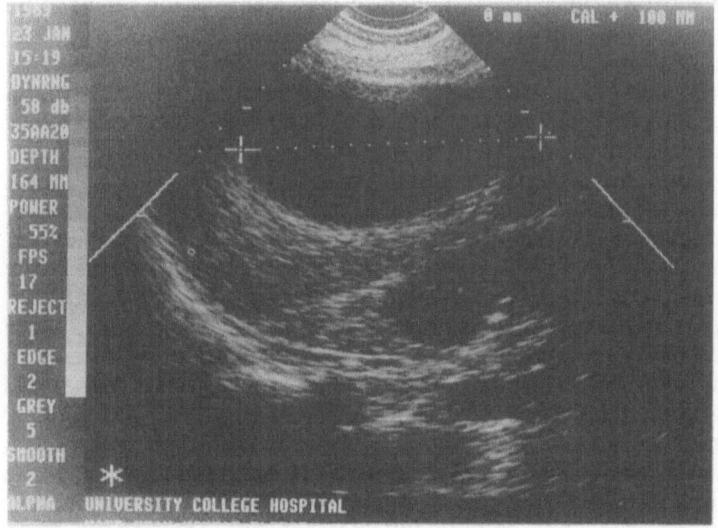

b

Fig. 6.4a,b. Ultrasound-scan of an amoebic liver abscess **a** before and **b** after chemotherapy. The diameter of the 'abscess' had increased slightly – which is the usual response following successful treatment.

answer must at present be *Yes* (Kovacz and Masur 1986); if and when determination of specific zymodemes (after culture) becomes a readily available diagnostic technique, individuals harbouring non-invasive zymodemes need not perhaps receive diloxanide (Sergeaunt 1987); however, this view has been challenged (Prasad and Virk 1987). The situation in Third World countries is different, and diloxanide is frequently not readily available. When limited funding prohibits treating all cyst-carriers, re-infection rates in the locality, sexual habits, etc., should perhaps be taken into account (Jackson 1987). A study carried out in India has suggested that in that country the cyst-carrier state usually resolves spontaneously (Nanda et al. 1984); however, far more data are required before this conclusion can be accepted at face value. *E histolytica* infections are common in male homosexuals but all seem to belong to non-invasive zymodemes (Sargeaunt et al. 1983; Allason-Jones et al. 1988) (see above); this finding is surprising and more information is required. Although many male homosexuals travel extensively, they frequently take courses of metronidazole; however, diloxanide is not widely used and presumably cysts of potentially invasive zymodemes must survive in the intestinal lumen in some of them. On the basis of their findings, Weber (1985) and Allason-Jones et al. (1988) have concluded that the cyst-carrier-state in homosexual men can be safely left untreated.

Other Colorectal Protozoan Infections

E polecki occasionally produces significant colonic pathology; although pig-to-man transmission is frequently suspected, man-to-man transmission seems to be important in Papua New Guinea (Desowitz and Barnish 1986; Rolston et al. 1986).

In certain parts of the world, e.g. Papua New Guinea, South-east Asia, and southern America, the large ciliated protozoan *Balantidium coli*, which also has a reservoir in pigs, is a significant human pathogen (Areán and Koppisch 1956). Dysentery is the usual form of presentation; anorexia, nausea and weight-loss are other associated symptoms. Colonic tenderness may be present. Although local complications (perforation, haemorrhage, shock, etc.) occasionally occur, metastatic spread to the liver and other organs is an extremely unusual event. Treatment is with tetracycline (500 mg qds for 10 days); iodoquinol, nitrimidazine and paromomycin are alternative agents but they are not widely used.

Although patients with a heavy *Giardia lamblia* infection (Cook 1980, 1985b) occasionally present with bloody diarrhoea, it is most likely that this is due to a colonic pathogen other than *G lamblia* itself. However, the possibility that this flagellated protozoon can cause colonic pathology *per se* has not been completely excluded. Treatment is with oral metronidazole, 2 g daily for 3 consecutive days, or tinidazole 2 g stat; ornidazole, nimorazole and mepacrine are also effective (Chap. 3) (Boreham et al. 1984). *Cryptosporidium* sp (Chap. 4) is predominantly a small-intestinal parasite, but colonic involvement has occasionally been reported, especially in AIDS (Casemore et al. 1985).

The remaining luminal protozoan parasites which involve the human colon are usually harmless commensals. Rarely, however, significant symptoms (and pathology) can result from a heavy infection especially in children; *Dientamoeba fragilis* is one example (Yang and Scholten 1977). There is also limited evidence that some of them might assume pathogenic qualities in AIDS patients (Rolston et al. 1986).

Trypanosoma cruzi causes Chagas' disease (Chap. 12); it is confined to Central and South America and is a further colonic protozoan parasite (Köberle 1968; Cook 1980); it is, however, mural rather than luminal, and megacolon forms the major problem in the *chronic* phase of the disease. Megaoesophagus and cardiomyopathy are other complications.

Helminthic Infections

Table 6.3 summarizes the major helminths which can produce colorectal disease. Cestodes, which are a relatively common problem in the small-intestine, do not feature in this list. *Trichuris trichiura* (the whipworm) and *Enterobius vermicularis* (the threadworm) dominate the scene (Cook 1980).

Table 6.3. Colorectal helminths

Nematodes	*Trichuris trichiura*
	Enterobius vermicularis
	Oesophagostomum sp
	Ternidens deminutus
	Strongyloides stercoralis
	Anisakis sp
Trematodes[a]	*Schistosoma mansoni*
	S. intercalatum
	S. mattheei
	S. japonicum
	S. mekongi

[a]These are not strictly colorectal because the adult worms live in the portal venous system of man; however, they all produce colorectal disease (Chap. 7).

Trichuris trichiura

T trichiura (the whipworm) is present throughout the world, but is especially abundant in the humid tropics. In some parts of Asia, prevalence rates in excess of 50% are reported; peak age incidence is 5 to 15 years. Both genetic and environmental factors are thought to be important (Cook 1988). Underlying malnutrition might be an important predisposing factor to infection, and this organism may be involved in the parasite ↔ malnutrition equation. In a study at Kuala Lumpur, Malaysia, nutritional status was significantly reduced in a group of children with heavy trichuriasis infection compared with controls (Gilman et al. 1983); improvement occurred after treatment.

Infection usually results from ingestion of infective eggs (transmitted by defaecation on to soil) from contaminated hands, food or drink; animal reservoirs do not seem to be important. The life-cycle is straightforward and adult worms mature in the caecum and ascending colon. The caecum is the major segment of the intestinal tract to be involved, although infection is sometimes present in the ileum also. In the rectum worms may adhere to rectal mucosa causing haemorrhage and ulceration. The adult worms obtain nourishment by liquefying mucosal cells (by their secretions) or by sucking the host's blood (approximately 0.005 ml per worm per day). Most infections are asymptomatic, but with heavy ones (i.e. 1000 worms or more) bloody diarrhoea with hypochromic anaemia and rectal prolapse may occur (Bundy 1986). Because infection with this helminth often occurs concurrently with hookworm (and *A lumbricoides*), hypochromic anaemia can be extremely severe. Crohn's disease may be simulated both clinically and radiologically (Sandler 1981). Appendicitis and peritonitis have also been reported. With very heavy infections, anorexia, diarrhoea (presumably resulting from impairment of colonic absorptive function), abdominal discomfort and weight-loss have been recorded. It seems probable that the overall impact of trichuriasis on health, especially in childhood, has been underestimated.

Diagnosis is by detection of ova in faecal samples; sigmoidoscopy or colonoscopy may reveal adult worms. Mebendazole is the treatment of choice and a single-dose regimen is usually effective (Kan 1983); albendazole and flubendazole have also been used. Recently, ivermectin has been claimed to give an 85% cure rate (Naquira et al. 1989).

Enterobius vermicularis

E vermicularis (the threadworm) is the only other nematode to cause major clinical problems in the lower intestinal tract. It is also world-wide in its distribution, and prevalence rates of up to 100% have been reported in some areas.

After ingestion, ova hatch in the upper intestine with liberation of larvae which migrate to the ileal region; as they detach they are passed to the anus where they shower sticky ova on to the perianal skin. Pruritus ani (Alexander-Williams 1983) is the major symptom. Appendicitis and vulvovaginitis are possible sequelae of infection. *E vermicularis* can produce eosinophilic granulomas in the colon, rectum and adjacent structures (Shiraki et al. 1974); extensive colorectal invasion by larval stages of this nematode has also been recorded (Bijlmer 1946). Migration of *E vermicularis* to ectopic sites can give rise to diagnostic difficulties (Chandrasoma and Mendis 1977): it has been reported as a cause of salpingitis (Saffos and Rhatigan 1977), hepatic granulomas (Mondou and Gnepp 1989) and a pulmonary nodule (Beaver et al. 1973). The granulomas have not infrequently been confused with those produced by *Schistosoma* sp. The complete life-cycle takes some 15 days or so. Infection often involves several individuals in a household; autoinfection can also be a major problem. Institutions for mentally handicapped people are frequently affected. Recently, *E vermicularis* infections have figured in the list of parasitic infections in the 'gay bowel' syndrome (Weller 1985).

Diagnosis is by demonstration of eggs in a faecal sample or perianal swab. Treatment is with mebendazole or one of the piperazine compounds. Single-dose mebendazole or albendazole regimens are usually effective (Cook 1989). Ivermectin has given an 85% cure rate in a study in Peru (Naquira et al. 1989). However, elimination of the infection from a household is often difficult; careful paring of fingernails under which eggs can lodge after defaecation, and close attention to hand-washing after defaecation are extremely important. Despite this, however, more than one treatment course, given to all members of the family simultaneously, is often required.

Other Colorectal Helminths

Of the lesser known colonic helminths, *Oesophagostomum* sp is important in East Africa, South-east Asia and South America (Anthony and McAdam 1972; Ross et al. 1989). The natural reservoir includes ruminants, monkeys and apes. Presentation is often with an appendicitis-like syndrome; an ileocaecal inflammatory mass may be present, masquerading as a tumour or *helminthoma*. Ileocaecal tuberculosis, Crohn's disease, appendicitis, colonic amoebiasis and schistosomiasis are important differential diagnoses. Cutaneous infection with this nematode has also been reported (Ross et al. 1989). *Ternidens deminutus* and *Strongyloides stercoralis* can produce colonic lesions. The life-cycle of *S stercoralis* is almost unique amongst colonic helminths because autoinfection occurs in the rectum and anal region (Chap. 5); larvae re-enter at these sites and the recurrent re-infection cycles can last for 40 years and more. Extensive colonic pathology caused by *S stercoralis* has been demonstrated in an immunologically competent woman at Texas, USA (Berry et al. 1983). Although it is usually considered to be a small-intestinal parasite (Chap. 3), *Anisakis* sp can also produce an appendicitis-like syndrome and/or colonic involvement (Rushovich et al. 1983; Lucas et al. 1985). The major source of infection is raw fish – obtained from sushi bars in some countries, including the USA (herring-worm disease).

The schistosomes are trematode parasites but not truly intestinal, because the adult worm-pairs actually reside in the portal system; they are reviewed in Chap. 7. They are capable of producing human colonic (and hepatic) disease. Eosinophilic colitis, like eosinophilic gastroenteritis in general (Cook 1980; Felt-Bersma et al. 1984) remains a confused subject; although a parasite is sometimes detected, most cases do not have such an aetiology and despite an extensive search a cause cannot be found (Lee et al. 1983).

The Tropical Colon

Many residents of tropical and subtropical countries exhibit minor changes in colonic morphology – tropical *colonopathy* (Mathan and Mathan 1985); it seems likely that colonic parasites, as well as bacteria and viruses, are involved in its production.

The Gay Bowel, and Colorectal Disease in AIDS

One estimate is that the anorectum is used for sexual fulfilment by between 2 and 2.5 million people in the United Kingdom alone (Weller 1985). Of the parasites involved, *E histolytica* and *E vermicularis* are clearly important. Most of the other protozoan infections are small-intestinal in origin and although they might appear in faecal samples are of limited relevance in the context of colonic disease.

Many parasites are now known to be present in the gastrointestinal tract of AIDS sufferers (Malebranche et al. 1983; Casemore et al. 1985; Cook 1989). With respect to the colon however, few, in addition to those involved in the gay bowel syndrome (see above) are of proven importance. *Cryptosporidium*, *Isospora belli* and *Sarcocystis* sp are predominantly small-intestinal parasites.

S stercoralis can produce generalized invasive disease (see above) and although it is occasionally important in African AIDS there are few well-documented reports of its presence.

Conclusions

Colorectal parasites are of relatively lesser importance numerically than those which involve the small-intestine. Protozoan infections are dominated by *Entamoeba histolytica*; amoebic colitis (dysentery) gives rise to significant morbidity and mortality especially in tropical and subtropical countries, and in travellers. Understanding of the invasive properties of this parasite is rapidly increasing. An important differential diagnosis is inflammatory bowel disease, especially non-specific ulcerative colitis. Many other pathogenic protozoa also involve the colon; these can be divided into luminal and mural, the latter being typified by *Trypanosoma cruzi* (Chagas' disease) (Chap. 12). The most important colorectal helminths are *Trichuris trichiura* (the whipworm) and *Enterobius vermicularis* (the threadworm). Whereas disease (rectal prolapse and haemorrhage) caused by the former is largely confined to children with heavy infections in tropical countries, the latter is common world-wide and eradication (especially in families) is often difficult. Although not true colorectal parasites (because the adults reside in the portal system) *Schistosoma mansoni* and some other schistosomes cause significant disease including colonic polyposis (Chap. 7). Other helminths are of lesser importance. Diagnosis of these infections can usually be made from a *fresh* faecal sample, preferably using a concentration technique (Allen and Ridley 1970). In invasive amoebiasis (and schistosomiasis) serology is now of great value. Proctoscopy has a clear place in diagnosis, but colonoscopy is only indicated in difficult and complicated cases. Although some of these protozoa and helminths are relatively common in homosexual men, it is perhaps surprising that few of them assume a major importance in AIDS sufferers.

References

Alexander-Williams J (1983) Pruritus ani. Br Med J 287:159–160
Allason-Jones E, Mindel A, Sargeaunt P, Katz D (1988) Outcome of untreated infection with *Entamoeba histolytica* in homosexual men with and without HIV antibody. Br Med J 297:654–657
Allen AVH, Ridley DS (1970) Further observations on the formol-ether concentration technique for faecal parasites. J Clin Pathol 23:545–546
Ambroise-Thomas P (1980) Amebiasis and other protozoal diseases. In: Houba V (ed) Immunological investigation of tropical parasitic diseases. Churchill Livingstone, Edinburgh, pp 75–83
Anthony PP, McAdam IWJ (1972) Helminthic pseudotumours of the bowel: thirty-four cases of helminthoma. Gut 13:8–16
Areán VM, Koppisch E (1956) Balantidiasis. A review and report of cases. Am J Pathol 32:1089–1115
Barker DC, Troup L, Maxwell LE (1976) Nutrition/invasion interaction migration of *Entamoeba*

invadens in response to varied carbohydrate stimuli. In: van den Bosshe H (ed) Biochemistry of parasites and host–parasite relationships. North-Holland, Amsterdam, pp 393–400

Bassily S, Farid Z, El-Masry NA, Mickhail EM (1987) Treatment of intestinal *E histolytica* and *G lamblia* with metronidazole, tinidazole and ornidazole: a comparative study. J Trop Med Hyg 90:9–12

Beaver PC, Kriz JJ, Lau TJ (1973) Pulmonary nodule caused by *Enterobius vermicularis*. Am J Trop Med Hyg 22:711–713

Beaver PC, Blanchard JL, Seibold HR (1988) Invasive amebiasis in naturally infected new world and old world monkeys with and without clinical disease. Am J Trop Med Hyg 39:343–352

Berry AJ, Long EG, Smith JH, Gourley WK, Fine DP (1983) Chronic relapsing colitis due to *Strongyloides stercoralis*. Am J Trop Med Hyg 32:1289–1293

Bijlmer J (1946) An exceptional case of oxyuriasis of the intestinal wall. J Parasitol 32:359–366

Boreham PFL, Phillips RE, Shepherd RW (1984) The sensitivity of *Giardia intestinalis* to drugs *in vitro*. J Antimicrob Chemother 14:449–461

Brumpt ME (1925) Etude sommaire de l'*Entamoeba dispar* a n.sp. amibe à kystes quadrinuclées, parasite de l'homme. Bull Acad Med Paris 94:943–952

Bundy DAP (1986) Epidemiological aspects of *Trichuris* and trichuriasis in Caribbean communities. Trans R Soc Trop Med Hyg 80:706–718

Casemore DP, Sands RL, Curry A (1985) *Cryptosporidium* species: a 'new' human pathogen. J Clin Pathol 38:1321–1336

Chandrasoma PT, Mendis KN (1977) *Enterobius vermicularis* in ectopic sites. Am J Trop Med Hyg 26:644–649

Cook GC (1980) Tropical gastroenterology. Oxford University Press, Oxford, pp 158–164, 381–393

Cook GC (1985a) Infective gastroenteritis and its relationship to reduced gastric acidity. Scand J Gastroenterol 20[Suppl 111]:17–23

Cook GC (1985b) Parasitic infection. In: Booth CC, Neale G (eds) Disorders of the small intestine. Blackwell Scientific Publications, Oxford, pp 283–298

Cook GC (1986a) The clinical significance of gastrointestinal helminths – a review. Trans R Soc Trop Med Hyg 80:675–685

Cook GC (1986b) Colorectal parasitic and mycotic infections. Ital J Gastroenterol 18:338–342

Cook GC (1988) Intestinal parasitic infections. Curr Opin Gastroenterol 4:113–123

Cook GC (1989) Parasitic infections of the gastrointestinal tract: a worldwide clinical problem. Curr Opin Gastroenterol 5:126–139

Councilman WT, Lafleur HA (1891) Amoebic dysentery. Johns Hopkins Hosp Rep 2:395–548

Desowitz RS, Barnish G (1986) *Entamoeba polecki* and other intestinal protozoa in Papua New Guinea highland children. Ann Trop Med Parasitol 80:399–402

Editorial (1985) Is that amoeba harmful or not? Lancet i:732–734

Ellyson JH, Bezmalinovic Z, Parks SN, Lewis FR (1986) Necrotizing amebic colitis: a frequently fatal complication. Am J Surg 152:21–26

Feingold C, Bracha R, Wexler A, Mirelman D (1985) Isolation, purification, and partial characterization of an enterotoxin from extracts of *Entamoeba histolytica* trophozoites. Infect Immun 48:211–218

Felt-Bersma RJF, Meuwissen SGM, Velzen D van (1984) Perforation of the small intestine due to eosinophilic gastroenteritis. Am J Gastroenterol 79:442–445

Gandhi BM, Irshad M, Acharya SK, Tandon BN (1988) Amebic liver abscess and circulating immune complexes of *Entamoeba histolytica* proteins. Am J Trop Med Hyg 39:440–444

Gilman RH, Chong YH, Davis C, Greenberg B, Virik HK, Dixon HB (1983) The adverse consequences of heavy *Trichuris* infection. Trans R Soc Trop Med Hyg 77:432–438

Gorbach SL (1982) Viral infections and inflammatory bowel disease. Gastroenterology 83:1318–1319

Greenwood BM, Whittle HC (1981) Immunology of medicine in the tropics. Edward Arnold, London, pp 178–210

Grundy MS, Voller A, Warhurst D (1987) An enzyme-linked immunosorbent assay for the detection of *Entamoeba histolytica* antigens in faecel material. Trans R Soc Trop Med Hyg 81:627–632

Harries AD, Myers B, Cook GC (1985) Inflammatory bowel disease: a common cause of bloody diarrhoea in visitors to the tropics. Br Med J 291:1686–1687

Healy GR (1986) Immunologic tools in the diagnosis of amebiasis: epidemiology in the United States. Rev Infect Dis 8:239–246

Hurst AF (1934) The clinical importance of achlorhydria. Br Med J 2:665–669

Istre GR, Kreiss K, Hopkins RS, Healy GR, Benziger M, Canfield TM, Dickinson P, Englert TR, Compton RC, Mathews HM, Simmons RA (1982) An outbreak of amebiasis spread by colonic irrigation at a chiropractic clinic. N Engl J Med 307:339–342

Jackson TFHG (1987) *Entamoeba histolytica* cyst passers – to treat or not to treat? South Afr Med J 72:657–658

Joyce MP, Ravdin JI (1988) Antigens of *Entamoeba histolytica* recognised by immune sera from liver abscess patients. Am J Trop Med Hyg 38:74–80

Kan SP (1983) Efficacy of single doses of mebendazole in the treatment of *Trichuris trichiura* infection. Am J Trop Med Hyg 32:118–122

Kean BH (1988) A history of amebiasis. In: Ravdin JI (ed) Amebiasis: human infection by *Entamoeba histolytica*. Churchill Livingstone, New York and Edinburgh, pp 1–10

Köberle F (1968) Chagas' disease and Chagas' syndromes: the pathology of American trypanosomiasis. Adv Parasitol 6:63–116

Kovacz JA, Masur H (1986) Protozoan infections of man: other infections. In: Campbell WC, Rew RS (eds) Chemotherapy of parasitic diseases. Plenum Press, New York, pp 139–158

Lalla F de, Rizzardini G, Cairoli GA, Rinaldi E, Santoro D, Ostinelli A (1988) Outbreak of amoebiasis in tourists returning from Thailand. Lancet ii:847

Lee FI, Costello FT, Cowley DJ, Murray SM, Srimankar J (1983) Eosinophilic colitis with perianal disease. Am J Gastroenterol 78:164–166

Lucas SB, Cruse JP, Lewis AHM (1985) Anisakiasis in the United Kingdom. Lancet ii:843–844

Lushbaugh WB, Hofbauer AF, Pittman FE (1984) Proteinase activities of *Entamoeba histolytica* cytotoxin. Gastroenterology 87:17–27

Malebranche R, Arnoux E, Guérin JM, Pierre GD, Laroche AC, Péan-Guichard C, Elie R, Morisset PH, Spira T, Mandeville R, Drotman P, Seemayer T, Dupuy J-M (1983) Acquired immunodeficiency syndrome with severe gastrointestinal manifestations in Haiti. Lancet ii:873–878

Manson P (1898) Abscess of the liver. In: Tropical diseases: a manual of the diseases of warm climates. Cassell, London, pp 343–378

Martínez-Palomo A (ed) (1986) Amebiasis. Elsevier, Amsterdam, p 269

Martínez-Palomo A (1987) The pathogenesis of amoebiasis. Parasitol Today 3:111–118

Mathan MM, Mathan VI (1985) Rectal mucosal morphologic abnormalities in normal subjects in southern India: a tropical colonopathy? Gut 26:710–717

Mirelman D (1987) Effect of culture conditions and bacterial associates on the zymodemes of *Entamoeba histolytica*. Parasitol Today 3:37–40

Mirelman D (1988) Ameba – bacterial relationship in amebiasis. In: Ravdin JI (ed) Amebiasis: human infection by *Entamoeba histolytica*. Churchill Livingstone, New York and Edinburgh, pp 351–369

Mirelman D, Bracha R, Chayen A, Aust-Kettis A, Diamond LS (1986a) *Entamoeba histolytica*: effect of growth conditions and bacterial associates on isoenzyme patterns and virulence. Exp Parasitol 62:142–148

Mirelman D, Bracha R, Wexler A, Chayen A (1986b) Changes in isoenzyme patterns of a cloned culture of nonpathogenic *Entamoeba histolytica* during axenization. Infect Immunol 54:827–832

Mondou EN, Gnepp DR (1989) Hepatic granuloma resulting from *Enterobius vermicularis*. Am J Clin Pathol 91:97–100

Nanda R, Baveja U, Anand BS (1984) Entamoeba histolytica cyst passers: clinical features and outcome in untreated subjects. Lancet ii:301–303

Naquira C, Jimenez G, Guerra JG, Bernal R, Nalin DR, Neu D, Aziz M (1989) Ivermectin for human strongyloidiasis and other intestinal helminths. Am J Trop Med Hyg 40:304–309

Nozaki T, Motta SRN, Takeuchi T, Kobayashi S, Sargeaunt PG (1989) Pathogenic zymodemes of *Entamoeba histolytica* in Japanese male homosexual population. Trans R Soc Trop Med Hyg 83:525

Parija SC, Kasinathan S, Rao RS (1989) Rapid indirect haemagglutination (rapid-IHA) using sensitized chick cells for serodiagnosis of amoebiasis at primary health centre level. J Trop Med Hyg 92:221–226

Prasad RN, Virk KJ (1987) *Entamoeba histolytica*: is it necessary to characterize pathogenic strains? Parasitol Today 3:352

Ravdin JI (ed) (1988). Amebiasis: human infection by *Entamoeba histolytica*. Churchill Livingstone, New York and Edinburgh, p 838

Ravdin JI (1989) *Entamoeba histolytica*: from adherence to enteropathy. J Infect Dis 159:420–429

Ravdin JI, Murphy CF, Salata RA, Guerrant RL, Hewlett EL (1985) N-acetyl-D-galactosamine-inhibitable adherence lectin of *Entamoeba histolytica*. I. Partial purification and relation to amebic virulence in vitro. J Infect Dis 151:804–815

Rogers L (1912) The rapid cure of amoebic dysentery and hepatitis by hypodermic injections of soluble salts of emetine. Br Med J i:1424–1425

Rogers L (1922) Amoebic liver abscess: its pathology, prevention and cure. Lancet i:463–469

Rolston KVI, Hoy J, Mansell PWA (1986) Diarrhea caused by 'nonpathogenic amoebae' in patients with AIDS. N Engl J Med 315:192

Ross RA, Gibson DI, Harris EA (1989) Cutaneous oesophagostomiasis in man. Trans R Soc Trop Med Hyg 83:394–395

Rushovich AM, Randell EL, Caprini JA, Westenfelder GO (1983) Omental anisakiasis: a rare mimic of acute appendicitis. Am J Clin Pathol 80:517–520

Saffos RO, Rhatigan RM (1977) Unilateral salpingitis due to *Enterobius vermicularis*. Am J Clin Pathol 67:296–299

Sandler M (1981) Whipworm infection in the colon and rectum simulating Crohn's colitis. Lancet ii:210

Sargeaunt PG (1987) The reliability of *Entamoeba histolytica* zymodemes in clinical diagnosis. Parasitol Today 3:40–43

Sargeaunt PG (1988) Zymodemes of *Entamoeba histolytica*. In: Ravdin JI (ed) Amebiasis: human infection by *Entamoeba histolytica*. Churchill Livingstone, New York and Edinburgh, pp 370–387

Sargeaunt PG, Williams JE, Grene JD (1978) The differentiation of invasive and non-invasive *Entamoeba histolytica* by isoenzyme electrophoresis. Trans R Soc Trop Med Hyg 72:519–521

Sargeaunt PG, Oates JK, Maclennan I, Oriel JD, Goldmeier D (1983) *Entamoeba histolytica* in male homosexuals. Br J Vener Dis 59:193–195

Sharma MP, Rai RR, Acharya SK, Ray JCS, Tandon BN (1989) Needle aspiration of amoebic liver abscess. Br Med J 299:1308–1309

Sheen IS, Chien CSC, Lin DY, Liaw YF (1989) Resolution of liver abscesses: comparison of pyogenic and amebic liver abscesses. Am J Trop Med Hyg 40:384–389

Shiraki T, Otsuru M, Kenmotsu M, Kihara T, Hisayasu N, Motoyama N (1974) Invasion of *Enterobius vermicularis* into the human tissues – a report of 4 cases of eosinophilic granulomas caused by adult *Enterobius* in the intestines and their adjacent tissues. Jap J Parasit 23:125–137

Shukla VK, Roy SK, Vaidya MP, Mehrotra ML (1986) Fulminant amebic colitis. Dis Colon Rectum 29:398–401

Speelman P, McGlaughlin R, Kabir I, Butler T (1987) Differential clinical features and stool findings in shigellosis and amoebic dysentery. Trans R Soc Trop Med Hyg 81:549–551

Strachan WD, Chiodini PL, Spice WM, Moody AH, Ackers JP (1988) Immunological differentiation of pathogenic and non-pathogenic isolates of *Entamoeba histolytica*. Lancet i:561–563

Sullam PM (1988) Amebiasis and giardiasis in homosexual men. In: Leech JH, Sande MA, Root RK (eds) Parasitic infections. Churchill Livingstone, New York and Edinburgh, pp 147–175

Tannich E, Horstmann RD, Knobloch J, Arnold HH (1989) Genomic DNA differences between pathogenic and nonpathogenic *Entamoeba histolytica*. Proc Natl Acad Sci USA 86:5118–5122

Vinayak VK, Sharma P (1989) Kinetics of the immune responses during the course of hepatic amoebic infection – an experimental study. Trans R Soc Trop Med Hyg 83:349–353

Walker E, Williams G (1985) ABC of healthy travel. British Medical Journal Publications, London, p 39

Walsh JA (1986) Problems in recognition and diagnosis of amebiasis: estimation of the global magnitude of morbidity and mortality. Rev Infect Dis 8:228–238

Wanke C, Butler T, Islam M (1988) Epidemiologic and clinical features of invasive amebiasis in Bangladesh: a case–control comparison with other diarrheal diseases and postmortem findings. Am J Trop Med Hyg 38:335–341

Weber J (1985) Sexually acquired parasitic infections in homosexual men. Parasitol Today 1:93–95

Weller IVD (1985) The gay bowel. Gut 26:869–875

Yang S (1989) Detection of *Entamoeba histolytica* trophozoites in liver pus by the indirect fluorescent antibody test for the aetiological diagnosis of amoebic liver abscess. Ann Trop Med Parasitol 83:253–255

Yang J, Scholten TO (1977) *Dientamoeba fragilis*: A review with notes on its epidemiology, pathogenicity, mode of transmission and diagnosis. Am J Trop Med Hyg 26:16–22

Chapter 7

Schistosomiasis: An Important Cause of Colonic, Hepatic and Urinary-Tract Disease

If anyone intentionally pollutes the water of another . . . let the injured party bring the cause before the warden of the city.

Plato (427-347 BC),
Laws, VIII, 845

Introduction

Schistosomiasis is a major world disease, one estimate being that 200 million people in 74 developing countries are infected (Rollinson and Simpson 1987). It is caused by several species of schistosome (see below) and has been known to affect man for many thousands of years (Nash et al. 1982; Laughlin 1984; Manson-Bahr and Bell 1987). It is a disease of great antiquity; schistosome eggs have been identified in Egyptian mummies from the twentieth dynasty (1200–1090 BC) and there is evidence that it was present in China at a similar period. The causative organism was first visualized by Bilharz (1853) whilst working in Cairo, Egypt. Differentiation of the three major human species was due to Manson in the early twentieth century. Katsurada (1904) described *S japonicum*. Pipe-stem fibrosis of the liver was first reported by Symmers (1904). The role of the snail (the intermediate host) was defined by Miyairi (1914) and confirmed by Leiper (1915). Actual rates for the prevalence of infection in Third World populations have received a great deal of attention. Figures have recently been produced for *S mansoni* infection in several developing countries: rural Zimbabwe (Chandiwana et al. 1987, 1988), Botswana (Friis and Byskov 1987), north-eastern Nigeria (Chikwem and Alaku 1987), Niger (Mouchet et al. 1988) and in a city population in the Dominican Republic (Vargas et al. 1987). In the Zimbabwe study (Chandiwana et al. 1988), 17.5% of the population tested was found to be infected (the comparable rate for *S haematobium* was 53.1%); age prevalence patterns showed a peak in the 10–20-year-old group. Transmission takes place throughout the year, unlike that in *S mattheei* and *S haematobium* infections, both of which have clear-cut seasonal peaks (Chandiwana et al. 1987). In a group of Botswana schoolchildren, 80.5% were found to be infected with *S mansoni* (Friis and Byskov 1987). In Niger, during a survey of a *S mansoni* focus in the south of the country, human infection with *S bovis* was also detected (Mouchet et al. 1988). In the report from the Dominican Republic, the overall prevalence of *S mansoni* was 11.8% (Vargas et al. 1987). Host–parasite relationships between *S mansoni* and its intermediate (*Biomphalaria arabica*) and definitive hosts have been further investigated in Saudi Arabia (Lwambo et al. 1987); transmission there is focal, and mainly in oases, where the water resources and human settlements are located. Recent reports of *S japonicum* infection have been made from northern Thailand (Bunnag et al. 1986) and the Philippines (Blas et al. 1986). One estimate is that there are 2.4 million cases in China, and 0.5 million in the Philippines (Viyanant and Upathan 1988).

Far from being brought under control, however, this group of infections is currently *increasing* in frequency as new dams and irrigation schemes are built, especially in Africa (Cook 1980) and as populations (from hunter/nomad to farmer) increase and become redistributed. In fact, schistosomiasis has been estimated to be the second most important tropical disease, after malaria, in terms of socioeconomic impact and effect on health. Apart from those actually infected, 500 to 600 million are potentially at risk. Throughout Africa, South America and the Middle-east (Cook 1986a) it remains a colossal health problem which requires concerted efforts for both prevention and cure. Indigenous cases of schistosomiasis have recently been documented in Papua New Guinea (Murthy et al. 1989) and India (Bidinger and Crompton 1989) respectively.

Although exposure to infection may be present throughout life (disease is not infrequently present at 6 years old) the maximum prevalence and intensity usually occur in the teenage period, following which they subsequently decline (Jordan and Webbe 1982). While circumstantial evidence suggests that some degree of immunity is acquired, hard scientific data are by no means easy to obtain. During infancy and childhood, bathing and playing in infected water is the most important means of infection, while washing overtakes these later in life. The precise extent and degree of morbidity resulting from chronic schistosomiasis is, however, difficult to evaluate scientifically. Excessive tiredness and non-specific signs and symptoms are extremely common. The overall importance of chronic mild diarrhoea, anaemia, hypoproteinaemia, dysuria and bacteriuria in a community is difficult to assess. Hepatosplenic (with ascites and fatal haemate-mesis) and renal (with chronic urinary obstruction and pyelonephritis) disease merely represents the tip of a large iceberg.

Diagnosis of all forms of the disease is ideally dependent upon detection of characteristic eggs in: urine, a faecal sample, or bladder-, liver-, or rectal-biopsy material. Concentration techniques are of value when dealing with urine-samples; specimens obtained between 10.00 am and 2.00 pm are most likely to be positive. Viability and quantification of eggs is important. Numerous serological tests have been used (Laughlin 1984). The ELISA now gives excellent (⩾90%) sensitivity and specificity; however, because conversion after successful treat-ment takes place very slowly (and does not become negative for 2–3 years) this is of very limited value in the assessment of cure (Tosswill and Ridley 1986). Ultrasonography is proving of considerable value in the diagnosis of Symmers' fibrosis (Homeida et al. 1988a).

Treatment of individuals with schistosomiasis has improved dramatically over the last decade (Webbe 1981; Jordan and Webbe 1982; Cook 1983, 1986a,b; Laughlin 1984; De Cock 1984). However, control of infection has made depressingly little progress (Jordan and Webbe 1982), with the exception of certain local eradication campaigns such as that at St Lucia (Jordan 1985). The sum total is that the cost of treatment is usually outside the reach of health budgets in Third World countries, while failure of control programmes allows the disease to increase. Whether chemotherapy should be given to individuals in infected areas is controversial; they will almost inevitably become re-infected.

Parasitology and Pathogenesis

Three species out of a very large group of trematodes produce most cases of human disease (man is the definitive host); *S mansoni* (inferior mesenteric vessels) and *S japonicum* (superior mesenteric vessels) cause colonic and hepatic problems, whereas *S haematobium* (bladder plexuses) produces urinary tract disease (Rollinson and Simpson 1987). Of lesser importance are *S intercalatum* and *S mattheei*, and *S mekongi* (which might be a variant of *S japonicum*). *S mansoni* has been detected in baboons, rodents and insectivores in Africa and South America, and *S japonicum* in dogs, cats, cattle, water buffaloes, pigs, horses, sheep and goats; the importance of these reservoirs is difficult to assess. *S haematobium* is present throughout much of Africa and the Middle-east, *S mansoni* Africa and South America, and *S japonicum* South-east Asia – including China, the Philippines, Indonesia, Laos, Thailand and Cambodia (Laughlin 1984).

Figure 7.1 summarizes the life-cycle. Adult worms (which can live for at least 30 years in the human portal venous system (Cook and Bryceson 1988)) vary from 6 to 17 mm in length and 0.4 to 1.0 mm diameter. Figure 7.2 shows a worm-pair of *S mansoni* as it would appear in the human portal circulation. A single worm-pair is capable of producing 300–2000 eggs per 24 hours. Eggs, which are deposited either in the colon or urinary tract, or transmitted to the liver parenchyma or another organ(s), provoke a granulomatous response which is host-produced and partially protective. The eggs of the three main species (70–175 μm × 40–70 μm) are readily identified: *S mansoni* has a lateral spine (Fig. 7.3), *S haematobium* a terminal one, whilst *S japonicum* is rounded with a small lateral hook. Morbidity correlates with the worm burden (and consequently egg output). Some eggs are excreted in urine (*S haematobium*) or faeces (*S mansoni* and *S japonicum*) and when deposited in fresh water the miracidium (Fig. 7.4) infects snails of the genus *Biomphalaria*; after development, cercariae (all of which appear similar, and are fish-like organisms with pear-shaped head and forked tail (Fig. 7.5)) are liberated; these infect man via intact skin, a single drop of water being theoretically sufficient to cause an infection. Egg-laying usually begins about 4–6 weeks after initial cercarial skin penetration. Following migration throughout the body, during which schistosomules (which are tailless) are produced, the adult worms mature in the portal system some 1–4 weeks after infection (see above); the factor(s) which determine the site of anchorage are unknown. Human

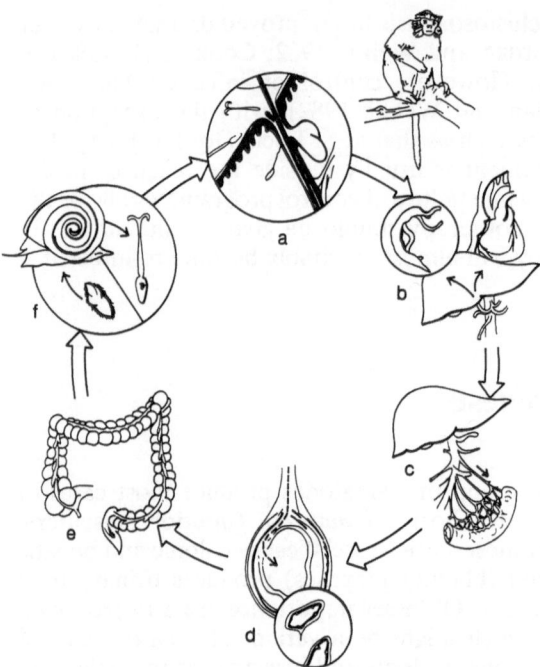

Fig. 7.1. Life-cycle of *Schistosoma mansoni*. (a) Cercaria penetrates human skin via a hair-follicle (its forked-tail is then lost) and becomes transformed into a schistosomule; (b) the schistosomule migrates to the lungs and liver, where adult(s) (12 mm in length × 1 mm diameter) are produced and, after maturing, begin mating; (c) worm-pairs migrate within the portal system to the colonic (and small-intestinal) venules where numerous eggs are produced; (d) eggs (130 µm in length × 60 µm wide) contain a miracidium which secretes proteases (this facilitates penetration through the venule wall, connective tissue and colonic wall); they are then deposited either in the colonic lumen or swept back into the pre-sinusoidal hepatic capillaries (in this event they depart from the life-cycle); (e) eggs remaining in the lumen are excreted in faeces and if deposited in freshwater continue the cycle; (f) in the extra-human cycle, the ciliated miracidium hatches, penetrates the snail host, transforms consecutively into a sporocyst and a cercaria (which lives for about a day during which time it swims around, using its forked-tail) which searches for a human host. [The best established non-human reservoir host is the baboon.]

infection, rarely severe, can be produced by about 20 species of non-human schistosomes (most of which infect birds or small animals); cercarial dermatitis may result.

Immunological aspects of *S mansoni* infection have been reviewed recently (Boros 1989) and several recent accounts refer to experimental studies of *S mansoni* infections. In a histological study of skin reactions to *S mansoni* schistosomules in baboons, varying degrees of vulnerability to the host's immunological attack were recorded (Seitz et al. 1987); in some of the lesions, a strong cellular response (in which eosinophils were visualized closely adherent to a schistosomule) was demonstrated. In the rat, protective immunity to *S mansoni* has been shown to be regulated by discrete subpopulations of T-lymphocytes (Phillips et al. 1987). The resultant granulomas (which reduce and confine the amount of tissue necrosis), are not pathognomonic unless the egg can be identified, and are similar for all species of schistosome (Laughlin 1984); collagen

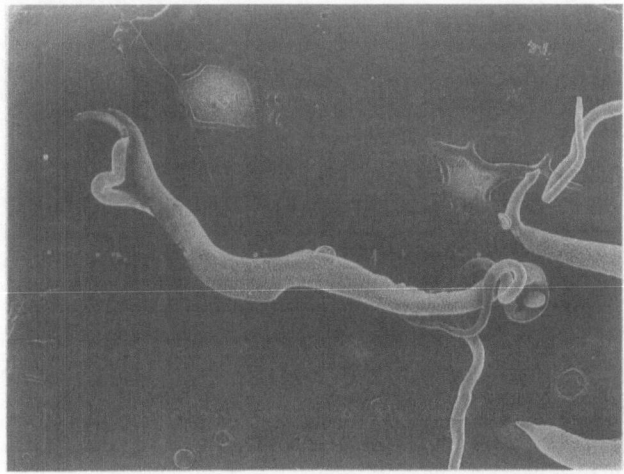

Fig. 7.2. Scanning electron-micrograph of an adult worm-pair of *Schistosoma mansoni* (× 14); the female is mostly hidden within the larger male.

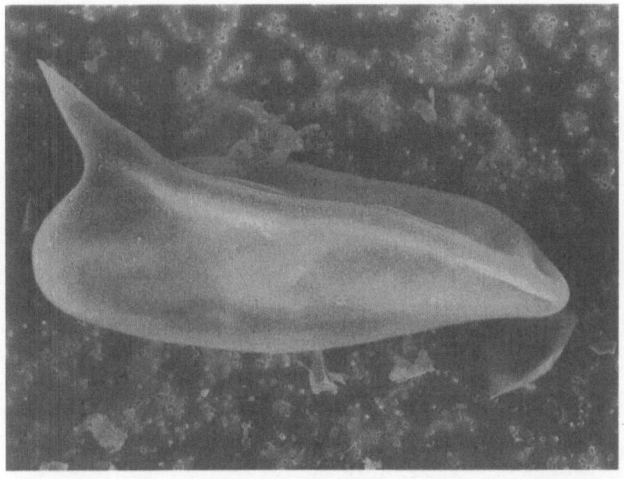

Fig. 7.3. Scanning electron-micrograph of an egg of *S mansoni* (× 700); note the lateral spine.

deposition and fibrosis account for most of the irreversible features of this group of diseases. The complex areas of immunity (to the different stages, i.e. cercaria, schistosomule, adult worm and egg) and immunopathology in experimental and human schistosomiasis have been addressed in two review articles (Butterworth 1987; Editorial 1987); these considerations are obviously important in the context of future vaccine development (see below). Antibody-dependent cell-mediated cytotoxicity is important in protection against the skin stages. Adult worms are protected by a 'camouflage' system (Laughlin 1984). The host granulomatous response may protect host-tissue from toxic egg secretions, but is

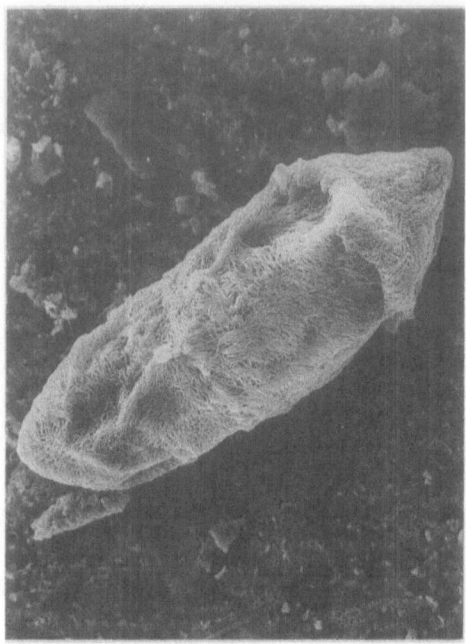

Fig. 7.4. Scanning electron-micrograph of a miracidium of *Schistosoma* sp (× 700).

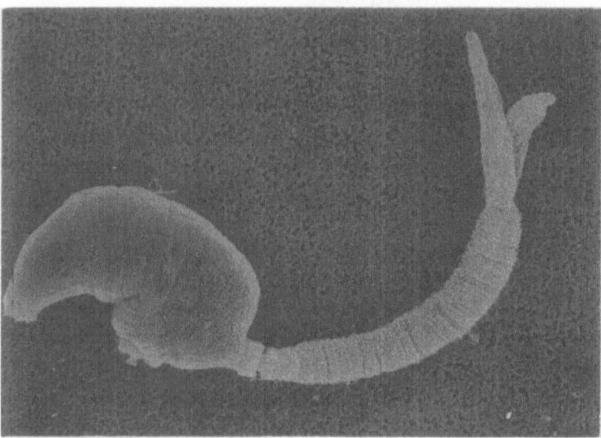

Fig. 7.5. Scanning electro-micrograph of a cercaria of *S japonicum* (× 600).

also obstructive to the local microcirculation; this response is modulated in chronic stages of the disease and is mediated by an antigen-specific suppressor T-lymphocyte response, localized antibodies, and/or immune-complexes. *S mansoni*-induced thrombocytopenia has been demonstrated in mice (Janitschke et al. 1987; Ngaiza and Doenhoff 1987); schistosomes may directly modulate platelet-mediated anti-parasite cytotoxicity reactions.

Acute Schistosomiasis (Katayama Fever)

Initial infection by cercariae present in infected water, usually goes unnoticed, although a localized, itchy dermatitis ('swimmer's itch') is an occasional sequel. However, after some 4 to 6 weeks, especially in the newly exposed (Chapman et al. 1988), an acute illness may ensue (Clarke et al. 1970; Zuidema 1981). This was first described in *Schistosoma japonicum* infections (acquired in the Katayama River valley in Japan) but can also occur with both *S mansoni* and less commonly *S haematobium*. Fever, hepatosplenomegaly, bronchospasm (comparable with hookworm pneumonitis), gastrointestinal symptoms and generalized urticaria are sometimes present and, if untreated, mortality is an occasional sequel. During the early stage, diagnosis may be difficult because an eosinophilia is usually absent, and schistosomal serology and faecal examination usually give negative results. It is important, therefore, to consider this syndrome in the differential diagnosis of a febrile illness in any individual who has recently been exposed to water possibily infected with cercariae. Although the severity of the syndrome bears some relationship to intensity of infection (Hiatt et al. 1979), this is not always so.

The pathogenesis of this acute disease is unclear: hypersensitivity, migration and/or maturation of schistosomules and the advent of egg production have been suggested to be important. Although an immune-complex basis has also been proposed, renal manifestations are very unusual. Host susceptibility might well be important. In management, caution is required in a severe case (see below).

Urinary Schistosomiasis

Manson (1898) devoted an entire chapter in the first edition of his monograph to: 'endemic haematuria' (bilharzia disease).

Clinical Aspects

The classical symptom of urinary schistosomiasis is terminal haematuria (Kibuka-musoke 1984; Laughlin 1984), associated with dysuria. Bladder pathology, which consists of sandy patches and narrowed ureteric orifices, increases with duration of infection. Urinary tract infection and pyelonephritis are common sequelae. Bladder calcification (seen on abdominal radiographs) is also a frequent finding in affected areas. Bladder carcinoma of squamous type is a long-term complication of infection, but this seems to have a geographical variation in incidence. It is, for example, common in Egypt (Kibukamusoke 1984). Several pathogenic mechanisms have been suggested (Laughlin 1984): (i) prolonged bladder irritation caused by egg granulomas, which produce hyperplasia and malignant change, (ii) urinary stasis, sepsis and urinary alkalinity consequent upon bladder obstruction, (iii) carcinogens resulting from the action of β-glucuronidase in the presence of urinary stasis, associated with alkalinity, and secondary bacterial action, and (iv) carcinogens produced by tryptophan metabolites in the presence of vitamin B_6 deficiency. Obstructive uropathy with hydronephroses and subsequent renal failure are serious complications that can result in uraemia. Recent evidence indicates that structural pathology (e.g. hydronephrosis) increases in untreated S *haematobium* infection despite the age-related reduction in egg burden (King et al. 1988); however, other manifestations (including haematuria) are related to urinary egg excretion at the time of diagnosis. An immune-complex glomerulo-nephritis is often present, but is usually asymptomatic and clinically insignificant. Nephrotic syndrome (sometimes associated with amyloid deposition) has been recorded in both *S haematobium* and also *S mansoni* infections (Kibukamusoke 1984).

Diagnosis

Urinary egg-count correlates significantly with the degree of proteinuria and haematuria (Mott et al. 1983). The overall incidence of abnormal intravenous urogram (IVU) examinations and calcified bladders in a population group correlates significantly with the prevalence of infection (Jordan and Webbe 1982). Figure 7.6 shows an IVU in an African man infected with *S haematobium*; the bladder is calcified, and bilateral hydroureters with early hydronephroses are present. Serology is of value (see above). Urinary LDH concentration, cytology and bladder biopsy are useful if a carcinoma is suspected.

Management

Chemotherapy is with praziquantel or metriphonate (which is considerably less expensive) (see below). In one study in Malawi, praziquantel, niridazole + metriphonate in combination, and metriphonate alone, caused a reduction in egg output at 6 months of 97%, 92% and 86% respectively (Pugh and Teesdale 1983). Secondary urinary tract infections, including pyelonephritis secondary to urinary schistosomiasis, require antibiotic treatment. Surgery may be indicated for obstructive uropathy. Bladder carcinoma may require cancer chemotherapy. Acute or chronic renal failure frequently requires either haemodialysis or renal transplant.

Colonic Schistosomiasis

S mansoni is the usual aetiological agent in Africa, South America and the Middle-east (Cook 1980). In Central and West Africa, *S intercalatum* and, in the Republic of South Africa, *S mattheei* are also important (Jordan and Webbe 1982). In South-east Asia, *S japonicum* is the usual species; it has now been eliminated from Japan. *S mekongi* also occurs in the lower Mekong River basin of South-east Asia. Likelihood of infection with *S mansoni* is greater in the dry

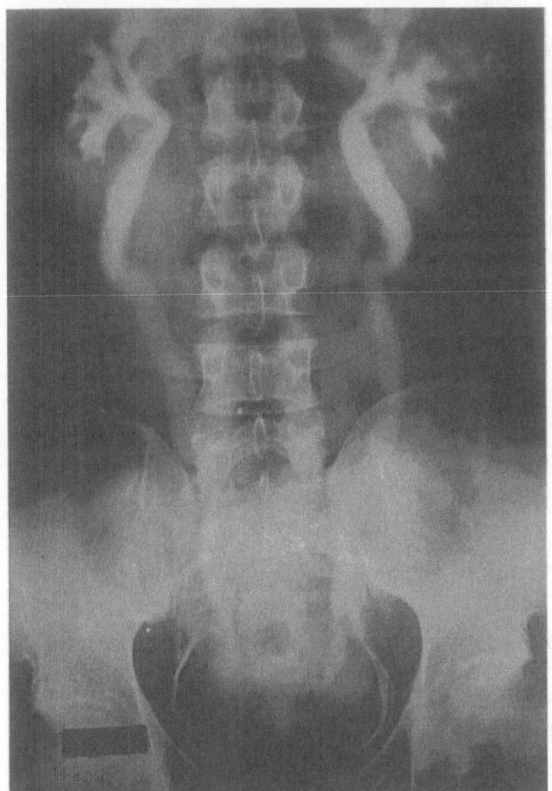

Fig. 7.6. Intravenous urogram in an African man with a *S haematobium* infection. The bladder is heavily calcified. Bilateral hydroureters with early hydronephroses are present.

season when the concentration of snails increases and flood-water is at a minimum (Jordan and Webbe 1982).

Clinical Aspects

In Egypt and Sudan, *S mansoni* often presents as intermittent bloody diarrhoea (Cook 1980; Laughlin 1984); this must be differentiated from other dysenteries and inflammatory bowel disease (Harries et al. 1985). Colonic polyp formation is an occasional sequel (Cook 1988a). Hypertrophic pulmonary osteoarthropathy is also a recognized complication and this is especially so in Egypt. The various complications of colonic disease – intussusception, rectal prolapse, anorectal fissures and abscesses – should be investigated and treated on their respective merits. Although evidence has been assembled that *S japonicum* infections are associated with an increased incidence of colonic carcinoma, such data are not forthcoming in the case of *S mansoni* infections or other species which involve the intestine (Cook 1980, 1986a,b,c).

Although the small-intestine can be involved, especially in *S japonicum* infection, significant clinical sequelae, e.g. malabsorption and protein-losing enteropathy are very unusual.

Diagnosis

Diagnosis is by visualizing viable eggs in a faecal sample or rectal-biopsy specimen. Serology (see above) is now of considerable value but its use is limited in areas where a very high percentage of the population is exposed to the disease. A nitrocellulose (NC) ELISA, which was originally used for the detection of viral and bacterial antigens has recently been adapted to demonstrate antibodies in patients with a parasitologically confirmed *S mansoni* infection (Janitschke et al. 1987): 100% sensitivity and specificity were recorded. The authors consider that this technique could be useful in developing countries, and that large-scale screening studies should be carried out to evaluate its value under field conditions.

Management

Praziquantel is the best available chemotherapeutic agent (see below); in *S mansoni* infections oxamniquine is also of value. There is some evidence that niridazole, which also has some anti-inflammatory properties, is of greater value when schistosomal colonic polyposis is also present.

Hepatosplenic Schistosomiasis

Hepatosplenic schistosomiasis is a corollary to the intestinal forms of infection, with *S mansoni* playing the major role in Africa, the Middle-east and South America (Cook 1980, 1986d). One estimate is that 100 million people are affected by this complication. The initial lesion is a granuloma which proceeds to fibrosis, and ultimately to the classical pipe-stem fibrosis of Symmers. The granulomas are pre-sinusoidal and produce portal fibrosis and hypertension; hepatocellular function is well preserved until late in the disease (unlike cirrhosis). Granuloma formation in the liver (Cheever et al. 1984) has been shown to be a protective host mechanism in experimental studies, as evidenced by the observation that in the presence of immunosuppression, granuloma formation in response to *S mansoni* ova is suppressed and extensive disease ensues (Moloney et al. 1982) (see above). Whether these observations are directly relevant to human disease is, however, questionable. Prevalence of hepatosplenomegaly bears a direct relationship to the underlying prevalence of infection in the population under study (Jordan and Webbe 1982). Figure 7.7 shows a young Egyptian man with very advanced hepatic involvement caused by *S mansoni*; decompensation, with portal hypotension and ascites has already occurred.

An association with the B hepatitis virus (HBV) carrier-state has been documented; this seems to be four or five times more common in people with

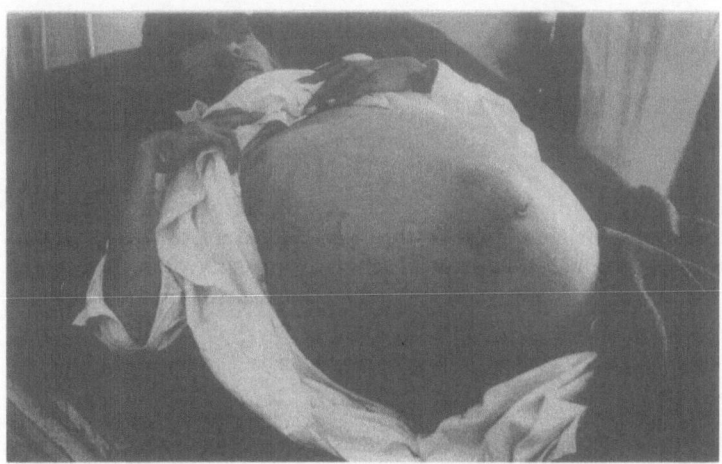

Fig. 7.7. Young Egyptian man (photographed in Cairo) with advanced pipe-stem fibrosis of the liver, which was complicated by portal hypertension and ascites. [Hepatocellular function is maintained longer than in hepatic cirrhosis, and this case therefore represents terminal disease.]

schistosomal hepatic disease caused by *S mansoni* infections, compared with those not infected (Bassily et al. 1983; Laughlin 1984; Cook 1986b); this association has not been established in *S japonicum* infections. HBV-associated macronodular cirrhosis may therefore complicate pipe-stem fibrosis. Co-existence of the two infections probably accounts in part at least, for decompensation in chronic disease. Although one recent study did not confirm this association (Larouzé et al. 1987), the bulk of evidence is supportive. Recent evidence has also been produced which throws some doubt upon a direct HBV-association (Madwar et al. 1989); in this study HBV-infected patients with uncomplicated schistosomiasis were both older and more likely to have received parenteral therapy in the past. It seems possible that individuals suffering from the two infections are: (i) more likely to be seeking medical care because they have symptoms associated with HBV, and (ii) have previously been infected with HBV iatrogenically. The anti-HB$_s$ response in infants born to mothers with an active *S mansoni* infection has been shown to be reduced (Ghaffar et al. 1989); this observation might well be important in HBV vaccination programmes in developing countries.

Clinical Aspects

Portal hypertension and bleeding oesophageal varices (which can often be controlled by sclerotherapy) are common sequelae to pipe-stem fibrosis (Cook 1980, 1986d). However, because hepatocellular function is well maintained in this entity, ascites and portal-systemic encephalopathy are late and often terminal complications. In the presence of a concurrent HBV infection, evidence of hepatocellular dysfunction may supervene earlier, and in this event a clinical differential diagnosis from alcoholic liver disease, veno-occlusive disease and other chronic hepatic diseases is important. Massive ascites signifies end-stage disease.

Diagnosis

Percutaneous liver-biopsy is of value in diagnosis. Barium swallow and/or endoscopy are necessary for delineation of the site and extent of oesophageal varices. Biochemical tests of hepatocellular function are usually well preserved. Serological tests (see above) are always positive in active hepatosplenic disease.

Management

Therapeutic agents currently used in hepatosplenic disease (see below) are not contraindicated in the presence of portal-systemic shunting, unlike niridazole. Treatment of complications should be undertaken on their respective merits. Precautions to prevent transmission of HBV infection to hospital and laboratory staff are clearly important.

Schistosomal Involvement of Other Organs

Portal-systemic collateral vessels allow eggs to bypass the liver and reach organs not normally accessible, e.g. lungs, spinal cord and brain. Cor pulmonale (which results from prolonged deposition of large numbers of eggs in the pre-arteriolar pulmonary circulation), can occur with *S mansoni*, *S japonicum* and *S haematobium* infections, and can be arrested by antischistosomal treatment; most cases of this complication have been reported from Egypt and Brazil. Radiological changes characterized by bronchopneumonitis may occur after treatment (Pedroso et al. 1987); these are possibly related to immune-complex deposition in the lungs. Severe bone and joint pain in hypertrophic osteoarthropathy may respond to corticosteroids. Central nervous system involvement is unusual, but when it does occur can produce a major clinical problem (Neves et al. 1973) (Chap. 8). Eggs can be deposited into any organ: *S haematobium* granulomas have, for example, been reported in the eye, and other organs affected include: the genitalia, pancreas, gall-bladder, peritoneum, omentum, stomach, duodenum (Contractor et al. 1988), heart, kidney and adrenals.

Salmonella sp infections are common in the presence of schistosomiasis; both infections should be treated simultaneously. The pathogenesis of salmonellosis in chronic schistosomiasis is unclear; there are three possibilities (Laughlin 1984): (i) abnormal survival of *Salmonella* sp as a result of immunological suppression resulting from schistosomiasis, (ii) physical attachment and proliferation of *Salmonella* sp on the integument or within the intestinal tract of the adult schistosome, with persisting haematogenous release, and (iii) a reduction in antigenic response to *Salmonella* sp lipopolysaccharide antigen in the presence of chronic schistosomiasis.

Chemotherapy of Schistosomiasis: A Review

Antimony (tartar emetic) was first used successfully by Christopherson (1918). Niridazole was introduced by Lambert (1964), hycanthone by Rosi et al. (1965), and oxamniquine by Richards and Foster (1969). Most of these older chemotherapeutic agents, including the antimony preparations, niridazole and hycanthone, should now be relegated to the therapeutic museum. Niridazole has a cure rate of 60%–90%, but possesses numerous side-effects and cannot be used in the presence of portal-systemic shunting. Hepatotoxicity is the major drawback with hycanthone, and mutagenic and carcinogenic properties are also of concern (De Cock 1984). However, these drugs have served their purpose and there is no doubt that, when used on a large scale, local prevalence rates of the disease have in some areas been reduced (Jordan and Webbe 1982).

Recent advances in, and indications for, chemotherapy have been reviewed (Laughlin 1984; Manson-Bahr and Bell 1987; Cook 1986c, 1988b, 1989). The recently introduced agents, which are administered orally, in some cases as a single dose, have revolutionized chemotherapy; cases in which liver damage is severe can now be treated; however, where the 'worm load' is very heavy development of bronchospasm and pulmonary infiltration a week or two after treatment may be a severe but transient event (see above). Most people with light infections do not experience significant problems; however, those not living in infected areas should receive treatment because a small minority will suffer CNS complications (Chap. 8).

Praziquantel has received widespread assessment in *S mansoni* infections. Although mild, a marked difference between the incidence of side-effects has been documented using different brands of this agent (Homeida et al. 1989); nausea, abdominal pain and vomiting are the major side-effects. Reports of a reduction in hepatosplenomegaly and even portal hypertension have been made after praziquantel administration (Morcos et al. 1985; Stephenson et al. 1985) (see below). In a large study in Sudan using ultrasonography (Homeida et al. 1988a), the prevalence of Symmers' fibrosis was shown to be between two and three times lower in a group of villagers who had been treated with praziquantel compared with another group who had not (Homeida et al. 1988b); this difference was even more marked in a younger (10–20-year-old) age group, in whom there was a dramatic reduction in the splenomegaly rate. In an experimental study using mice, praziquantel did *not*, however, have a significant effect on hepatic fibrosis in *S japonicum* infections (Cheever and Deb 1989). In *S mansoni* infections, clinical evaluation of the overall value of oxamniquine (a tetrahydroquinoline compound) (15–60 mg/kg given over 3 days) indicates that a cure is produced in >80% and reduction in egg excretion in >90% of individuals (Foster 1987). Side-effects consist of drowsiness and dizziness, although fever and convulsions have been recorded. Praziquantel and oxamniquine have been compared in *S mansoni* infections (Da Silva et al. 1986; Gryseels et al. 1987). In a double-blind trial in Brazil, cure rates of 79% and 84%, after praziquantel and oxamniquine respectively, were recorded (Da Silva et al. 1986); furthermore, in those who were not cured, the mean reduction in faecal egg-count was 93% and 84% respectively. Neither difference was significant statistically; a similar incidence of side-effects was recorded after use of both agents. However, in mass treatment campaigns in Burundi, praziquantel (given as a 40 mg/kg single dose) was considered superior to oxamniquine because it was cheaper and more acceptable, but not on account of a better anti-parasite effect (Gryseels et al. 1987). In a comparison between these two agents in Ethiopia, praziquantel was also favoured (Taddese and Zein 1988); experience there was comparable with that in Burundi. Although a synergistic effect between praziquantel and oxamniquine in *S mansoni* infections has been noted, this combination was not considered to have a curative advantage in a study in Zimbabwe (Creasey et al. 1986). The long-term effects of treatment and re-treatment of *S mansoni* infections using both oxamniquine and praziquantel have been studied in Kenya (Sturrock et al. 1987b); beneficial effects of treating even a limited section of a community at intervals of a year or more, without necessarily stopping transmission, have been recorded. Two reports have, however, drawn attention to oxamniquine resistance in *S mansoni* when this agent is used for mass chemotherapy (Coles et al. 1987; Yeang et al. 1987); resistance has been documented in Kenya, Brazil and Liberia. Further evidence of the value of oxamniquine in the treatment of *S mansoni* colonic polyposis has been reported from Cairo, Egypt (Ayad El-Masry et al. 1986); however, overall resolution is slower than with niridazole. A higher dose of praziquantel (60 mg/kg in two divided doses on 1 day) is required in *S japonicum* infections.

The mode of action of praziquantel (and most other schistosomicides) is still not clearly understood; evidence for an immune-dependent action has been documented in experimental studies in mice (Doenhoff et al. 1987). The effect of praziquantel on the larval stages of *S japonicum* has been studied (Ming and Combes 1987); while mature and almost mature cercariae are rapidly killed by this agent, young cercarial embryos and sporocysts are not. In an in vitro investigation, increased exposure of parasite antigens at the surface of adult male parasites has been documented (Harnett and Kusel 1986). Tegumental repair in *S mansoni* after in vivo praziquantel has been studied in the mouse (Shaw and Erasmus 1987). In the other human intestinal schistosome infection *S japonicum*, an in vitro study has further evaluated the effect of praziquantel on the larval stages (Yi and Combes 1987).

Using metriphonate (an organophosphate compound which has anti-cholinesterase activity) in *S haematobium* infection, three treatment regimens were compared in a study in Somalia: (1) 10 mg/kg once daily, (2) 5 mg/kg three times during one day, and (3) 7.5 mg/kg three times during one day (Aden-Abdi et al. 1987). Unlike regimen 2, regimens 1 and 3 produced toxic side-effects. After 4–6 weeks, reduction in egg-count was between 96% and 100% after regimens 1 and 2, but this was not evaluated after regimen 3. The authors concluded that a short course at low dosage is probably more effective, safer and better tolerated than a high dose one. A large review of metriphonate (10 mg/kg body-weight given three times at bi-weekly intervals) usage in areas with a *S haematobium* mono-infection has confirmed both its efficacy and safety (Feldmeier and Doehring 1987). Nausea, vomiting and bronchospasm are rare side-effects. Its cost is low.

In urinary tract infections with *S haematobium*, the influence of the interval between doses on the response to the formerly used agent niridazole has been evaluated (Abdu-Aguye and Lege-Oguntoye 1986); results after two were superior to those after three 'divided' daily doses, but this did not attain statistical significance. Praziquantel has also been further evaluated in urinary schistosomiasis in Nigeria (Chuks Ejezie and Okeke 1987); at the dose used (20–30 mg/kg), 99.1% of infections were cleared, all were reduced in intensity, and there were only minimal side-effects. Low dose praziquantel regimens (single dose of 10–30 mg/kg body-weight) have been compared with a standard 40 mg/kg dose in a study in Kenya (King et al. 1989); whereas after 2–3 months the *cure-rate* in *S haematobium* infection was 84% with the 40 mg regimen, rates of 26%, 68% and 78% were reported after the 10, 20 and 30 mg/kg regimens. However, there was no significant difference between 20 and 40 mg/kg doses in terms of mean post-treatment intensity of infection, or post-treatment prevalence of haematuria or proteinuria; the authors argue, therefore, that although not acceptable for individual treatment, the 20 mg/kg regimen might have a value in large-scale population-based chemotherapy programmes.

Clinical deterioration during chemotherapy when carried out in the acute stage of schistosomiasis (Katayama fever) has been documented in three patients with a *S mansoni* infection treated in London (Harries and Cook 1987); it seems wise, therefore, to delay chemotherapy until the acute phase of the disease has passed, or alternatively to give a corticosteroid 'cover' (Gelfand et al. 1981; Harries and Cook 1987). Experimental evidence has been produced which is consistent with this observation (Lambertucci et al. 1989); using a murine model, a combination of a schistosomicide and a corticosteroid produced an inhibition in fecundity which was significantly greater (and synergistic) than when the former was used alone.

Further work on the use of oltipraz in *S mansoni* infection has been reported (Homeida et al. 1986); however, as lately pointed out, clinical trials with this agent have now been suspended because of late-onset toxicity (Sturrock 1987). Experimentally, 9-acridanone-hydrazone compounds have been shown to be curative in *S mansoni* infections in baboons (Sturrock et al. 1987a); in this study, a successful chemotherapeutic result significantly correlated with the ELISA antibody concentration. Amoscanate has also undergone trial but this agent has CNS and hepatotoxic side-effects which will almost certainly limit its use (Jordan and Webbe 1982).

Prevention and Control

Attempts at snail control have used molluscicidal (niclosamide has been most widely used) and biological agents, and environmental modification. Efforts at reducing water contact and contamination have involved programmes aimed at providing safe domestic water supplies and facilities for sanitary disposal of excreta. Control, based on a combination of health education (stressing avoidance of contact with water that is likely to be infected, prevention of contamination of water, and early recognition of symptoms) along with low-cost diagnostic techniques and modern drugs, has achieved a relative degree of success in Brazil, Egypt and the Sudan. The major objective is to reduce the prevalence of heavy infection and to maintain it at a level which is not a public health hazard.

All successful eradication programmes have to date used a multifaceted approach (Jordan 1985). Both mass chemotherapy and targeted population chemotherapy have been used; this approach involves identifying and treating moderate to heavy excreters only, and this obviously involves more time, energy, technology and equipment. The problems encountered in control have been summarized in relation to the southern province of Saudi Arabia (Sinha and Lambourne 1987); simultaneous reduction of man–water contact (by supplying clean water to the villages) and periodic chemotherapy can result in satisfactory control. The value of repeated mass treatment of *S mansoni* infection in hyperendemic areas of Brazil has been evaluated (Kloetzel and Schuster 1987); sanitation, vector control and health education are obviously important additional strategies. In rural Zambia, a re-survey for *S mansoni* infection in a community after selective mass chemotherapy with praziquantel had been discontinued, has shown that infection and resultant morbidity rapidly returned to the pre-treatment level (Sukwa et al. 1988).

Vaccination has received a great deal of attention. Although studies in domestic animals using attenuated cercarial and schistosomule vaccines seem promising (Hoffman et al. 1981; Webbe 1981), a human vaccine seems a very long way off. Paramyosin has been considered to function as a vaccine antigen; it is released from the parasite, and elicits a T-lymphocytic-dependent cell-mediated response (Sher and Pearce 1988). Epidemiological implications for an effective vaccine have been summarized in a recent review article (Mott 1987); if or when a cheap and safe vaccine becomes available, careful epidemiological assessments will be required in the design of field trials to evaluate its efficacy.

Conclusions

Schistosomiasis affects an estimated 200 million people in 74 developing countries of the world; a further 500–600 million are potentially at risk. Far from being on the decline, this ancient disease is increasing in prevalence as more irrigation schemes and dams are constructed. For the individual with one of these infections, diagnosis has recently become far simpler, and chemotherapy much more effective (with fewer side-effects). However, far greater attention to prevention and control of these diseases is required; more financial support is required in Third World countries. Work on a possible vaccine is in train but it is likely that a safe and effective preparation is still very many years away.

References

Abdu-Aguye I, Lege-Oguntoye L (1986) Influence of the dosing interval on the response of urinary schistosomiasis to therapy with niridazole. East Afr Med J 63:635–639

Aden-Abdi Y, Gustafsson LL, Elmi SA (1987) A simplified dosage schedule of metrifonate in the treatment of *Schistosoma haematobium* infection in Somalia. Eur J Clin Pharmacol 32:437–441

Ayad El-Masry N, Farid Z, Bassily S, Kilpatrick ME, Watten RH, Girgis NI (1986) Oxamniquine treatment for schistosomal polyposis: a 1–2 year follow-up study. J Trop Med Hyg 89:19–21

Bassily S, Dunn MA, Farid Z, Kilpatrick ME, El-Masry NA, Kamel IA, Alamy M El, Murphy BL (1983) Chronic hepatitis B in patients with schistosomiasis mansoni. J Trop Med Hyg 86:67–71

Bidinger PD, Crompton DWT (1989) A possible focus of schistosomiasis in Andhra Pradesh, India. Trans R Soc Trop Med Hyg 83:526

Bilharz TM (1853) Ein Beitrag zur Helminthographia humana aus brieflichen Mittheilungen des Dr Bilharz in Cairo, nebst Bemerkungen von CT v Siebold. Z Wiss Zool 4:53–76

Blas BL, Cabrera BD, Santos AT, Noseñas JS (1986) An attempt to study the case fatality rate in *Schistosoma japonicum* infection in the Philippines. Southeast Asian J Trop Med Publ Health 17:67–70

Boros DL (1989) Immunopathology of *Schistosoma mansoni* infection. Clin Microbiol Rev 2:250–269

Bunnag T, Impand P, Sornmani (1986) *Schistosoma japonicum*-like infection in Phichit Province, Northern Thailand: a case report. Southeast Asian J Trop Med Publ Health 17:189–193

Butterworth AE (1987) Immunity in human schistosomiasis. Acta Trop 44[suppl 12]:31–40

Chaffar YA, Kamel M, El-Sobsky M, Bahnasy R, Strickland GT (1989) Response to hepatitis B vaccine in infants born to mothers with schistosomiasis. Lancet ii:272

Chandiwana SK, Christensen NØ, Frandsen F (1987) Seasonal patterns in the transmission of *Schistosoma haematobium*, *S mattheei* and *S mansoni* in the highveld region of Zimbabwe. Acta Trop 44:433–444

Chandiwana SK, Taylor P, Clarke V de V (1988) Prevalence and intensity of schistosomiasis in two rural areas in Zimbabwe and their relationship to village location and snail infection rates. Ann Trop Med Parasitol 82:163–164

Chapman PJC, Wilkinson PR, Davidson RN (1988) Acute schistosomiasis (Katyama fever) among British air crew. Br Med J 297:1101

Cheever AW, Deb S (1989) Persistence of hepatic fibrosis and tissue eggs following treatment of *Schistosoma japonicum* infected mice. Am J Trop Med Hyg 40:620–628

Cheever AW, Duvall RH, Hallack TA (1984) Differences in hepatic fibrosis and granuloma size in several strains of mice infected with *Schistosoma japonicum*. Am J Trop Med Hyg 33:602–607

Chikwem JO, Alaku OS (1987) A retrospective study of nine years' hospital records of schistosomiasis in north-eastern Nigeria. Trans R Soc Trop Med Hyg 81:383–384

Christopherson JB (1918) The successful use of antimony in bilharziosis. Lancet ii:325–327

Chuks Ejezie G, Okeke GCE (1987) Chemotherapy in the control of urinary schistosomiasis in Nigeria. J Trop Med Hyg 90:149–151

Clarke V de V, Warburton B, Blair DM (1970) The Katayama syndrome: report on an outbreak in Rhodesia. Cent Afr Med J 16:123–126

Coles GC, Mutahi WT, Kinoti GK, Bruce JI, Katz N (1987) Tolerance of Kenyan *Schistosoma mansoni* to oxamniquine. Trans R Soc Trop Med Hyg 81:782–785

Contractor QQ, Benson L, Schulz TB, Contractor TQ, Kasturi N (1988) Duodenal involvement in *Schistosoma mansoni* infection. Gut 29:1011–1012

Cook GC (1980) Schistosomal involvement of the liver. Intestinal schistosomiasis. In: Tropical gastroenterology. Oxford University Press, Oxford, pp 141–149, 394–405

Cook GC (1983) The tropical liver. In: Jewell DP, Shepherd HA (eds) Topics in gastroenterology 11. Blackwell Scientific Publications, Oxford, pp 175–190

Cook GC (1986a) Schistosomiasis: a major world scourge with few signs of hope! Ann Saudi Med 6:237–241

Cook GC (1986b) Colorectal parasitic and mycotic infections. Ital J Gastroenterol 18:338–342

Cook GC (1986c) The clinical significance of gastrointestinal helminths – a review. Trans R Soc Trop Med Hyg 80:675–685

Cook GC (1986d) Tropical infections and the liver. In: Triger DR (ed) Proceedings of advanced medicine conference. Royal College of Physicians of London. Baillière Tindall, London, pp 193–202

Cook GC (1988a) Intestinal parasitic infections. Curr Opin Gastroenterol 4:113–123

Cook GC (1988b) Chemotherapy of parasitic infections. Curr Opin Infect Dis 1:423–438

Cook GC (1989) Parasitic infections of the gastrointestinal tract: a worldwide clinical problem. Curr Opin Gastroenterol 5:126–139

Cook GC, Bryceson ADM (1988) Longstanding infection with *Schistosoma mansoni*. Lancet i:127

Creasey AM, Taylor P, Thomas JEP (1986) Dosage trial of a combination of oxamniquine and praziquantel in the treatment of schistosomiasis in Zimbabwean schoolchildren. Cent Afr J Med 32:165–167

De Silva LC, Zeitune JMR, Rosa-Eid LMF, Lima DMC, Antonelli RH, Christo CH, Saez-Alquezar A, Carbone A de C (1986) Treatment of patients with Schistosomiasis mansoni: a double blind clinical trial comparing praziquantel with oxamniquine. Rev Inst Med Trop São Paulo 28:174–180

De Cock KM (1984) Human schistosomiasis and its management. J Infect 8:5–12

Doenhoff MJ, Sabah AAA, Fletcher C, Webbe G, Bain J (1987) Evidence for an immune-dependent action of praziquantel on *Schistosoma mansoni* in mice. Trans R Soc Trop Med Hyg 81:947–951

Editorial (1987) Immunopathology of schistosomiasis. Lancet ii:194

Feldmeier H, Doehring E (1987) Clinical experience with metrifonate: review with emphasis on its use in endemic areas. Acta Trop (Basel) 44:357–368

Foster R (1987) A review of clinical experience with oxamniquine. Trans R Soc Trop Med Hyg 81:55–59

Friis H, Byskov J (1987) *Schistosoma mansoni*: intensity of infection and morbidity among schoolchildren in Matlapaneng, Ngamiland, Botswana. Trop Geog Med 39:251–255

Gelfand M, Clark V de V, Bernberg H (1981) The use of steroids in the earlier hypersensitivity stage of schistosomiasis. Cent Afr Med J 27:219–221

Ghaffar YA, Kamel M, El-Sobky M, Bahnasy R, Strickland GT (1989) Response to hepatitis B vaccine in infants born to mothers with schistosomiasis. Lancet ii:272

Gryseels B, Nkulikyinka L, Coosemans MH (1987) Field trials of praziquantel and oxamniquine for the treatment of schistosomiasis mansoni in Burundi. Trans R Soc Trop Med Hyg 81:641–644

Harnett W, Kusel JR (1986) Increased exposure of parasite antigens at the surface of adult male *Schistosoma mansoni* exposed to praziquantel *in vitro*. Parasitology 93:401–405

Harries AD, Cook GC (1987) Acute schistosomiasis (Katayama fever): clinical deterioration after chemotherapy. J Infect 14:159–161

Harries AD, Myers B, Cook GC (1985) Inflammatory bowel disease: a common cause of bloody diarrhoea in visitors to the tropics. Br Med J 291:1686–1687

Hiatt RA, Sotomayor ZR, Sanchez G, Zambrana M, Knight WB (1979) Factors in the pathogenesis of acute schistosomiasis mansoni. J Infect Dis 139:659–666

Hoffman DB, Phillips SM, Cook JA (1981) Vaccine development for schistosomiasis: report of a workshop. Am J Trop Med Hyg 30:1247–1251

Homeida MMA, Ali HM, Sulaiman SM, Bennet JL (1986) Oltipraz: administration with food increases its anti-schistosomal activity. Trans R Soc Trop Med Hyg 80:908–910

Homeida M, Ahmed S, DaFalla A, Suliman S, Eltom I, Nash T, Bennett JL (1988a) Morbidity associated with *Schistosoma mansoni* infection as determined by ultrasound: a study in Gezira, Sudan. Am J Trop Med Hyg 39:196–201

Homeida MA, Fenwick A, DeFalla AA, Suliman S, Kardaman MW, El Tom I, Nash T, Bennett JL (1988b) Effect of antischistosomal chemotherapy on prevalence of Symmers' periportal fibrosis in Sudanese villages. Lancet ii:437–440

Homeida MMA, Eltom SM, Sulaiman SM, Ali HM, Bennett JL (1989) Tolerance of two brands of praziquantel. Lancet ii:391

Janitschke K, Reinhold A, Bode L (1987) Nitrocellulose dot-ELISA for serodiagnosis of schistosomiasis. Trans R Soc Trop Med Hyg 81:956–958

Jordan P (1985) Schistosomiasis: the St Lucia project. Cambridge University Press, Cambridge.

Jordan P, Webbe G (eds) (1982) Schistosomiasis: epidemiology, treatment and control. Heinemann Medical Books, London.

Katsurada F (1904) The aetiology of a parasitic disease. Ijo Shimbun no. 669:1325–1332

Kibukamusoke JW (ed) (1984) Schistosomiasis: the kidney and the urinary tract. In: Tropical nephrology. Citforge, Canberra, pp 85–141

King CH, Keating CE, Muruka JF, Ouma JH, Houser H, Arap Siongok TK, Mahmoud AAF (1988) Urinary tract morbidity in Schistosomiasis haematobia: associations with age and intensity of infection in an endemic area of Coast Province, Kenya. Am J Trop Med Hyg 39:361–368

King CH, Wiper DW, Stigter KV de, Peters PAS, Koech D, Ouma JH, Arap Siongok TK, Mahmoud AAF (1989) Dose-finding study for praziquantel therapy of *Schistosoma haematobium* in Coast Province, Kenya. Am J Trop Med Hyg 40:507–513

Kloetzel K, Schuster NH (1987) Repeated mass treatment of schistosomiasis mansoni: experience in hyperendemic areas of Brazil. I. Parasitological effects and morbidity. Trans R Soc Trop Med Hyg 81:365–370

Lambert CR (1964) Chemotherapy of experimental *Schistosoma mansoni* infections with a nitro-thiazole derivative, CIBA 32, 644–Ba. Ann Trop Med Parasitol 58:292–303

Lambertucci JR, Modha J, Curtis R, Doenhoff M (1989) The association of steroids and schistosomicides in the treatment of experimental schistosomiasis. Trans R Soc Trop Med Hyg 83:354–357

Larouzé B, Dazza MC, Gaudebout C, Habib M, Elamy M, Cline B (1987) Absence of relationship between *Schistosoma mansoni* and hepatitis B virus infection in the Qalyub Governate, Egypt. Ann Trop Med Parasitol 81:373–375

Laughlin LW (1984) Schistosomiasis. In: Strickland GT (ed) Hunter's tropical medicine, 6th edn. Saunders, Philadelphia, pp 708–740

Leiper RT (1915) Report on the results of the bilharzia mission in Egypt, 1915. J R Army Med Corps 25:1–55, 147–192, 253–267

Lwambo NJS, Upatham ES, Kruatrachue M, Viyanant V (1987) The host–parasite relationship between the Saudi Arabian *Schistosoma mansoni* and its intermediate and definitive hosts. I. *S mansoni* and its local snail host *Biomphalaria arabica*. Southeast Asian J Trop Med Publ Health 18:156–165

Madwar MA, El Tahawy M, Strickland GT (1989) The relationship between uncomplicated schistosomiasis and hepatitis B infection. Trans R Soc Trop Med Hyg 83:233–236

Manson P (1898) Endemic haematuria (bilharzia disease). In: Tropical diseases: a manual of the diseases of warm climates. Cassell, London, pp 498–508

Manson-Bahr PEC, Bell DR (1987) Manson's tropical diseases, 19th edn. Baillière Tindall, London, pp 448–485

Ming Yi X, Combes C (1987) Effect of praziquantel on larval stages of *Schistosoma japonicum*. Trans R Soc Trop Med Hyg 81:645–650

Miyairi K, Suzuki M (1914) Der Zwischenwirt des *Schistosomum japonicum* Katsurada. Mitt Med Fak Univ Kyushu 1:187–197

Moloney NA, Doenhoff MJ, Webbe G, Hinchcliffe P (1982) Studies on the host–parasite relationship of *Schistosoma japonicum* in normal and immunosuppressed mice. Parasite Immunol 4:431–440

Morcos SH, Khayyal MT, Mansour MM, Saleh S, Ishak EA, Girgis NI, Dunn MA (1985) Reversal of hepatic fibrosis after praziquantel therapy of murine schistosomiasis. Am J Trop Med Hyg 34:314–321

Mott KE (1987) Epidemiological considerations for development of a schistosome vaccine. Acta Trop 44[suppl 12]:13–20

Mott KE, Dixon H, Osei-Tutu E, England EC (1983) Relation between intensity of *Schistosoma haematobium* infection and clinical haematuria and proteinuria. Lancet i:1005–1008

Mouchet F, Develoux M, Magasa MB (1988) *Schistosoma bovis* in human stools in Republic of Niger. Trans R Soc Trop Med Hyg 82:257

Murthy DP, Igo JD, Lutz SA, Cooke RA (1989) A probable endemic case of schistosomiasis from Papua New Guinea. Med J Aust 150:162

Nash TE, Cheever AW, Ottesen EA, Cook JA (1982) Schistosome infections in humans: perspectives and recent findings. NIH conference. Ann Intern Med 97:740–754

Neves J, Marinho RP, Araujo PK de, Raso P (1973) Spinal cord complications of acute schistosomiasis mansoni. Trans R Soc Trop Med Hyg 67:782–792

Ngaiza JM, Doenhoff MJ (1987) *Schistosoma mansoni*-induced thrombocytopenia in mice. Trans R Soc Trop Med Hyg 81:655–656

Pedroso ERP, Lambertucci JR, Greco DB, Rocha MO da C, Ferreira CS, Raso P (1987) Pulmonary schistosomiasis mansoni: post-treatment pulmonary clinical–radiological alterations in patients in the chronic phase: a double-blind study. Trans R Soc Trop Med Hyg 81:778–781

Phillips SM, Walker D, Abdel-Hafex SK, Linette GP, Cought L, Perrin PJ, El Fathelbab N (1987) The immune response to *Schistosoma mansoni* infections in inbred rats. VI. Regulation by T cell subpopulations. J Immunol 139:2781–2787

Pugh RN, Teesdale CH (1983) Single dose oral treatment in urinary schistosomiasis: a double-blind trial. Br Med J 286:429–432

Richards HC, Foster R (1969) A new series of 2-aminomethyltetrahydroquinoline derivatives displaying schistosomicidal activity in rodents and primates. Nature 222:581–582

Rollinson D, Simpson AJG (eds) (1987) The biology of schistosomes from genes to latrines. Academic Press, London, p 472

Rosi D, Peruzzotti G, Dennis EW, Berberian DA, Freele H, Archer S (1965) A new active metabolite of 'Miracil D'. Nature 208:1005–1006

Seitz HM, Cottrell BJ, Sturrock RF (1987) A histological study of skin reactions of baboons to *Schistosoma mansoni* schistosomula. Trans R Soc Trop Med Hyg 81:385–390

Shaw MK, Erasmus DA (1987) *Schistosoma mansoni*: structural damage and tegumental repair after *in vivo* treatment with praziquantel. Parasitology 94:243–254

Sher A, Pearce EJ (1988) Schistosomiasis vaccine. Nature 334:478

Sinha NP, Lambourne A (1987) Schistosomiasis control in the southern province of Saudi Arabia. J R Soc Health 107:79

Stephenson LS, Latham MC, Kinoti SN, Oduori ML (1985) Regression of splenomegaly and hepatomegaly in children treated for *Schistosoma haematobium* infection. Am J Trop Med Hyg 34:119–123

Sturrock RF (1987) Oltipraz withdrawn from clinical trials. Trans R Soc Trop Med Hyg 81:528

Sturrock RF, Bain J, Webbe G, Doenhoff MJ, Stohler H (1987a) Parasitological evaluation of curative and subcurative doses of 9-acridanone-hydrazone drugs against *Schistosoma mansoni* in baboons, and observations on changes in serum levels of anti-egg antibodies detected by ELISA. Trans R Soc Trop Med Hyg 81:188–192

Sturrock RF, Bensted-Smith R, Butterworth AE, Dalton PR, Kariuki HC, Koech D, Mugambi M, Ouma JH, Arap Siongok TK (1987b) Immunity after treatment of human schistosomiasis mansoni. III. Long-term effects of treatment and retreatment. Trans R Soc Trop Med Hyg 81:303–314

Sukwa TY, Boatin BA, Wurapa FKW (1988) A three year follow-up of chemotherapy with praziquantel in a rural Zambian community endemic for schistosomiasis mansoni. Trans R Soc Trop Med Hyg 82:258–260

Symmers W St C (1904) Note on a few form of liver cirrhosis due to the presence of the ova of *Bilharzia haematobia*. J Pathol Bacteriol 9:237–239

Taddese K, Zein ZA (1988) A comparison between the efficacy of oxamniquine and praziquantel in the treatment of *Schistosoma mansoni* infections on a sugar estate in Ethiopia. Ann Trop Med Parasitol 82:175–180

Tosswill JHC, Ridley DS (1986) An evaluation of the ELISA for schistosomiasis in a hospital population. Trans R Soc Trop Med Hyg 80:435–438

Vargas M, Gomez Perez J, Malek EA (1987) Schistosomiasis mansoni in the Dominican Republic; prevalence and intensity in the city of Higuey by coprological and serological methods. Trop Geogr Med 39:244–250

Viyanant V, Upatham ES (1988) Schistosomiasis japonica: epidemiology and genetic aspects. Southeast Asian J Trop Med Publ Health 19:139–150

Webbe G (1981) The six diseases of WHO. Schistosomiasis: some advances. Br Med J 283:1104–1106

Webbe G (1987) Treatment of schistosomiasis. Eur J Clin Pharmacol 32:433–436

Yeang FSW, Marshall I, Huggins M (1987) Oxamniquine resistance in *Schistosoma mansoni*: fact or fiction? Ann Trop Med Parasitol 81:337–339

Yi XM, Combes C (1987) Effect of praziquantel on larval stages of Schistosoma japonicum. Trans R Soc Trop Med Hyg 81:645–650

Zuidema PJ (1981) The Katayama syndrome; an outbreak in Dutch tourists to the Omo National Park, Ethiopia. Trop Geogr Med 33:30–35

Chapter 8

Some Parasitoses Involving the Central Nervous System*

Have not you maggots in your brains?

Francis Beaumont (1584–1616) & John Fletcher (1579–1625),
Women Pleased, III, iv

Introduction

This chapter deals with the various parasitoses of the central nervous system (CNS) in order of taxonomic classification (Table 8.1). When viewed in a world context, *Plasmodium falciparum* is probably the most common protozoan, and neurocysticercosis the most important helminthic infection to produce severe cerebral disease. Many clinical (Bia and Barry 1986; Kennedy and Johnson 1987; Cook 1990), pathological (Brown and Voge 1982) and therapeutic (Leech et al. 1988) aspects of parasitic (both protozoan and helminthic) infections of the central nervous system have been reviewed lately. This chapter therefore gives a broad overview of this important group of human infections, but excludes parasitic infections of the CNS which are common in the acquired immuno-deficiency syndrome (AIDS) (Cook 1987; Leech et al. 1988; Pons et al. 1988) of which *Toxoplasma gondii* infection in the most important, and also neuro-cysticercosis; these are covered in Chapters 9 and 10 respectively.

Protozoan Infections

Cerebral Malaria (*Plasmodium falciparum* Infection)

Introduction

Only one of the four species of *Plasmodium* to infect man (reviewed in Chap. 1) is capable of causing cerebral disease, i.e. *P falciparum*. Many aspects of the

---

*NB Chapters 9 and 10 should be read in conjunction with this one.

Table 8.1. Taxonomic classification of the major protozoan and helminthic infections of the central nervous system

Protozoan	Cerebral malaria (*Plasmodium falciparum* infection) (Chap. 1)
	Trypanosomiasis
	African trypanosomiasis (*Trypanosoma brucei* sp)
	South American trypanosomiasis (Chagas' disease) (Chap. 12)
	Amoebic meningoencephalitis (*Naegleria* and *Acanthamoeba* sp)
	Entamoeba histolytica cerebral abscess
	Toxoplasma gondii infection (Chap. 9)
Nematode	Eosinophilic meningoencephalitis
	Angiostrongylus cantonensis
	Gnathostoma spinigerum
	Toxocariasis (visceral larva migrans)
	Trichinella spiralis
	The human filariases
	Loa loa
	Dracunculus medinensis
	Nematodes and immunosuppression
	Strongyloides stercoralis
Trematodes	Schistosomiasis
	S mansoni
	S haematobium
	S japonicum
	Paragonimiasis
Cestodes	Neurocysticercosis (Chap. 10)
	Coenuriasis
	Hydatid disease

pathophysiology, clinical features, and management of this potentially lethal complication have been reviewed (Wernsdorfer and McGregor 1988). In substantial areas of the tropics and subtropics, CNS involvement caused by this protozoan parasite is associated with a vast toll of morbidity and mortality – especially in infants and children (Tharavanij et al. 1984; Bruce-Chwatt 1985; Spencer 1986). Estimates for the mortality rate vary from 20% to 50% (Macpherson et al. 1985). Cerebral involvement (including coma) is especially common in individuals who have not previously been exposed to the parasite; in Africa, well-nourished children are apparently more susceptible than malnourished ones (this might be related to body iron status (Hershko et al. 1988)). Cerebral malaria is also common in pregnancy, where both foetal and maternal morbidity are high; the reason(s) for this is not entirely clear but is probably associated with a relative immunosuppression. Patients with *severe* cerebral malaria seem to have reduced humoral responses (Tharavanij et al. 1984); while there is some evidence that corticosteroid administration might predispose to a *severe P falciparum* infection, there is no good evidence that this observation can be extrapolated to the immunosuppression which results from HIV infection. It is vital that the clinical diagnosis should be made early; delay is frequently associated with mortality.

Parasitology and Pathogenesis

The parasitological factors involved in severe malaria are summarized in Chap. 1. At post-mortem examination, the cerebral capillaries and venules are packed with parasitized erythrocytes. Therefore, various theories for the pathophysiology of this potentially lethal complication of *P falciparum* infection have evolved (Macpherson et al. 1985; Warrell 1987). Underlying thromboses within the cerebral vessels, and disseminated intravascular coagulation (DIC) have both been invoked but these suggestions have now been largely discarded. 'Sludging' of parasitized red cells within the microcirculation, in association with large quantities of malarial pigment (and resultant ischaemia), has also been incriminated (White 1986). The importance of cerebral oedema was the basis for a further hypothesis which gained considerable support; as a result dexamethasone was widely administered until a controlled trial showed it to be valueless (Fishman 1982; Warrell et al. 1982) (see below). [In contrast to the human evidence, limited experimental work indicates that pre-treatment of *P berghei*-infected hamsters with dexamethasone prevents some of these severe pathological consequences (Franz et al. 1988).] It is presently considered that neither increased cerebral capillary permeability nor oedema (Looareesuwan et al. 1983a) are important in pathogenesis. A local immune-complex vasculitis of the cerebral microvasculature has also been suggested as being important; however, in a fatal case of cerebral malaria, although the endothelium is in fact abnormal (on electron-microscopic examination), there is very little evidence of perivascular inflammatory infiltrate and certainly no evidence of immune-complex deposition in the cerebral vessels. Overall it seems unlikely, therefore, that such processes are directly involved in the pathogenesis of cerebral malaria (Macpherson et al. 1985).

Recently, there has been renewed interest in microvascular obstruction by non-deformable, spherical, parasitized erythrocytes (a *mechanical* hypothesis) (Igarashi et al. 1987; Aikawa 1988); however, this does not explain why the majority of red cells in cerebral capillaries (as visualized at post-mortem in fatal cases of the disease) contain *mature* parasites whereas in peripheral blood most are young 'ring' forms; nor does it account for sequestration in venules. *Adherence* of parasitized red-cells to the vascular endothelium ('cytoadherence') has also received a great deal of attention (Miller 1989); this phenomenon has been shown to be stage-specific, i.e. although mature trophozoites and schizonts are adherent, immature 'ring' forms are not; this phenomenon has been shown to be mediated by splenic function. Membrane protrusions ('knobs') on erythrocytes are associated with cytoadherence (Macpherson et al. 1985; Igarashi et al. 1987; Aikawa 1988); these consist of submembranous accretions of a parasite-derived histidine-rich protein (in which expression of a strain-variable high-molecular-weight glycoprotein takes place) on the cell surface. However, endothelial cytoadherence is now known to take place in the absence of knobs (Udomsangpetch et al. 1989). Adherence can be inhibited by a monoclonal antibody (33G2) which might constitute a useful adjunct in the treatment of complicted *P falciparum* malaria. One of the receptors has recently been shown to be: intercellular adhesion molecule-1 (ICAM-1) (Berendt et al. 1989). An endothelial ligand, possibly associated with thrombospondin, might also be involved (Warrell et al. 1988). The magnitude of sequestration, i.e. the ratio of parasitized cells in the cerebral capillaries and venules compared with that in peripheral blood (and the subsequent intensity of packing), is greater in the brain than in any other organ (Macpherson et al. 1985); this undoubtedly accounts in part at least, for the fact that coma is such a prominent feature in severe *P falciparum* infection. Obviously, the vascular occlusion which does occur must be largely reversible, otherwise neurological recovery would be incomplete; a mild reduction in microvascular flow on a permanent basis does seem likely, however. [Sequestration of parasitized erythrocytes can be reversed in the *Aotus* monkey by infusion of strain-specific antibody; this could form a potential basis for a new therapeutic approach in human cerebral malaria.] Cerebral lactate production is significantly increased in cerebral malaria (which is reflected in a raised CSF lactate concentration (White et al. 1985)); this presumably reflects anaerobic glycolysis (Warrell et al. 1988) (and reduced oxygen supply to the brain) (White et al. 1985), but unfortunately it is presently impossible to distinguish between host- and parasite-derived lactate. To what extent the coma of cerebral malaria is of *metabolic* origin – resulting from anaerobic glycolysis rather than mechanical factors – remains unclear. The Bolivian squirrel monkey has recently emerged as a useful model for the study of severe human *P falciparum* infection (Whiteley et al. 1987).

A further important feature of severe *P falciparum* malaria is hypoglycaemia (this is especially common in pregnancy; Chap. 1), which can itself produce severe cerebral anoxia; when quinine is administered chemotherapeutically this may act as an exacerbating factor because this agent directly stimulates the pancreatic β-cells.

Clinical Aspects

A severe headache is usual, and this is followed by increasing drowsiness, confusion, delirium and coma; hallucinations may also be present. Usually, but by no means always, the history obtained is of fever for several days; in children especially, the history can be extremely short. One or more *grand mal* fits may have occurred, following which coma has supervened. Convulsions (indistinguishable from 'febrile' ones) are especially common in young children with complicated malaria; whether they predispose to epilepsy in later life remains unknown. Focal epilepsy is not uncommon. Other accompanying signs which are present in a severe *P falciparum* infection are summarized in Chap. 1.

The level of coma often fluctuates; however, if hypoglycaemia is present concurrently, progressive deepening (which may be irreversible) is usual. The duration of coma is very variable; indigenous children in an endemic area usually recover within 48 hours, as do most adults; however, unconsciousness may last for many days. Retinal haemorrhages (which are reversible on recovery) are present in a high percentage of cases (Looareesuwan et al. 1983b); exudates are unusual, however, and papilloedema rare. Evidence of meningeal irritation is absent. Transient eye movements may be noted; the corneal reflexes are usually intact. Fixed closure of the jaws (which may make intubation difficult) and tooth grinding are common. One-third of cases have a jaw jerk. There may be muscular 'twitchings' and jerky or rhythmic movements of the head, neck and extremities. Muscle tone, tendon reflexes and plantar responses are all variable; abdominal reflexes are usually absent. Hiccoughs may be present. Evidence of autonomic involvement (apart from orthostatic hypotension) is absent. Fits (usually isolated) may occur after recovery.

Viral encephalitis and bacterial meningitis (both of which can co-exist with cerebral malaria) are important clinical differential diagnoses.

Diagnosis

Diagnostic techniques are summarized in Chap. 1. Cases of cerebral malaria have occasionally been recorded in which *P falciparum* parasites were not demonstrable in a peripheral blood film; some of these (especially in malarious areas of the world) had, however, already received some form of antimalarial chemotherapy. CSF pressure is usually normal, or may even be low; although clear, the fluid may be jaundiced. In 50% of cases the protein is elevated, but is rarely greater than 200 mg/dl; the lactate concentration is related inversely to the glucose concentration (when the CSF lactate concentration is >6 mmol/1 the prognosis is usually extremely poor). On microscopy, <10 cells/ l (most often all lymphocytes) are usually present.

Various EEG changes have been recorded, but no direct correlation can be made between them and either the clinical state or the ultimate prognosis. CT-scanning is usually normal, although evidence of cerebral oedema may sometimes be present terminally. Areas of either increased or decreased attenuation are occasionally present in a CT-scan; their nature is obscure and does not correlate with the clinical abnormalities.

Management

No preventive or chemoprophylactic regimen for *P falciparum* infection can now be considered anything like 100% protective (Chap. 1) (Cook 1986, 1988a); therefore cerebral malaria must always be considered a possibility (this applies to individuals who have made every attempt to avoid infection) following exposure to an infected area even if the clinical presentation is only mildly suggestive. An early diagnosis is important prognostically. Table 8.2 summarizes various

Table 8.2. Chemotherapeutic regimens for use in the treatment of cerebral malaria (Cook 1986, 1988a)

Agent[a]	Dose during first 4 h	Subsequent dose	Duration of course (days)
Quinine dihydrochloride (300 mg/ml)	20 mg/kg[b]	10 mg/kg (max. 600 mg) 8-hourly	7
Quinidine gluconate	15 mg/kg	7.5 mg/kg 8-hourly	7
Chloroquine sulphate (40 mg/ml)	5 mg/kg[c]	5 mg/kg 8-hourly	5
'Fansidar'[de]		3 tablets	1
Mefloquine[d]	0.75g	0.75 g	1
Doxycycline[d]		100 mg bd	7
Tetracycline[d]		250 mg 6-hourly	7

[a]The intravenous route should *always* be used; failing this deep intramuscular injection is second best.
[b]A minority of physicians use 10 mg/kg, but this is *not* recommended.
[c]This should be continued at the same constant rate during the next 4 hours.
[d]These regimens should *follow* the above-mentioned ones especially in patients who contracted their infection in South-east Asia; they are *not* adequate by themselves.
[e]One tablet ≡ pyrimethamine 25 mg + sulfadoxine 500 mg.

chemotherapeutic regimens which have been used in cerebral malaria; when available, quinine should always be used unless there is good evidence of widespread resistance in the vicinity. For general measures in management, see Chap. 1. Nursing on the side with frequent turning is necessary to reduce the chance of vomiting and aspiration. Eyelids should be lightly taped to prevent corneal abrasions. Corticosteroids are *not* indicated (see above). Fits are common and can be controlled with phenobarbitone (3.5 mg/kg given prophylactically as a single intramuscular dose (White et al. 1988)); convulsions should be treated with intravenous benzodiazepines or intramuscular paraldehyde.

Other differential diagnoses of coma should always be considered; the fact that *P falciparum* trophozoites are present in a peripheral blood film does not necessarily imply that the coma is a direct consequence of this. Every patient must be subjected to a detailed clinical examination at least once daily; the level of consciousness must be recorded, chest and urinary infections sought, and the intravenous line frequently inspected for evidence of sepsis.

Prognosis

The overall mortality rate in cerebral malaria varies enormously in different reports; it is dependent on many factors including definition (and depth) of coma, and the standards involved in management. Some investigators have defined cerebral malaria as an unrousable coma in the presence of a peripheral parasitaemia consisting of asexual forms of *P falciparum*, when other identifiable causes of unconsciousness are absent. Others have introduced a time factor (e.g. 6 hours in coma following a fit). The presence or absence of hypoglycaemia is clearly of crucial importance. Provided the level of unconsciousness does not deepen, the prognosis is generally good. Several clinical and laboratory indices have been shown to be useful (Chap. 1):

1. *Magnitude of parasitaemia*, i.e. the percentage of erythrocytes parasitized (in a blood film, or per unit volume of blood). A parasitaemia >20% carries a poor prognosis, and at >50% the survival rate is low.

2. *Other organ involvement*. Co-existent evidence of cardiovascular, pulmonary, hepatic, or renal involvement, and coagulation abnormalities (sometimes there is evidence of multi-organ involvement) all lower the chance of recovery. When renal function is severely impaired this is a particularly serious complication.

3. *Laboratory evidence*. A high CSF lactate concentration (see above), raised serum aspartate aminotransferase concentration, hypoglycaemia, metabolic acidosis, and presence of a coagulopathy usually indicate a grave prognosis. When the serum creatinine concentration at admission is >3 mg/dl, the mortality rate is around 50%

Provided survival occurs neurological recovery is usually complete; the sole exception is probably when hypoglycaemia has been present for several hours. Transient problems, e.g., psychoses, intermittent course tremor, cerebellar signs (Senanayake 1987), extrapyramidal manifestations, and VI nerve palsy are well documented. There are numerous old clinical reports of persisting neurological and psychiatric abnormalities, but the accuracy of a number of these should be seriously questioned. When neurological damage is in fact present after recovery from cerebral malaria, an underlying cause should always be sought (Currie and Krause 1989).

Trypanosomiasis

These protozoan infections have a limited geographical distribution, and are considered with the 'exotic' infections (Chap. 12); however, African trypanoso-miasis exerts such a profound effect on the central nervous system that a description is included here. South American trypanosomiasis is covered in Chap. 12; that account should be read in conjunction with this chapter.

The history, parasitology and early stages of African trypanosomiasis (*Trypa-nosoma brucei* sp) are outlined in Chap. 12. Invasion of the CNS (which follows a more insidious course in a *T b gambiense* infection than one caused by *T b rhodesiense*) produces a meningoencephalitis resulting in mental and physical lethargy, coma and, when untreated, death.

Parasitology and Pathogenesis

Meningoencephalitis may supervene following extensive lymphatic involvement and pancarditis (Chap. 12) (Poltera 1980). Perivascular infiltration, associated with prominent neuroglial proliferation, is most marked in the pia-arachnoid of the brain and spinal cord (Brown and Voge 1982). Oedema may be present, together with haemorrhages and granulomas; cerebral degeneration results from an endarteritis, which is followed by thromboses. Lymphophagocytosis, and the presence of morular or Mott cells (modified plasma cells – up to 20 μm in diameter – which contain large eosinophilic inclusions consisting of IgG) (Brown and Voge 1982) can be demonstrated in the meninges; these cells produce IgM which diffuses locally into the CSF. In some experimental studies in *T brucei* infection, stripping of ependymal cells from the ventricular surface of the brain has been demonstrated, and intracellular trypomastigotes are present in the remaining cells (Ormerod and Hussein 1986); this suggests an important relationship between the parasite and the ependymal cell. It might in fact shelter the trypanosome from the action of chemotherapeutic agents (Raseroka and Ormerod 1985, 1987). There is only minimal demyelination. The pathogenesis of trypanosomal encephalopathy has received attention using a murine model (Jennings et al. 1987, 1989); it has been suggested that following the removal of non-CNS trypanosomes by chemotherapy, the immune system directs its attack at those few organisms which crossed the blood–brain barrier soon after infection. This could explain, in part at least, the value of a corticosteroid 'cover' during melarsoprol treatment in the prevention of encephalopathy (see below).

Clinical Aspects

Clinically, CNS involvement follows some 3 to 4 weeks after a *T b rhodesiense* infection, but may take many months or years in the case of *T b gambiense* (Molyneux et al. 1984). There may be initial evidence of a change in behaviour and personality; however, the major symptoms and signs result from a diffuse meningoencephalitis in which the predominant involvement is towards the base of the brain. Indifference, lassitude and daytime somnolence may be present. Extrapyramidal signs (with tremors of the tongue and fingers); fasciculations in the muscles of the limbs, face, lips and tongue; choreiform or oscillatory movements of the arms, head, neck and trunk; increasing tonicity or muscular rigidity may follow. Speech becomes indistinct; cerebellar ataxia produces difficulty in walking; headache and papilloedema reflect cerebral oedema. There may be a backache and neck stiffness. Parkinson's disease may be mimicked. Later, fits which are sometimes followed by local paralyses, euphoria, mania and somnolence may supervene. In a heavily infected individual, the trypanosomes can consume 25 g glucose per hour, which must make a significant contribution to the degree of somnolence in the 'sleeping sickness' (Southwood 1987). Cranial nerve palsies and long tract signs are uncommon. Progressive mental deterioration, generalized pruritus, wasting, and dribbling with increasing immobility and ultimately coma, constitute the final downhill pathway. Death usually occurs as a result of intercurrent infection or malnutrition.

Diagnosis

This is outlined in Chap. 12. CSF pressure may be increased; it may contain >25 mg/dl protein (with an elevated IgM concentration), have a cell count >5 leucocytes per mm^3, and in addition morular cells of Mott may be present (Molyneux et al. 1984). A definitive diagnosis rests on the demonstration of trypanosomes in the CSF. Differential diagnoses when CNS involvement is present include: viral encephalitis, CNS tumours, psychoses, and meningitis caused by other infections which provoke a mononuclear response in the CSF.

Management

The management of this infection before the onset of CNS involvement is outlined in Chap. 12. When CNS involvement is present, melarsoprol ('Mel B') – which superseded the widespread use of tryparsamide (Thomson 1989) – is indicated; on account of its toxicity this compound should not, however, constitute the first line of attack in the *absence* of CNS involvement. In view of limited experimental evidence indicating that all *T b rhodesiense* infections result in a degree of CNS involvement (with persisting infection in the choroid plexuses (see above)), some physicians consider that melarsoprol should always be given following the suramin course. Three courses of three successive or alternate-day injections (of a 3.6% solution in propylene glycol) separated by an interval of one week between each course should be given; several dose-regimens (total dose ≡ 20 g/kg) have been used, one of which (for a 60 kg adult) is: 2.5, 3.0 and 3.5 ml, followed by 3.5, 4.0, and 4.5 ml, and a further 5.0, 5.0 and 5.0 ml. Relapses after melarsoprol treatment are due either to parasite resistance or to a shift of the parasites within the CNS (Poltera 1980). Local reactions and a Jarisch–Herxheimer reaction are occasional sequelae, but more importantly a reactive encephalopathy (occasionally fatal and occurring during the first course) has been reported; most of these reactions have, however, been reported in very sick, often malnourished, individuals who have frequently had very advanced disease. In a recent large prospective randomized clinical trial, the addition of prednisolone (1 mg/kg) body weight daily (maximum 40 mg) to the therapeutic regimen used in *T b gambiense* infections significantly reduced the incidence of melarsoprol-induced encephalopathy ($P<0.002$) (Pepin et al. 1989). Rarely, a haemorrhagic encephalopathy has been reported; abdominal pain, vomiting, albuminuria, and an exfoliative dermatitis are also encountered. α-Difluoromethylornithine (eflornithine, DFMO) – an ornithine decarboxylase inhibitor – has recently been subjected to clinical trial, especially in *T b gambiense* infections (McCann et al. 1987; Cook 1988b); even in late-stage disease (and CNS involvement) results have so far been encouraging (Chap. 12). In one study (Pepin et al. 1987), all of 21 patients who completed a course of treatment showed complete clearance of CNS trypanosomes, with a return of CSF to normal, and no evidence of relapse during a 6–30 month follow-up period.

If CNS involvement is severe and/or CSF protein content is >40 mg/dl when treatment is commenced the prognosis is usually bad. Serial CSF examination is necessary in follow-up; a relapse is reflected by an elevation of cell count, followed by a raised IgM concentration, despite the fact that the patient may remain asymptomatic. If there are good grounds for suspecting a recrudescence, a further treatment course is always indicated.

Amoebic Meningoencephalitis

Primary amoebic meningoencephalitis (PAM) is the most common manifestation of infection with the free-living amoebae: *Naegleria* sp and *Acanthamoeba* sp (Warhurst 1985; Carter 1972; Brown and Voge 1982; Duma 1984; Bia and Barry 1986; Rondanelli 1987). These organisms are ubiquitous in nature and are free-living in soil and water where they are readily found. Infection usually takes place via the nasal mucus membrane and cribiform plate. PAM, which was first described by Fowler and Carter (1965) in Australia can pursue acute, subacute or chronic courses depending on: the responsible pathogen, incubation period, and length of illness; the disease is almost invariably fatal. Some evidence indicates an increased frequency of infection in the debilitated and immunosuppressed individual (Martinez 1987). Although three cases of *Acanthamoeba* sp infection have been reported in association with AIDS it is too early to draw a conclusion as to whether this constitutes an 'opportunistic' infection in that disease (Chap. 2).

Acute PAM is most often caused by *N fowleri* but occasionally by *Acanthamoeba* sp. Contact with warm freshwater in lakes or parks (the Roman baths at Bath have recently been infected) is the cause of *N fowleri* infection, although dust-borne spread has been reported. The source of *Acanthamoeba* sp infection is frequently unknown, but seems to be more common in the immunosuppressed individual. Incubation period is 5–7 days. Clinically, the disease is very similar to acute purulent bacterial meningitis; an abrupt onset of severe frontal headache associated with fever, nausea and vomiting is often accompanied by fits; olfactory involvement is common. Signs of meningeal involvement are often present and the patient may be confused, obtunded or comatose. Death usually occurs within 72 hours. Subacute or chronic disease is usually caused by *Acanthamoeba* sp (usually *A castellanii* or *A polyphaga*). Incubation period is >7 days and the clinical course, which is more common in immunosuppressed individuals, varies from weeks to months. Focal fits and localizing neurological signs are common. The disease is invariably fatal. Ophthalmic, pulmonary, otitic and sinus involvement, sometimes proceeding to CNS involvement, are other presentations.

When caused by *Naegleria* sp (Duma et al. 1971), amoebae can be readily demonstrated and isolated from CSF; glucose concentration is often very low (<10 mg/dl); a neutrophilia is usually present, and red blood cells are occasionally seen. These findings are frequently absent, however, in subacute and chronic disease. Serological tests are of no use in the acute disease. CT-scanning is of value in identifying (using an immunofluorescent technique) and localizing focal lesions. Isolation and identification of the organism is usually not difficult provided specimens are kept at room temperature and *not* frozen (Bia and Barry 1986).

Experimental and clinical aspects of chemotherapy have been reviewed (Thong and Ferrante 1987); numerous agents have been tested. In acute disease (caused by *Naegleria* sp), intravenous amphotericin B must be started without delay; slow administration (≥ 1 hour) of 1 mg/kg per day should be reached by the second day of chemotherapy, and continued for 10 days. Miconazole and rifampicin have been used but their value has not been established; limited evidence suggests that amphotericin B and miconazole are synergistic (Duma 1984; Bia and Barry 1986). There is no satisfactory treatment for *Acanthamoeba*-induced CNS disease; if the lesion is single, surgical excision occasionally gives a satisfactory result. Flucytosine and sulphonamides have been administered but their value is in doubt. There is currently no vaccine.

Entamoeba Histolytica Cerebral 'Abscess'

Invasive amoebiasis is primarily a colorectal or hepatic disease (Chap. 6). Spread of *E histolytica* to the brain takes place via the haematogenous route; liver and/or pulmonary disease is usually, but not always, present concurrently (Lenshoek et al. 1958; Brown and Voge 1982; Wolfe 1984). Cerebral involvement is a rare event, but should always be suspected in a patient suffering from invasive hepatic amoebiasis who undergoes either mental or neurological deterioration, including convulsions. Lesions, which are not true abscesses (they are in fact necrotic areas of neural tissue and may be single or multiple), may occur in any area within the brain; the left hemisphere is apparently more often affected than the right. Larger lesions consist of necrotic areas which contain yellowish-green material with an occasional haemorrhage; co-existent meningeal involvement resembles on clinical grounds other types of acute purulent meningitis. Smaller lesions consist of minute areas of 'softening' with petechial haemorrhages. In a large study, 17 out of 210 autopsies carried out at Mexico City on individuals with invasive amoebiasis (all had hepatic disease) revealed evidence of cerebral involvement (Lombardo et al. 1964); the diagnosis was confirmed histologically in 11 of them. In that series, most 'abscesses' were multiple and varied in size from petechial haemorrhages to large necrotic areas (up to 5 cm in diameter); meningeal lesions were present in six cases.

The presence of a lesion(s) can be confirmed by a CT-scan; in addition ultrasonography or CT-scanning of the liver, and/or chest radiography usually demonstrates evidence of invasive amoebiasis there also. Amoebic serology is almost always positive, although in a minority of cases seroconversion will not have occurred at the time of clinical presentation; the immunofluorescent antibody test (IFAT), cellulose acetate precipitation (CAP) and counter-current immunoelectrophoresis (CIE) are usually all positive, the former at very high titre. Detection of trophozoites and/or cysts of *E histolytica* in a faecal sample (Chap. 6) neither confirms nor refutes the diagnosis, especially when the individual has previously undergone travel to a tropical or subtropical location. *E histolytica* trophozoites are *not* found in the CSF. Aspiration of necrotic material and/or a biopsy from the affected area occasionally shows *E histolytica* trophozoites.

Treatment consists of metronidazole (800 mg three times daily for 10 days by the oral or, if necessary, intravenous route); this should be followed by diloxanide furoate (500 mg three times daily for 10 days) to eliminate cysts of potentially invasive *E histolytica* zymodemes from the colonic lumen (Chap. 6). Response to this regimen is, however, frequently far from satisfactory. Surgical intervention, or aspiration (under CT-control) is usually indicated to remove necrotic material (Lenshoek et al. 1958). Except in cases which are diagnosed very early the prognosis is poor; also, cerebral lesions are frequently 'silent' and not diagnosed until autopsy.

Nematode Infections

Animal nematodes, i.e. those which are 'foreign' and have not achieved any degree of adaptation to *Homo sapiens* occasionally produce severe CNS disease: *Angiostrongylus cantonensis*, *Gnathostoma spinigerum*, *Toxocara canis*, *Capillaria hepatica* and *Trichinella spiralis* fall into this category. Two human filariases (*Loa loa* and *Dracunculus medinensis*) also produce human CNS disease but only rarely. In many ways the most dramatic illness of all can be caused by *Strongyloides stercoralis*, but almost always in the presence of immunosuppression (Chap. 5). In addition to the infections covered in this section, two cases of *Micronema deletrix*, a saprophagous nematode infection which can cause fatal meningoencephalitis, have been reported (Brown and Voge 1982).

Eosinophilic Meningoencephalitis

The term eosinophilic meningoencephalitis usually refers to infection caused by the rat lungworm *Angiostrongylus cantonensis*. The rare condition eosinophilic myeloencephalitis which results from a *Gnathostoma spinigerum* infection, however, presents in a similar way. Other infections which should be taken into account in a list of differential diagnoses include: acute cysticercosis, paragonimiasis and toxocariasis (Smit 1963); rarely, *Ascaris lumbricoides* and *S stercoralis* (during their migratory cycles) and also *Fasciola hepatica* can cause an eosinophilic meningitis. Another example, albeit a rare one, is schistosomiasis (see below).

The diagnosis of this group of CNS infections is difficult; unless larvae can be demonstrated in the brain or meninges (at biopsy or post-mortem) the diagnosis is essentially a clinical one. Treatment of these nematode infections is overall unsatisfactory; albendazole, which has not yet been adequately evaluated, may prove to be the best chemotherapeutic agent. These infections are frequently difficult to diagnose, and management is often based on probabilities, taking an accurate geographical history into account. The following is an illustrative case-report:

A 40-year-old English banker developed an acute illness – with 'flu-like symptoms and headache – following a raw fish meal in Hong Kong. This was followed by weakness and decreased sensation in both legs, followed by urinary retention. CT-scan showed extensive cerebral oedema and three intra-cerebral mass-lesions; CSF was under increased pressure and contained a large number of eosinophils. Following evacuation to London, a biopsy of one of the lesions showed a heavy infiltration with histiocytes and plasma cells. The clinical possibilities considered were infection with *G spinigerum* and *A cantonensis*. He was treated with a 28-day course of albendazole; serological test for *G spinigerum* was negative. Although the spastic paraparesis remained, sensation in both legs, bladder and colorectum was beginning to return when he was discharged from hospital for rehabilitation. *Comment*: This man contracted eosinophilic meningitis following a raw fish meal in South-east Asia. Although a definitive diagnosis could not be established a nematode infection seems certain.

Angiostrongylus cantonensis Infection

Although this parasite is widespread throughout the tropics, human infection most commonly occurs in South-east Asia, Papua New Guinea, the Pacific, and Australia. The adult helminth is a delicate filariform nematode which measures 17–25 mm in length; it is neurotropic and requires a period of development in the brain of its definitive host, despite the fact that the adults inhabit the pulmonary arteries of a wide range of rodents (Bunnag 1984). Eggs are laid in the pulmonary capillaries, where they lodge and subsequently hatch; the resultant larvae enter alveolar spaces, migrate into the trachea, and then enter the gastrointestinal tract; following excretion in faeces, they infect intermediate hosts (snails and slugs). When ingested by the rat, larvae migrate to the brain and thence to the pulmonary arteries, thus completing the life-cycle; it is at this latter point in the cycle that man can become an *incidental* host by accidentally ingesting the larvae in raw or undercooked dishes containing snails, crabs, prawns or slug-contaminated vegetables. In man, cerebral congestion and small haemorrhages may be present; larvae of *A cantonensis* can be recovered from meninges, blood vessels or perivascular spaces on the surface of the brain and spinal cord, and rarely the eyes (Brown and Voge 1982). A local reaction consists of lymphocytes, plasma cells, macrophages and eosinophils.

The incubation period is 6–15 days; most cases occur during the rainy season. Severe occipital and bitemporal headache, nausea, vomiting, neck stiffness and sensory impairment may be present (Punyagupta et al. 1975). Fever is, however, uncommon. There may be evidence of meningitis, radiculitis and/or encephalitis (Bia and Barry 1986). Motor weakness, localized paraesthesiae and cranial nerve involvement have also been recorded; haemorrhages and retinal detachment may be present in ocular disease.

A peripheral eosinophilia is inconstant. An ELISA has been developed but its availability in routine practice is limited. CSF pressure is usually raised, and the fluid turbid (>500 leucocytes/mm^3); in most cases eosinophils (Punyagupta et al. 1975; Brown and Voge 1982), and sometimes larvae are present (Brown and Voge 1982).

Analgesics and corticosteroids may relieve symptoms, but there is no specific chemotherapy (thiabendazole seems to be ineffective) (Brown and Voge 1982; Editorial 1988); the disease is usually self-limiting in 4–6 weeks (Punyagupta et al. 1975). Fatalities are rare. A recent report has documented the successful use of albendazole, provided it was administered within 15 days after infection, in a mouse model (Hwang and Chen 1988). Prevention depends on proper cooking of edible snails, especially the giant African snail *Achatina fulica* (Editorial 1988), and thorough washing of all salad vegetables.

Gnathostoma spinigerum Infection

Although most reports of this infection have come from Asia (notably Thailand (Bunnag et al. 1970) and Japan), sporadic cases occur in the Middle-east, Europe, Africa and the Americas. Human infection is acquired through consumption of raw or undercooked flesh of intermediate hosts which contain encysted larvae; it is also possible that drinking-water infected with *Cyclops* sp can convey infection.

Male adults which are 11–25 mm and females 25–50 mm in length, lie coiled in a mass in the stomach wall of domestic and wild cats and dogs (Bunnag et al. 1970); eggs are extruded and excreted in faeces. In freshwater, the larvae hatch and infect *Cyclops* sp in which they undergo development and are ingested by a fish, frog, snake or bird; when these animals are eaten by the definitive host the parasites localize to the stomach and mature in 3–12 months. Man is an *incidental* host in whom the life-cycle is not completed; the worms are migratory and can involve any organ (Brown and Voge 1982) with the production of necroses, haemorrhages and an eosinophilic infiltration. The brain, spinal cord, choroid plexuses and eye may all be affected (Bunnag et al. 1970); in the latter, subconjunctival oedema, haemorrhages and retinal damage can occur.

Clinically, a creeping eruption, migratory swellings (which are intensely itchy) (Fig. 8.1), low-grade fever, abdominal pain, tender hepatomegaly, pneumonitis, and peripheral eosinophilia may be present; other signs and symptoms depend on the system involved. Neurologically, severe agonizing nerve-root pain with paralysis of the extremities and sensory impairment may occur; cerebral haemorrhage(s) (sometimes massive) may also be present (Bunnag et al. 1970; Brown and Voge 1982). Eye involvement is unusual. There is a relatively high fatality rate (Bunnag et al. 1970; Brown and Voge 1982). The diagnosis is frequently difficult, and other helminthic diseases (see above) must be carefully considered; this particular myeloencephalitis should be clinically distinguishable from that caused by *A cantonensis*.

CSF is often xanthochromic (or frankly bloody) with an eosinophilic pleocytosis (leucocyte count >500 cells/mm^3). Serological studies are rarely conclusive. Definitive diagnosis depends on identifying the worm(s) at biopsy or post-mortem.

Antihistamines and corticosteroids are useful for symptomatic relief of the cutaneous swellings; surgical excision of a subcutaneous worm (for confirmation

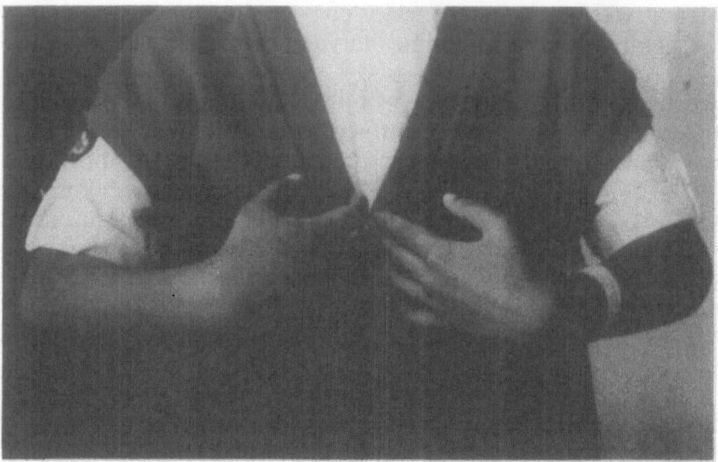

Fig. 8.1. A 5-year-old Bangladeshi boy who complained of transient, migratory swelling usually involving the dorsum of the hands. One of these subcutaneous swellings is shown on the right hand. Peripheral blood eosinophil count was 1.99×10^9/l. Serological test for *G spinigerum* was strongly positive.

of the diagnosis) is occasionally feasible. In Thailand recent trials using albendazole have given encouraging results (Chap. 3). Mebendazole has been claimed to be effective (Brown and Voge 1982). Prevention consists of avoiding uncooked or poorly cooked freshwater fish, chicken, birds, snakes and other intermediate hosts (Bunnag et al. 1970); untreated drinking water should also be avoided.

Toxocariasis (Visceral Larva Migrans)

Toxocara canis is a common and important canine zoonosis; it occurs worldwide and is covered in Chap. 11 (Cook 1989). Its major importance in human disease is that it occasionally causes a retinal lesion (which is almost always unilateral) (ocular larva migrans) which leads to blindness in a child who usually keeps and/ or plays with a pet dog (Gillespie 1987). However, CNS involvement (Schantz and Glickman 1978; Glickman and Schantz 1981) occasionally occurs as part of the migratory cycle – *visceral larva migrans*; an eosinophilic meningitis and convulsions have been reported (Gould et al. 1985). *T canis* has been demonstrated in an intradural extramedullary space-occupying lesion of the spinal cord (Russegger and Schmutzhard 1989). In the CNS, a transient encephalitis (with fits) can occur. In addition to Jacksonian or generalized fits, ataxia, paresis, and diabetes insipidis have been recorded (Brown and Voge 1982). In a post-mortem examination of a case of CNS toxocariasis in a 2½-year-old infant (Hill et al. 1985), larvae, which were surrounded by a giant cell reaction, were detected in the pons, right frontal lobe, and white matter of the cerebellum.

The possibility has been raised on several occasions that *T canis* (and possibly other migratory nematodes also) can by mechanical means introduce pathogenic viruses (including poliomyelitis and Japanese B encephalitis) to the brain (Brown and Voge 1982); evidence for this is, however, based largely on circumstantial evidence. Reports of laboratory investigations when CNS involvement is present are scanty (Schantz and Glickman 1978; Glickman and Schantz 1981); however, an eosinophilic pleocytosis in the CSF can be expected. For the available evidence on efficacy of chemotherapy, see Chap. 11.

Other Causes of Visceral Larva Migrans

Rarely this syndrome is caused by *Capillaria hepatica* infection (Cook 1989); this parasite is confined to South-east Asia. Occasionally granulomata are found incidentally in brain tissue at either operation or post-mortem; *Ascaris lumbricoides*, and various ascarids of dog or cat origin have also occasionally been identified (Brown and Voge 1982). Any human small-intestinal nematode which undergoes a migratory cycle can in fact produce cerebral lesions.

Trichinella spiralis Infection

Trichinellosis (or trichinosis) consists of infection by the nematode *Trichinella spiralis*, which is acquired in man by ingestion of muscle of wild animals or domestic pigs (Murrell and Nelson 1984). The disease is a major problem in the USA, Mexico, Chile and some other southern American countries; of the tropical countries affected, Thailand, Kenya, Tanzania and Senegal all harbour the disease. Arctic polar bears also carry the infection.

Following an initial intestinal phase (Chap. 3), the invasive stage begins 7–9 days later and involvement of skeletal muscles usually dominates the clinical picture. Other organ (including the myocardium and CNS (Brown and Voge 1982)) involvement is only rarely prominent; in the latter, meningeal irritation may simulate meningitis, while intracranial haemorrhage is an occasional accompaniment (Bia and Barry 1986). Dizziness, ataxia, hysteria and psychoses may be present; in a severe infection, fits, monoparesis and coma may ensue. Rarely, CNS involvement proves fatal (Gay et al. 1982; Bia and Barry 1986). A peripheral blood and/or CSF eosinophilia is usually present. The CSF may be xanthochromic (Brown and Voge 1982). An ELISA is of value. Muscle-biopsy frequently confirms the diagnosis (Bia and Barry 1986); enzymes may be elevated. Corticosteroids are indicated if cerebral oedema is present (Brown and Voge 1982); thiabendazole (50 mg/kg for 5 days) and mebendazole both have a degree of efficacy.

The Human Filariases

Filarial infections (Chap. 12) do not often involve the CNS. However *Loa loa* and *Dracunculus medinensis* (the guinea worm) occasionally produce significant problems. *Onchocerca volvulus* has a profound effect on the eye, but brain and spinal cord pathology has not been well documented (erosion of the skull by a nodule(s) (Chap. 12) rarely produces epilepsy); microfilariae can sometimes be demonstrated in CSF in a heavy infection (Chap. 12) (Brown and Voge 1982). A suggestion that *Dipetalonema perstans* can produce significant CNS pathology rests mostly upon anecdotal evidence (Brown and Voge 1982).

The most serious complication of loaiasis is a meningoencephalitis (the subarachnoid space can contain many microfilariae, and they may also be present in CSF) (Brown and Voge 1982; Negesse et al. 1985). An encephalitis (often accompanied by retinal haemorrhages) results from an allergic reaction to dead and dying microfilariae which obstruct the cerebral capillaries; this rarely proves fatal (Negesse et al. 1985). The mechanism by which occlusive thrombi form around *L loa* microfilariae is unclear. This syndrome has usually been associated with treatment (and killing of microfilariae) with diethylcarbamazine (DEC). Loaiasis tends to be considered the least important of the human filariases and it is therefore important to appreciate that this serious complication is a possibility.

In a small proportion of cases of *Dracunculus medinensis* infection, instead of bursting through subcutaneous tissue, the worm penetrates a joint(s) – rarely within the vertebral column; a spinal extradural abscess with neurological damage may then result. Paraplegia, with subsequent mortality, has been reported on several occasions (Muller 1971; Brown and Voge 1982). Surgical intervention and antibiotics are frequently necessary to deal with this complication of the disease.

Nematode Involvement of the CNS in the Presence of Immunosuppression – *Strongyloides stercoralis* Infection

Strongyloidiasis is covered in Chap. 5. Central nervous system involvement occurs as part of the 'hyperinfection syndrome'. The usual sequel is meningitis, which is caused by *E coli* and/or larvae of *S stercoralis*; both organisms can usually be detected in CSF (Ower and Wamukota 1976; Bia and Barry 1986; Smallman et al. 1986). This can masquerade as a cerebral vasculitis. Larvae are deposited throughout the CNS (via haematogenous spread resulting in small infarcts), and perivascular spaces (leading to involvement of dura, subarachnoid spaces and meninges) (Neefe et al. 1973; Owor and Wamukota 1976). They can usually be detected in faecal samples. In addition to the CNS findings, a peripheral eosinophilia (Bia and Barry 1986) (sometimes also detectable in CSF (Vishwanath et al. 1982)) is an inconsistent finding. An ELISA is of value; serological tests for filariasis often give a false-positive result.

Trematode Infections

Schistosomiasis

Only two of the human schistosomiases are generally considered to cause significant CNS disease (Bia and Barry 1986): *Schistosoma mansoni* (which produces predominantly cord lesions) and *S japonicum* (brain lesions). However, there can be no doubt that *S haematobium* (the cause of urinary tract disease) also produces CNS pathology, which usually consists also of spinal cord involvement and myelitis (Scrimgeour and Gajdusek 1985; Cosnett and Dellen 1986). The colonic, hepatic and urinary sequelae of this infection are covered in Chap. 7.

S mansoni and S haematobium Infection

CNS involvement (which is overall very unusual compared with other organ involvement) occurs at one of three stages during the life-cycle (Scrimgeour and Gajdusek 1985; Bia and Barry 1986): (i) acute schistosomiasis (Katayama fever) (Scrimgeour and Gajdusek 1985); (ii) deposition of ova in the brain or, more importantly, the spinal cord; and (iii) an aberrant adult schistosome or worm-pair(s) is conveyed to the brain or cord – where continuous egg production can occur (Pittella and Lana-Peixoto 1981; Bambirra et al. 1984); this latter event is extremely unusual. The resultant lesions are a reflection of the host reaction to the eggs; in the CNS they consist of: space-occupying lesions (Scrimgeour and Gajdusek 1985), obstruction, and later the consequences of scarring (e.g. fits); cerebral haemorrhage is a rare complication.

The most common CNS complication of *S mansoni* infection is transverse myelitis (Scrimgeour and Gajdusek 1985; Bia and Barry 1986; Cosnett and Dellen 1986); in addition to a peripheral blood eosinophilia the CSF shows a pleocytosis (often without eosinophils) and an elevated protein concentration. Anterior spinal artery occlusion (Siddorn 1987), a granulomatous multiple-root syndrome, intrathecal granuloma formation, and myelitis have also been recorded (Bia and Barry 1986); a case involving total myelonecrosis of the spinal cord below T4 has been documented. Although eggs are frequently deposited in the brain (especially when cardiopulmonary involvement is also present) they rarely produce symptoms unless the infection is very heavy (Pittella and Lana-Peixoto 1981; Scrimgeour and Gajdusek 1985). However, in a study (from Egypt) using CT-scanning, cortical atrophy was documented in a high percentage (36%) of patients with a chronic *S mansoni* infection (Khalil et al. 1986). For reasons which are not entirely clear, astrocytes within the cerebral cortex show significant proliferation in hepatosplenic schistosomiasis (Pittella 1981); similar changes have been recorded in individuals in the presence of cirrhosis.

Diagnosis is dependent on detection of the characteristic eggs in a faecal sample, rectal or liver biopsy – specimen or other biopsy (urine or bladder wall in the case of *S haematobium* infection) (Chap. 7); the ELISA, which is highly sensitive and specific, does not differentiate between the various species of schistosome. CSF serology is usually positive. Myelography is of value diagnostically. Chemotherapy in a *S mansoni* infection is similar whether CNS disease is present or not and consists of praziquantel (a single dose of 40–50 mg/kg body-weight) or oxamniquine (15–30 mg/kg body-weight on 1 or 2 days) (Chap. 7). As an alternative, metriphonate (10 mg/kg body-weight in alternate weeks, on three occasions) can be used in a *S haematobium* infection. When CNS involvement is suspected, a corticosteroid 'cover' is usually recommended. Successful results following chemotherapy of CNS involvement have been documented (Efthimiou and Denning 1984; Cosnett and Dellen 1986). Surgical decompression is occasionally necessary. The following is an illustrative case-report of *S mansoni* involvement of the CNS:

A 31-year-old English woman developed an acute systemic illness and fever, rigors, diarrhoea and vomiting, and a maculopapular rash (trunk and upper arms) about 2 weeks after a safari holiday in

Botswana and Zimbabwe; she had canoed on the Zambesi. 12 days later she developed a severe frontal headache (which was worse in the mornings), memory impairment, mental blunting, vomiting and severe urgency of micturition. She was pyrexial (37.4 °C), vague, disorientated and had a significant memory loss for the previous two months. There was blurring of the nasal margins of both optic discs, a right facial weakness, and drift of her outstretched forearms with a triceps and right hip and knee flexion weakness; both plantar responses were extensor and there was a left-sided palmomental reflex. Other systems were normal except that she had several spider naevi. Total polymorphonuclear leucocyte and eosinophil counts were 9.7 and 1.2 $\times$ 10^9/l respectively; CSF eosinophil count was 12%; CT-scan showed diffuse swelling and a left frontal lucency with surrounding enhancement. She was treated with praziquantel (to 'cover' schistosomiasis and neurocysticercosis (Chap. 10)), albendazole (for a possible nematode infection involving the CNS) and dexamethasone. She steadily improved and at 10 days after admission, was neurologically normal. A faecal sample at this time showed *S mansoni* eggs, and a *Schistosoma* sp ELISA was positive in serum and CSF. ELISA for *Gnathostoma* sp IgG was negative. Serological tests for *Trichinella spiralis*, *Toxocara canis*, cysticercosis and *Trypanosoma bruci* sp were negative. Serum bilirubin on admission was normal; ALT 124 iu/l, GT 286 iu/l, and alkaline phosphatase 356 iu/l. At discharge, the latter indices were 110, 197 and 252 iu/l respectively. *Comment:* In retrospect it seems most likely that the initial episode represented acute schistosomiasis (Chap. 7), and that the neurological sequelae were caused either by granuloma formation around eggs which had bypassed the liver, or resulted from an egg-laying worm pair(s) in the CNS. Recovery was ultimately complete.

S japonicum Infection

The life-cycle and clinical presentation are similar to those of a *S mansoni* infection (Chap. 7). However cerebral involvement is more common (Warren 1978); the reason for this is unclear. In a study from the Philippines, generalized and Jacksonian fits, and psychomotor epilepsy were common, while EEG abnormalities were present in 51 (68%) out of 75 infected patients (Bia and Barry 1986). There is reasonably good evidence, however, that spinal cord involvement is less common than in *S mansoni* and *S haematobium* infections (Marcial-Rojas and Fiol 1963). Diagnosis of a *S japonicum* infection is similar to that of *S mansoni*; treatment is with praziquantel (see above); oxamniquine is ineffective.

Paragonimiasis

The genus *Paragonimus* comprises several species of lung fluke (Markell and Goldsmith 1984); the most common is *P westermani*, which has a reservoir in freshwater crayfish and crabs (and other animals, which include several mammalian species) in South-east Asia, the Indian subcontinent, the Philippines, Indonesia and Papua New Guinea. Other species, which produce similar clinical manifestations, are present in parts of Africa (especially the West), and South and Central America. [Another trematode, *Alaria*, has also been reported to produce CNS involvement: petechiae in the cortex and white matter, subarachnoid haemorrhage, and spinal cord involvement (Brown and Voge 1982).] Infection is usually acquired by ingestion of encysted metacercariae in crayfish and crabs; after excystation in the small-intestine they proceed to the lungs where maturation of adult worms occurs in 5–6 weeks; they live for at least 6–7 years as cysts in the bronchial tree. The life-cycle is completed when they are coughed up, or swallowed and excreted in faeces; after deposition in freshwater, free-swimming miracidia are liberated, which in turn infect a suitable snail host where cercariae (which invade the viscera of crayfish and crabs) are produced. Most human infections are asymptomatic, although a cough (with rusty sputum), chronic pulmonary disease (including chronic bronchitis, bronchiectasis, pleural effusion and fibrosis) may occur; pleural adhesions and calcification are late events (Markell and Goldsmith 1984; Bia and Barry 1986). Pulmonary tuberculosis is often simulated.

Flukes occasionally develop in the brain and spinal-cord (children are especially vulnerable) which are ectopic sites; invasion seems to take place via the soft tissues of the neck and through the large foramina, including the jugular foramen. Clinically, cysts are most often present in the temporal and occipital (and also parietal) lobes; signs of a space-occupying lesion (Oh 1968) with epilepsy and paresis may result; optic atrophy and papilloedema (Oh 1968) is less common. Headache, visual disturbances, hemiplegia, mental deterioration, nausea and vomiting may also occur (Bia and Barry 1986). Invasion of the vertebral canal is a rare event and spinal-cord compression, with resultant paralysis, a possible sequel. Other syndromes include: meningitis, subacute progressive encephalopathy, chronic brain syndrome, a 'tumour-like' presentation and cerebral infarction (Oh 1968; Bia and Barry 1986). Transverse myelitis has been documented.

Diagnostically, *P westermani* eggs may be detected in sputum, faeces, pleural fluid or cutaneous lesions; adults can be removed surgically and identified. Serology is of value. CSF usually shows an elevated protein concentration with a mononuclear pleocytosis; in a minority of cases eosinophils are present; there may be evidence of haemorrhage (Madrigal et al. 1982; Bia and Barry 1986). A wide spectrum of CT-findings has been documented; these include ventricular dilatation. Cerebral involvement can be accompanied by intracranial calcification (Oh 1968; Brown and Voge 1982). Chemotherapy is with bithionol (30–50 mg/kg body-weight in divided doses on alternate days for 10–15 doses); a high success rate has also been reported with praziquantel (25 mg/kg body-weight given three times on a single day). Cerebral lesions may require drainage or surgical removal (Madrigal et al. 1982).

Cestode Infections

Neurocysticercosis

This important parasitic disease is reviewed in Chap. 10.

Coenuriasis

This zoonotic disease of man is caused by the larval stage of *Taenia (multiceps)* sp (McGreevy and Nelson 1984). Neurocoenuriasis produces clinical manifestations which are very similar to those of neurocysticercosis (Chap. 10) (Brown and Voge 1982). Although a rare disease overall, occasional cases have been reported from the UK, France, Africa, North America, and Brazil (Benger et al. 1981). The adult worms are present in the small-intestine of dogs and other canids;

proglottides, which are excreted in faeces, disintegrate with the production of many free eggs – which, when ingested by man, develop into coenuri in the CNS and skeletal muscles. The sheep is the major intermediate host (Brown and Voge 1982).

In man, a single intracranial space-occupying lesion (2–6 cm in diameter) may be present in the cerebrum, ventricles, posterior horn of the lateral ventricle, brain stem or spinal cord (Brown and Voge 1982); alternatively the cranial nerves may be involved (McGreevy and Nelson 1984). Ophthalmic involvement has also been recorded. Subcutaneous cysts may be present, as in cysticercosis. The value of serology is limited, cross-reactions occurring between cysticercosis and hydatid disease (Brown and Voge 1982). CT-scanning is of value in delineating an intracranial cyst(s). A definitive diagnosis depends on surgical removal and parasitological confirmation. No chemotherapeutic agent is of proven efficacy. However, evidence has been presented which indicates that praziquantel is of value in an animal model – an Asiatic primate (Price et al. 1989). Prevention should be aimed at treating dogs with praziquantel or niclosamide, thus reducing the environmental contamination with eggs.

Hydatid Disease

This infection is reviewed in Chap. 11. The liver is most often affected (60%) and this is followed by the lungs (25%) and other organs, which include the brain (<1%) (Brown and Voge 1982) and rarely the spinal cord; 80% of cysts are solitary. Although cerebral (and spinal cord and ocular) cysts sometimes produce symptoms in children, clinical presentation is usually in young adults. Presenting symptoms and signs depend on the site of the cyst(s); the disease should be suspected in any individual with a space-occupying lesion (within the CNS or elsewhere), who has lived in an area where the disease is endemic. Rupture of a cyst into the subarachoid space has been recorded (Abdulla et al. 1988). Vertebral involvement (a common site for a bone lesion) can result in cord compression (Bia and Barry 1986). An important differential diagnosis is neurocysticercosis (see Chap. 10); however, in that infection cysts are usually more numerous.

Parasite identification can be confirmed by examination of a cyst(s) removed either at surgery or post-mortem. A single fluid-filled cavity is surrounded by a translucent white membrane which contains opaque dots representing scoleces, brood capsules, and hydatid 'sand'; the scolex has four spherical suckers, a rostellum, and two rows of hooks. A novel approach to diagnosis has recently been reported (Hira et al. 1988): fine needle aspiration of hydatid cysts in 11 patients yielded fluid which contained characteristic hooklets. Although none of the cysts in this small series involved the CNS, there seems no reason why this technique should not be applicable in this situation also. Although no complications arose from the procedure, confirmation of safety is obviously necessary; aspiration of a hydatid cyst has always been viewed as being potentially hazardous due to the possibility of spillage and/or an anaphylactoid response to leaking fluid. Serology is now of great value in diagnosis (Chap. 11). CT-scanning is an invaluable technique for localization of both cerebral and vertebral disease (Bia and Barry 1986; Cook 1989). Figure 8.2 gives an example of intracranial hydatidosis.

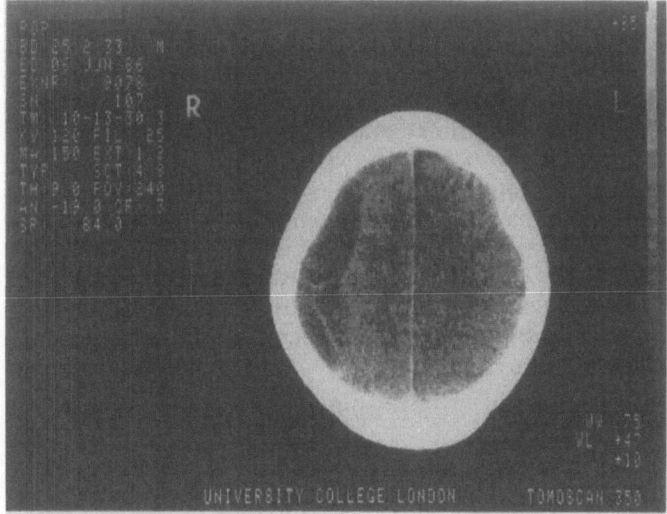

Fig. 8.2. Intracranial (loculated) hydatid cyst in a 53-year-old Nigerian man. The cyst is located at the surface of the right cerebral hemisphere, and there are minute specks of calcification in its walls; a gross shift of the mid-line structures is also shown.

Until recently management was always surgical (Brown and Voge 1982; Bia and Barry 1986); whereas cysts in most organs were initially injected to kill the protoscoleces, those in the brain and spinal cord were dissected out with great care but usually without prior treatment lest neural tissue should be damaged. Over the last decade the benzimidazole compounds have been introduced (Chap. 11); they continue to undergo evaluation (Wilson et al. 1987; Todorov et al. 1988). Praziquantel also possesses protoscolicidal properties, but has not yet been subjected to adequate clinical trial and its efficacy is currently impossible to ascertain. Therefore, results of large, multicentre, controlled trials of albendazole (Davis et al. 1986) and praziquantel, or both, are keenly awaited in disease involving the CNS as well as other organs. Some intracranial and spinal cord cysts will presumably always require surgery but only after prior albendazole and/or praziquantel treatment. Prognosis of CNS disease obviously depends to a considerable extent on the site of the cyst(s).

Conclusions

Parasitic infections should always be considered in the differential diagnosis of CNS disease in an individual who has had either recent (e.g. *P falciparum* malaria with cerebral involvement, or African trypanosomiasis) or past (e.g. neurocysticercosis, hydatid disease or schistosomiasis) exposure to a part of the world where standards of hygiene and sanitation are less than excellent. Therefore, a precise and detailed travel history is mandatory. Certain dietary items (e.g. raw fish and/

or vegetables from South-east Asia) are now readily available in many temperate countries (including the UK), having arrived by air transport; therefore, a history of overseas travel is no longer required before a diagnosis of a parasitic disease involving the CNS is a possibility. When there is evidence of immunosuppression (for any reason), the *S stercoralis* hyperinfection syndrome should be seriously considered. If an HIV infection (or AIDS) co-exists, there must be a strong possibility that *T gondii* is the causative factor.

Whilst diagnosis and treatment have improved significantly during the last few years, major problems still exist with some infections (e.g. gnathostomiasis and coenuriasis). While a high 'index of suspicion' must always be maintained for a CNS parasitic infection, the possibility that a disease entity has nothing to do with present and/or past tropical or subtropical exposure should also be considered; lymphomas of the CNS are but one example.

References

Abdulla K, Tapoo AK, Agha HSA (1988) Ruptured cerebral hydatid cyst: a case report. J Trop Med Hyg 91:302–305

Aikawa M (1988) Human cerebral malaria. Am J Trop Med Hyg 39:3–10

Bambirra EA, De Souza Andrade J, Cesarini I, Rodrigues PA, Drummond CASA (1984) The tumoral form of schistosomiasis: report of a case with cerebellar involvement. Am J Trop Med Hyg 33:76–79

Benger A, Rennie RP, Roberts JT, Thornley JH, Scholten T (1981) A human coenurus infection in Canada. Am J Trop Med Hyg 30:638–644

Berendt AR, Simmons DL, Tansey J, Newbold CI, Marsh K (1989) Intercellular adhesion molecule-1 is an endothelial cell adhesion receptor for *Plasmodium falciparum*. Nature 341:57–59

Bia FJ, Barry M (1986) Parasitic infections of the central nervous system. Neurol Clin 4:171–206

Brown WJ, Voge M (1982) Neuropathology of parasitic infections. Oxford University Press, Oxford, p 240

Bruce-Chwatt LJ (1985) Essential malariology, 2nd end. Heinemann, London p 452

Bunnag T (1984) Angiostrongyliasis: eosinophilic meningitis. In: Strickland GT (ed) Hunter's tropical medicine, 6th edn. Saunders, Philadelphia, pp 700–702

Bunnag T, Comer DS, Punyagupta S (1970) Eosinophilic myeloencephalitis caused by *Gnathostoma spinigerum*: neuropathology in nine cases. J Neurol Sci 10:419–434

Carter RF (1972) Primary amoebic meningo-encephalitis: an appraisal of present knowledge. Trans R Soc Trop Med Hyg 66:193–208

Cook GC (1986) *Plasmodium falciparum* infection: problems in prophylaxis and treatment in 1986. Q J Med 61:1091–1115

Cook GC (1987) Opportunistic parasitic infections associated with the acquired immune deficiency syndrome (AIDS): parasitology, clinical presentation, diagnosis and management. Q J Med 65:967–983

Cook GC (1988a) Prevention and treatment of malaria. Lancet i:32–37

Cook GC (1988b) Chemotherapy of parasitic infections. Curr Opin Infect Dis 1:423–438

Cook GC (1989) Canine-associated zoonoses: an unacceptable hazard to human health. Q J Med 70:5–26

Cook GC (1990) Protozoan and helminthic infections of the central nervous system. In: Kass EH, Weller TH, Wolff SM, Tyrrell DAJ (eds) Handbook of infectious diseases. B.C. Decker, Toronto (in press)

Cosnett JE, Dellen JR van (1986) Schistosomiasis (Bilharzia) of the spinal cord: case reports and clinical profile. Q J Med 61:1131–1139

Currie BJ, Krause VL (1989) Focal neurological signs in cerebral malaria accounted for by preceding neurological damage. J Trop Med Hyg 92:276–278

David A, Pawlowski ZS, Dixon H (1986) Multicentre clinical trials of benzimidazolecarbamates in human echinococcosis. Bull WHO 64:383–388

Duggan AJ, Hutchinson MP (1966) Sleeping sickness in Europeans: a review of 109 cases. J Trop Med Hyg 69:124–131

Duma RJ (1984) Free-living amebic infections. In: Strickland GT (ed) Hunter's tropical medicine 6th edn. Saunders, Philadelphia, pp 502–505

Duma RJ, Rosenblum WI, McGehee RF, Jones MM, Nelson EC (1971) Primary amebic meningoencephalitis caused by *Naegleria*. Ann Intern Med 74:923–931

Editorial (1988) Escargots and eosinophilic meningitis. Lancet ii:320

Efthimiou J, Denning D (1984) Spinal cord disease due to *Schistosoma mansoni* successfully treated with oxamniquine. Br Med J 288:1343–1344

Fishman RA (1982) Steroids in the treatment of brain edema. N Engl J Med 306:359–360

Fowler M, Carter RF (1965) Acute pyogenic meningitis probably due to *Acanthamoeba* sp: a preliminary report. Br Med J ii:740–742

Franz DR, Lim TS, Baze WB, Arimbalam S, Lee M, Lewis GE (1988) Pathologic activity of *Plasmodium berghei* prevented but not reversed by dexamethasone. Am J Trop Med Hyg 38:249–254

Gay T, Pankey GA, Beckman EN, Washington P, Bell KA (1982) Fatal CNS trichinosis. JAMA 247:1024–1025

Gillespie SH (1987) Human toxocariasis. J Appl Bacteriol 63:473–479

Glickman LT, Schantz PM (1981) Epidemiology and pathogenesis of zoonotic toxocariasis. Epidemiol Rev 3:230–250

Gould IM, Newell IS, Green SH, George RH (1985) Toxocariasis and eosinophilic meningitis. Br Med J 291:1239–1240

Hershko C, Peto TEA, Weatherall DJ (1988) Iron and infection. Br Med J 296:660–664

Hill IR, Denham DA, Scholtz CL (1985) *Toxocara canis* larvae in the brain of a British child. Trans R Soc Trop Med Hyg 79:351–354

Hira PR, Shweiki H, Lindberg LG, Shaheen Y, Francis I, Leven H, Behbehani K (1988) Diagnosis of cystic hydatid disease: role of aspiration cytology. Lancet ii:655–657

Hwang K-P, Chen E-R (1988) Larvicidal effect of albendazole against *Angiostrongylus cantonensis* in mice. Am J Trop Med Hyg 39:191–195

Igarashi I, Oo MM, Stanley H, Reese R, Aikawa M (1987) Knob antigen deposition in cerebral malaria. Am J Trop Med Hyg 37:511–515

Jennings FW (1987) Chemotherapy of late-stage trypanosomiasis: the effect of nitrothiazole compounds. Trans R Soc Trop Med Hyg 81:616

Jennings FW, McNeil PE, Ndung'u JM, Murray M (1989) Trypanosomiasis and encephalitis: possible aetiology and treatment. Trans R Soc Trop Med Hyg 83:518–519

Kennedy PGE, Johnson RT (eds) (1987) Infections of the nervous system. Butterworth, London, p 284

Khalil HH, Wahab MA el, Deeb A el, Ayad W, Hamdy E, Badawi T, Halawani N el, Khalil T, Seddik Z, Belal A (1986) Cerebral atrophy: a schistosomiasis manifestation? Am J Trop Med Hyg 35:531–535

Leech JH, Sande MA, Root RK (eds) (1988) Parasitic infections. Churchill Livingstone, New York and Edinburgh, p 364

Lenshoek CH, Baumann C, Wielenga DK (1958) Brain abscess due to *Entamoeba histolytica*. Arch Chir Neerl 10:34–40

Lombardo L, Alonso P, Arroyo LS, Brandt H, Mateos JH (1964) Cerebral amebiasis: report of 17 cases. J Neurosurg 21:704–709

Looareesuwan S, Warrell DA, White NJ, Sutharasamai P, Chanthavanich P, Sundaravej K, Juel-Jensen BE, Bunnag D, Harinasuta T (1983a) Do patients with cerebral malaria have cerebral oedema? A computed tomography study. Lancet i:434–437

Looareesuwan S, Warrell DA, White NJ, Chanthavanich P, Warrell MJ, Chantaratherakitti S, Changswek C, Chongmankongcheep L, Kanchanaranya C (1983b) Retinal hemorrhage, a common sign of prognostic significance in cerebral malaria. Am J Trop Med Hyg 32:911–915

Macpherson GG, Warrell MJ, White NJ, Looareesuwan S, Warrell DA (1985) Human cerebral malaria: a quantitative ultrastructural analysis of parasitized erythrocyte sequestration. Am J Pathol 119:385–401

Madrigal RB, Rodríguez-Ortiz B, Solano GV, Obando EMO, Sotela PJR (1982) Cerebral hemorrhagic lesions produced by *Paragonimus mexicanus*: report of three cases in Costa Rica. Am J Trop Med Hyg 31:522–526

Marcial-Rojas RA, Fiol RE (1963) Neurologic complications of schistosomiasis: review of the literature and report of two cases of transverse myelitis due to *S mansoni*. Ann Intern Med 59:215–230

Markell EK, Goldsmith R (1984) Paragonimiasis. In: Strickland GT (ed) Hunter's tropical medicine, 6th edn. Saunders, Philadelphia, pp 755–758

Martinez AJ (1987) Pathogenesis of free-living amebic infections. In: Rondanelli EG (ed) Amphizoic amoebae: human pathology. Piccin Nuova Libraria, Padua, pp 149–160

McCann PP, Bitonti AJ, Bacchi CJ, Clarkson AB (1987) Use of difluoromethylornithine (DFMO, eflornithine) for late-stage African trypanosomiasis. Trans R Soc Trop Med Hyg 81:701

McGreevy PB, Nelson GS (1984) Coenuriasis. In: Strickland GT (ed) Hunter's tropical medicine, 6th edn. Saunders, Philadelphia, pp 782–783

Miller LH (1989) Binding of infected red cells. Nature 341:18

Molyneux DH, Raadt P de, Seed JR (1984) African human trypanosomiasis. In: Gilles HM (ed) Recent advances in tropical medicine 1. Churchill Livingstone, Edinburgh, pp 39–62

Muller R (1971) Dracunculus and dracunculiasis. Adv Parasitol 9:73–151

Murrell KD, Nelson GS (1984) Trichinosis. In: Strickland GT (ed) Hunter's tropical medicine, 6th edn. Saunders, Philadelphia, pp 689–695

Neefe LI, Pinilla O, Garagusi VF, Bauer H (1973) Disseminated strongyloidiasis with cerebral involvement: a complication of corticosteroid therapy. Am J Med 55:832–838

Negesse Y, Lanoie LO, Neafie RC, Connor DH (1985) Loiasis: 'Calabar' swellings and involvement of deep organs. Am J Trop Med Hyg 34:537–546

Oh SJ (1968) Ophthalmological signs of cerebral paragonimiasis. Trop Geogr Med 20:13–20

Ormerod WE, Hussein MS-A (1986) The ventricular ependyma of mice infected with Trypanosoma brucei. Trans R Soc Trop Med Hyg 80:626–633

Owor R, Wamukota WM (1976) A fatal case of strongyloidiasis with Strongyloides larvae in the meninges. Trans R Soc Trop Med Hyg 70:497–499

Pepin J, Milord F, Guern C, Schechter PJ (1987) Difluoromethylornithine for arseno-resistant Trypanosoma brucei gambiense sleeping sickness. Lancet ii:1431–1433

Pepin J, Milord F, Guern C, Mpia B, Ethier L, Mansinsa D (1989) Trial of prednisolone for prevention of melarsoprol-induced encephalopathy in Gambiense sleeping sickness. Lancet i:1246–1250

Pittella JEH (1981) Astrocytes of the cerebral cortex in hapatosplenic schistosomiasis mansoni and in liver cirrhosis: a morphological, quantitative and karyometric study. Virchows Arch [A] 390:229–241

Pittella JEH, Lana-Peixoto MA (1981) Brain involvement in hepatosplenic schistosomiasis mansoni. Brain 104:621–632

Poltera AA (1980) Immunopathological and chemotherapeutic studies in experimental trypanosomiasis with special reference to the heart and brain. Trans R Soc Trop Med Hyg 74:706–715

Pons VG, Jacobs RH, Hollander H (1988) Nonviral infections of the central nervous system in patients with the acquired immunodeficiency syndrome. In: Rosenblum ML, Levy RM, Bredesen DE (eds) AIDS and the nervous system. Raven Press, New York, pp 263–283

Price TC, Dresden MH, Alvarado T, Flanagan J, Chappell CL (1989) Coenuriasis in a spectacled langur (Presbytis obscura): praziquantel treatment and the antibody response to cyst antigens. Am J Trop Med Hyg 40:514–520

Punyagupta S, Juttijudata P, Bunnag T (1975) Eosinophilic meningitis in Thailand: clinical studies of 484 typical cases probably caused by Angiostrongylus cantonensis. Am J Trop Med Hyg 24:921–931

Raseroka BH, Ormerod WE (1985) Protection of the sleeping sickness trypanosome from chemotherapy by different parts of the brain. E Afr Med J 62:452–458

Raseroka BH, Ormerod WE (1986) The trypanocidal effect of drugs in different parts of the brain. Trans R Soc Trop Med Hyg 80:634–641

Rondanelli EG (ed) (1987) Amphizoic amoebae: human pathology. Piccin Nuova Libraria, Padua, p 279

Russegger L, Schmutzhard E (1989) Spinal toxocaral abscess. Lancet ii:398

Schantz PM, Glickman LT (1978) Toxocaral visceral larva migrans. New Engl J Med 298:436–439

Schmidt H, Bafort JM (1985) African trypanosomiasis: treatment-induced invasion of brain and encephalitis. Am J Trop Med Hyg 34:64–68

Scrimgeour EM, Gajdusek DC (1985) Involvement of the central nervous system in Schistosoma mansoni and S haematobium infection. Brain 108:1023–1038

Senanayake N (1987) Delayed cerebellar ataxia: a new complication of falciparum malaria? Br Med J 294:1253–1254

Siddorn JA (1978) Schistosomiasis and anterior spinal artery occlusion. Am J Trop Med Hyg 27:532–534

Smallman LA, Young JA, Shortland-Webb WR, Carey MP, Michael J (1986) Strongyloides *stercoralis* hyperinfestation syndrome with *Escherichia coli* meningitis: report of two cases. J Clin Pathol 39:366–370

Smit AM (1963) Eosinophilic meningitis. Trop Geogr Med 15:225–232

Southwood TRE (1987) The natural environment and disease: an evolutionary perspective. Br Med J 294:1086–1089

Spencer HC (1986) Epidemiology of malaria. In: Strickland GT (ed) Clinics in tropical medicine and communicable diseases 1. Saunders, London, 1:1–28

Tharavanij S, Warrell MJ, Tantivanich S, Tapchaisri P, Chongsa-Nguan M, Prasertsiriroj V, Patarapotikul J (1984) Factors contributing to the development of cerebral malaria. I. Humoral immune responses. Am J Trop Med Hyg 33:1–11

Thomson KDB (1989) Tryparsamide. Lancet ii:573

Thong YH, Ferrante A (1987) Experimental pharmacology. In: Rondanelli EG (ed) Amphizoic amoebae: human pathology. Piccin Nuova Libraria, Padua, pp 251–272

Todorov T, Vutova K, Petkov D, Balkanski G (1988) Albendazole treatment of multiple cerebral hydatid cysts: case report. Trans R Soc Trop Med Hyg 82:150–152

Udomsangpetch R, Aikawa M, Berzins K, Wahlgren M, Perlmann P (1989) Cytoadherence of knobless *Plasmodium falciparum*-infected erythrocytes and its inhibition by a human monoclonal antibody. Nature 338:763–765

Vishwanath S, Baker RA, Mansheim BJ (1982) *Strongyloides* infection and meningitis in an immunocompromised host. Am J Trop Med Hyg 31:857–858

Warhurst DC (1985) Pathogenic free-living amoebae. Parasitol Today 1:24–28

Warrell DA (1987) Pathophysiology of severe falciparum malaria in man. Parasitology 94:S53–S76

Warrell DA, Looareesuwan S, Warrell MJ, Kasemsarn P, Intaraprasert R, Bunnag D, Harinasuta T (1982) Dexamethasone proves deleterious in cerebral malaria: a double-blind trial in 100 comatose patients. New Engl J Med 306:313–319

Warrell DA, White NJ, Veall N, Looareesuwan S, Chanthavanich P, Phillips RE, Karbwang J, Pongpaew P (1988) Cerebral anaerobic glycolysis and reduced cerebral oxygen transport in human cerebral malaria. Lancet ii:534–538

Warren KS (1978) Schistosomiasis japonica. Clin Gastroenterol 7:77–85

Wernsdorfer WH, McGregor I (eds) (1988) Malaria: principles and practice of malariology (2 vols). Churchill Livingstone, Edinburgh, p 1818

White NJ (1986) Pathophysiology. In: Strickland GT (ed) Clinics in tropical medicine and communicable diseases 1. Saunders, London, pp 55–90

White NJ, Warrell DA, Looareesuwan S, Chanthavanich P, Phillips RE, Pongpaew P (1985) Pathophysiological and prognostic significance of cerebrospinal-fluid lactate in cerebral malaria. Lancet i:776–778

White NJ, Looareesuwan S, Phillips RE, Chanthavanich P, Warrell DA (1988) Single dose phenobarbitone prevents convulsions in cerebral malaria. Lancet ii:64–66

Whiteley HE, Everitt JI, Kakoma I, James MA, Ristic M (1987) Pathologic changes associated with fatal *Plasmodium falciparum* infection in the Bolivian squirrel monkey (*Saimiri sciureus boliviensis*). Am J Trop Med Hyg 37:1–8

Wilson JF, Rausch RL, Mc Mahon BJ, Shantz PM, Trujillo DE, O'Gorman MA (1987) Albendazole therapy in alveolar hydatid disease: a report of favorable results in two patients after short-term therapy. Am J Trop Med Hyg 37:162–168

Wolfe MS (1984) Amebiasis. In: Strickland GT (ed) Hunter's tropical medicine, 6th edn. Saunders, Philadelphia, p 477–495

Chapter 9

Toxoplasma gondii Infection: A Feline Zoonosis with Potential Dangers for the Unborn Foetus and AIDS Sufferer

The young disease, that must subdue at length,
Grows with his growth, and strengthens with his strength.

Alexander Pope (1688–1744),
An Essay on Man

Introduction

Toxoplasmosis is a world-wide zoonotic infection which is caused by the protozoan parasite *Toxoplasma gondii* (Cook 1990); it produces a generalized disease but the central nervous system frequently bears the major brunt. Many other animals in addition to man are affected (Frenkel 1984; Kwantes 1987; Manson-Bahr and Bell 1987; Dubey and Beattie 1988). The domestic cat and other felines constitute the definitive host (Elliot et al. 1985; Paradisi et al. 1989); between 30% and 80% of domestic cats are affected. The life-cycle usually involves the cat, together with several small rodents and birds (the intermediate host) (Kwantes 1987); man and other large mammals (*T gondii* is a major cause of abortion in sheep) may suffer serious disease but they play no part in the cycle. The acute infection is usually asymptomatic, but a febrile illness (often accompanied by lymphadenopathy) and cardiac, cerebral, ophthalmic, pulmonary and/or hepatic involvement may occur. Foetal infection (which results from transplacental transmission) can result in serious congenital defects (McCabe and Remington 1983; Couvreur and Desmonts 1988; McCabe and Remington 1988); recrudescence of an established (latent) infection in the presence of immunosuppression (most importantly that caused by AIDS) constitutes a very serious 'opportunistic' event (McCabe and Remington 1983, 1988; Editorial 1989; Cook 1987). Human disease results from ingestion of (i) oocysts passed in feline faeces (usually via soil contamination), or (ii) tissue cysts in infected meat; rarely, blood tachyzoites are responsible (see below).

Although first accurately described in a northern African rodent, *Ctenodactylus gondii* – at Tunisia – in 1908, and named by Nicolle and Manceaux (1909), *T gondii* was not associated with human retinal disease until 1923 when Jankû, an ophthalmologist working at Prague, described choroidoretinitis which followed an intrauterine infection in an 11-month-old child (Kwantes 1987; Couvreur and Desmonts 1988). It seems possible that Laveran had previously observed the parasite in Java sparrows (*Padda oryzivora*) in 1900 (Pinkerton and Weinmann 1940). Wolf, Cowen and Paige reported a fatal case of infantile granulomatous encephalitis which was caused by a protozoan parasite (which was subsequently confirmed by Sabin to be *T gondii*) in 1939 (Wolf et al. 1939; Kwantes 1987). Although Castellani had suggested in 1913 that *Toxoplasma* sp could probably cause a generalized human infection, the first detailed description of an adult case was made (at post-mortem) by Pinkerton and Weinman in 1940 in a Peruvian patient at Lima who had concurrently suffered from bartonellosis (Pinkerton and Weinman 1940). In 1948, Sabin and Feldman devised a serological test, which remains in use today (see below) (Sabin and Feldman 1948); this contribution allowed epidemiological studies to get underway.

Epidemiology

Substantial variations occur in prevalence rates in different populations (as determined by serological testing). Overall, about 30% of *Homo sapiens* is probably infected, but local rates range from 5% to 90% (Manson-Bahr and Bell 1987). In the UK and USA, approximately 10% of the population possesses IgG antibody at 10 years, 20% at 20 years, and 50% at 70 years of age (Kwantes 1987). However, in Costa Rica, up to 30% of children have already been infected at 5 years old (Frenkel 1984), and in France about 80%–85% at 20 years (McCabe and Remington 1983; Kwantes 1987). In Paris, the rate is very high in French men and women, but those with a Spanish, Portuguese or north African origin have a prevalence of about 50% (Frenkel 1984). Whilst high rates are usually associated with frequent ingestion of undercooked meat, low ones are usually found where there is a relatively low density of domestic cats (and intermediate hosts) and the soil is dry – making prolonged survival of viable oocysts less likely. Undercooked meat seems to be commonly eaten in France, Germany and parts of the Arab world (Frenkel 1984). Raw eggs do not transmit infection (Couvreur and Desmonts 1988). In tropical and subtropical countries, contaminated soil seems a more important source of infection (Ruiz and Frenkel 1977; Frenkel and Ruiz 1981) and a high proportion of children become infected early in life (Ahmed et al. 1988; Paradisi et al. 1989), whereas in 'developed' countries infected meat is usually a more likely source and seroconversion occurs more often in adult life (Bannister 1982). Incidence of infection in the pregnant woman depends on: (i) prevalence of *T gondii* in the community, (ii) frequency of contact with one of the sources of infection, and (iii) the number of pregnant women in the community who have not previously developed immunity (as a consequence of a prior infection (see above)) (Couvreur and Desmonts 1988). Obviously the risk is markedly increased in women migrating from a community of low prevalence to one where the infection is widespread (e.g. from the UK to France) (Couvreur and Desmonts 1988). The antibody status of the neonate is similar to that of its mother, with the exception that IgM antibody (which does not cross the placental barrier) is absent; however, the IgG titre decreases to zero during the first 6 months of life unless an acute infection occurs meanwhile.

Parasitology and Pathogenesis

T gondii undergoes a sexual cycle (schizogony) and gametogony (isosporan phase) in the enterocyte of the domestic cat (a definitive host), but only an asexual cycle (toxoplasmic phase) in man (Manson-Bahr and Bell 1987). During the latter, the trophozoite form, the tachyzoite (endozoite or toxoplasma (4×1.5 μm)) parasitizes nucleated cells (especially those within the reticuloendothelial system) to form 'pseudocysts' in the acute stage; the bradyzoite (cystozoite or merozoite) forms tissue cysts in the chronic stage of the disease. Electron-microscopy shows the trophozoite to contain a central nucleus and a complicated system of organelles which are enclosed within a double-membrane; there are no flagella or cilia, and locomotion is by body flexion (Kwantes 1987). In a study aimed at *T gondii* strain-characterization, three isoenzyme patterns were detected amongst seven strains examined (Darde et al. 1988); whether or not this bears a relationship to biological behaviour remains to be determined. Studies are in progress to unravel molecular details of *T gondii* (Boothroyd et al. 1988).

The life-cycle of *T gondii* was slow to unravel. Figure 9.1 summarizes the major events in the cycle. In 1967, Hutchison and his co-workers (Hutchison et al. 1968) demonstrated that after ingestion of a *T gondii*-infected mouse or bird (Peach et al. 1989), cats shed an infective stage (identified as consisting of oocysts (9×13 μm)) in their faeces; up to 10 million oocysts may be passed per 24 hours for 7–20 days (McCabe and Remington 1983; Kwantes 1987). One estimate is that the 5 million pet cats in Britain kill 70 million small animals and birds annually (Young 1989). Following ingestion of tissue cysts (bradyzoites) in muscle and brain, almost 100% of cats shed oocysts, whereas only 16%–20% do so after ingesting oocysts or tachyzoites ($2–4 \times 6–7$ μm); the pre-patent periods are 3–10 and 19–48 days, respectively. Oocysts (which sporulate after 3–4 days) remain viable in moist soil for up to a year or more. Kittens are the most important source of infection (Frenkel and Ruiz 1981) and oocyst-shedding continues for long periods after infection; immunity from disease occurs after 7–20 days (Manson-Bahr and Bell 1987).

A series of epidemiological studies, many of them carried out in Costa Rica, made major contributions to the important role of cats in the transmission of this disease (Hutchison et al. 1968; Frenkel and Dubey 1972; Ruiz and Frenkel 1977; Teutsch et al. 1979; Ruiz and Frenkel 1980a,b; Frenkel and Ruiz 1981); evidence for faecally-spread oocyst ingestion in transmission soon became overwhelming. However, the earthworm is a significant transport host and not only conveys infected oocysts to a wider area, but also infects birds which ingest it (Frenkel

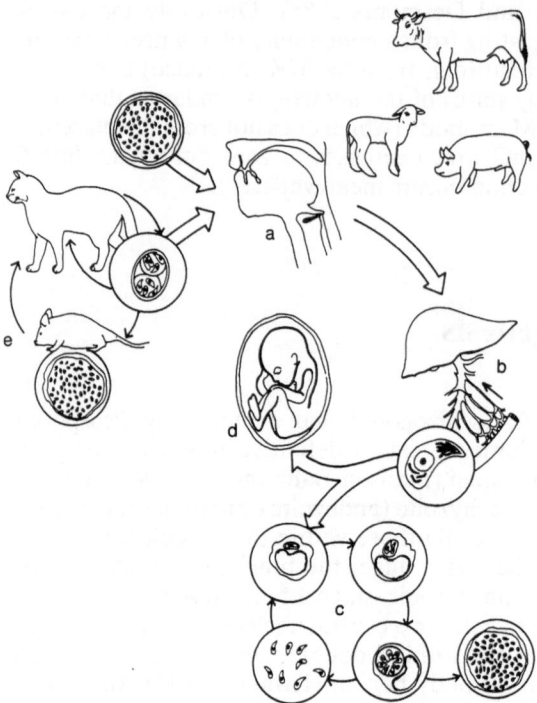

Fig. 9.1. Life-cycle of *Toxoplasma gondii*. (a) Infection occurs when pseudocysts (3–100 μm diameter) (containing numerous bradyzoites) in raw or undercooked meat (many mammalian species can be infected), or oocysts (in cat faeces) are ingested; (b) after the cyst wall has been eroded by digestion enzymes, bradyzoites and sporozoites emerge, penetrate the small-intestinal mucosa, and after haematogenous transport infect hepatic Kupffer cells and parenchymal; (c) macrophages transport *T gondii* throughout all organs and tissues ('rosettes' of tachyzoites are produced), and pseudocysts (in which numerous bradyzoites are produced) are formed; these can lie dormant for many years; (d) transplacental infection of the foetus can occur; (e) in the feline host, the sexual cycle is initiated by ingestion of an infected rodent or bird (the intermediate host) which contains pseudocysts or oocysts. [The asexual cycle can also take place in the cat.]

1984; Ruiz and Frenkel 1980b). It is probable that flies, cockroaches and other insects also spread oocysts within the environment (McCabe and Remington 1983; Frenkel 1984). An epidemic of acute *T gondii* infection in soldiers undergoing training in the Panama jungles was traced to oocyst-contaminated drinking water (Benenson et al. 1982); infected jungle cats were presumed to be the source. Transmission of the tissue cyst to man (a dead-end host) is usually via infected mutton, pork or goat-meat; up to 25% of mutton and pork may contain cysts (McCabe and Remington 1983).

When the initial infection occurs during pregnancy (in the human, sheep or goat) transplacental infection gives rise to a 30%–50% rate of foetal involvement (Editorial 1989); however, if previous infection has occurred (i.e. before pregnancy) maternal antibodies protect the foetus completely. Danger to the foetus is therefore much greater in countries with a low prevalence of the disease, because the initial infection is statistically more likely to be *during* pregnancy (see below); in a country where the disease is common (e.g. France) most women in the 20–30 year age group already possess immunity. In Britain about 2–3 women per 1000 appear to be infected during pregnancy (Editorial 1989). *T gondii* can also be isolated from other tissues (e.g. peripheral blood in symptomatic patients), and can be transmitted or reactivated by organ, especially cardiac (cysts are frequently present in both myocardium and bone marrow) transplantation (Löwenberg et al. 1983; Hirsch et al. 1984; Jehn et al. 1984; Ackerman et al. 1986; Fisher et al. 1987; McCabe and Remington 1988). Fatal cerebral *T gondii* infection (encephalitis) has been reported in patients with leukaemia, aplastic anaemia and Burkitt's lymphoma, and after allogeneic bone-marrow transplant (Löwenberg et al. 1983; Hirsch et al. 1984; Jehn et al. 1984; Ackerman et al. 1986; Fisher et al. 1987); toxoplasmal serology is frequently negative (see below). Infection has rarely resulted from laboratory accidents (McCabe and Remington 1983).

Following human ingestion, invasion of the small-intestinal enterocytes takes place, and there is widespread dissemination of tachyzoites to lymph-glands (via lymphatics) and other organs (via haematogenous spread). Cell-to-cell and haematogenous spread, within monocytes and granulocytes, is important (Frenkel 1984). The mechanism of cell penetration has received attention (Saffer et al. 1989); it seems likely that phospholipase A_2 (PLA_2) is important as is the case with the cytopathogenicity of *Entamoeba histolytica*. Tachyzoites multiply (dividing every 5–12 hours) in all nucleated cells – especially the macrophages of the reticuloendothelial system – with destruction of the host cell; entry to adjacent cells results in focal necrosis. A type III antigen–antibody reaction between host-antibody (which seeps through the vessel wall) and parasite-antigen causes intravascular thrombosis and infarction (Manson-Bahr and Bell 1987). Therefore, significant cell-destruction occurs before effective immunity has been established; myocarditis, myositis, encephalitis, focal hepatitis and interstitial pneumonia can ensue. In the lymph-glands, there is usually preservation of architecture with follicular hyperplasia (collections of enlarged epithelioid cells with abundant pale cytoplasm and prominent nucleoli are present) and a paucity of organisms. Histology is often diagnostic in the acute disease. In the chronic stage, cysts rupture with the production of bradyzoites which elicit a type IV reaction accompanied by round cell infiltration, granuloma formation and tissue necrosis (Manson-Bahr and Bell 1987). When recrudescence of infection occurs in the immunosuppressed individual numerous tachyzoites are present in those organs in which cellular immunity is most severely compromised: brain, retina and lung. Congenital *T gondii* infection arises when the foetus becomes infected after a short lag period, following placental infection. The rate of placental infection depends upon the trimester of pregnancy in which the infection occurs (it being more likely that placentitis will follow when infection occurs late), and on whether the woman has been treated with spiramycin (Couvreur and Desmonts 1988). In an infected placenta chronic inflammation is present in the decidua capsularis, with focal lesions in the villi (Couvreur and Desmonts 1988); tachyzoites are only rarely found, and the precise mechanism of transmission to the foetus is poorly understood. Foetal infection is either generalized (myocarditis, hepatitis and pneumonia are serious complications) or localized within the CNS. In the former, the lesions (which ultimately fibrose) consist of a mononuclear inflammatory reaction with tachyzoites at the periphery. In the latter, an active encephalitis with microglial nodules, scattered infarcts and periventricular necrosis is characteristic; obstruction, with accumulation of *T gondii* antigen in the lateral and third ventricles, may result from an ependymitis of the aqueduct.

Humoral immunity is important initially, and IgG antibody reaches a maximum concentration 2 months after infection; this persists for life. IgM antibody appears before IgG, and disappears before the latter reaches a peak. Whilst these events clear tachyzoites from blood, tissue bradyzoites (in brain and muscle) remain unaffected (Manson-Bahr and Bell 1987). In chronic infection, CMI forms the basis of the immune response and is transferred by lymphocytes; this receives recurrent reinforcement throughout life because bradyzoites 'escape' from tissue cysts (in brain, retina, skeleton and myocardium) from time to time. The type IV allergic reaction (see above) is especially important in the retina; it is also responsible for focal encephalitis and myositis. While the CMI response is usually adequate to destroy the released bradyzoites, in the immunosuppressed individual tachyzoites exhibit renewed proliferation.

Clinical Aspects

The clinical presentation depends on the age at which infection occurs, and the immune status of the host; prior to the AIDS epidemic, the two major patterns of disease in the UK were: (i) a glandular form (accompanied by a high antibody concentration), and (ii) an ocular, or late form (a lower antibody concentration) (Bannister 1982).

Acute Acquired *T gondii* Infection in the Immunointact Individual

Glandular disease accounted for 27.5% of newly reported cases of *T gondii* infection in England and Wales between 1976 and 1980 (Bannister 1982). The incubation period after ingestion of oocysts lies between 7 and 17 days; however, the vast majority of infections are symptomless and inapparent (Frenkel 1984; Manson-Bahr and Bell 1987). Fever, headache and lymphadenopathy are the most common presenting features; presence of the latter (most often involving the cervical glands) differs with sex and age at the time of infection: in childhood, the male : female ratio is 3 : 1, whereas the corresponding figures for adolescence and adulthood are 1 : 1 and 1 : 3, respectively (Kwantes 1987). One or more glands may be involved which are firm, discrete and 'rubbery', but non-tender. One estimate is that 15% of cases of unexplained lymphadenopathy are caused by toxoplasmosis (Elliot et al. 1985). Hepatosplenomegaly may be present in addition. Symptoms can continue with a varying degree of malaise and fatigue for up to several months (Kwantes 1987). Less frequently, myalgia, sore-throat, a maculo-papular or urticarial rash, and arthralgia co-exist; pneumonia, hepatitis (sometimes accompanied by jaundice), myocarditis (occasionally associated with pericarditis), and encephalitis have also been recorded, the latter two complications resulting in occasional mortality. Differential diagnoses include: infectious mononucleosis (EBV), cytomegalovirus (CMV), syphilis, brucellosis, leptospirosis, glandular tuberculosis, lymphoma or Hodgkin's disease, leukaemia, visceral larva migrans, African trypanosomiasis and visceral leishmaniasis (Kala-azar) (Frenkel 1984; Manson-Bahr and Bell 1987). Features which overlap with lymphoma are persistent lymphadenopathy, splenomegaly and a Coombs negative haemolytic anaemia; the possibility of a dual diagnosis should also be considered. The polymorphonuclear leucocyte count is either normal or slightly reduced, with a relative lymphocytosis and monocytosis (with the occasional presence of atypical cells). In prolonged disease, a normochromic, normocytic anaemia may develop. Serum transaminase concentrations are often mildly elevated. IgG and IgM antibodies are elevated; serial estimations are valuable (see below). A lymph-node biopsy-specimen shows follicular hyperplasis (see above). Chest radiography is either normal, or reveals evidence of an interstitial pneumonia.

Foetal Infection

Most infections acquired during pregnancy are asymptomatic; however, in a minority (perhaps 10%) of women, posterior cervical lymph-glands may be enlarged (McCabe and Remington 1983; Kwantes 1987). The magnitude of this problem is difficult to assess. During the period 1975–1980, 91 cases of congenital infection were reported in England, Wales and Northern Ireland (Hall 1983); however, using very strict criteria only 34 of them were certain examples of in utero infection. In Scotland, a prospective study carried out between 1975 and 1977 has indicated that the incidence there is not less than 1 in 2000 births (Williams et al. 1981); a retrospective study carried out for the 10-year period 1976–1986 revealed, however, only 27 cases during which time 224 cases of ophthalmic involvement (which usually results from congenital infection) were documented (Chatterton et al. 1989). The latter figure might well be due to lack of recognition and/or poor reporting.

In the USA, between 1 : 1000 and 1 : 8000 of live-births have evidence of having been infected with T $gondii$ in utero (McCabe and Remington 1988). Approximately 30%–50% of foetuses infected in utero ultimately undergo a significant pathological event which presents either at birth or later in life (Frenkel 1984; Kwantes 1987; Manson-Bahr and Bell 1987; Williams et al. 1981); although the severity of foetal damage is usually greatest when infection is acquired in the first trimester a significant danger still exists, and indeed the overall incidence is greatest, in the third (Kwantes 1987; Couvreur and Desmonts 1988; McCabe and Remington 1988).

Whilst only about 10% of children with a congenital infection manifest severe disease in the neonatal period, most of the remainder develop problems later in life (Wilson et al. 1980). Abortion, intrauterine growth retardation, prematurity (Kasper and Kass 1988), still-birth and neonatal death are all recognized sequelae. Of those severely affected, a minority develop a generalized disease: splenomegaly, hepatomegaly, jaundice, fever, anaemia, lymphadenopathy, pneumonia and a papular or purpuric rash (Manson-Bahr and Bell 1987). CNS involvement may also occur (Couvreur and Desmonts 1988): Sabin's tetrad consists of internal hydrocephalus, convulsions, cerebral calcification (Frenkel 1984; Couvreur and Desmonts 1988) and choroidoretinitis (this complication, which is not necessarily present at birth, subsequently develops in about 75%–90% of cases); microcephaly, ocular nystagmus, strabismus, cataract, deafness, optic atrophy, hypothermia and abnormal CSF are other sequelae of an in utero infection (Frenkel 1984; Manson-Bahr and Bell 1987). Retinal lesions are usually bilateral and involve the macular region; they may be obscured at retinoscopy by an intense vitreous inflammatory exudate. Necrotizing choroidoretinitis should be differentiated from that caused by syphilis and tuberculosis. In most severe cases, disease is recognized at birth, and neural damage usually results in early death; however, evidence of infection (including mental retardation, spastic paresis, psychomotor disturbances, and visual and auditory abnormalities) may not appear until a few months or even years later.

There is no way of predicting the ultimate outcome, but chemotherapy (see below) undoubtedly offers some hope (McCabe and Remington 1988). In one prospective study, 70% of infants who were infected at the time of birth appeared normal, 20% had minor abnormalities, and a further 10% had serious disabilities (see above) (Elliot et al. 1985); it is likely that most of those who were asymptomatic at birth developed ophthalmological or neurological sequelae later. In a careful follow-up study in the USA, 22 (92%) out of 24 infants born with an asymptomatic *T gondii* infection ultimately (i.e. at mean age 8.5 years) developed sequelae; this usually consisted of choroidoretinitis although four became mentally retarded (Wilson et al. 1980). Nine out of 11 cases of congenital *T gondii* infection diagnosed at Amsterdam, Holland, developed new lesions, usually choroidoretinitis during a 20-year follow-up study (Koppe et al. 1986). There are probably no acceptable reports of more than one affected foetus/infant being born to the same woman (Kwantes 1987; Couvreur and Desmonts 1988); a previous infection almost always renders lasting immunity to subsequent foetuses (see above).

Ocular Involvement

During the period 1976–1980, 60% of newly reported cases of *T gondii* infection in England and Wales involved eye complications (Bannister 1982). The peak incidence of ocular *T gondii* involvement occurs in the 10–34 age group where it accounts for up to 50% of cases of uveitis (Elliot et al. 1985); although nearly always a result of reactivation of an in utero infection (Wilson et al. 1980; Koppe et al. 1986; Chatterton et al. 1989), primary infection in adult life is rarely responsible. Whilst frequently not recognized until later in life it virtually always results from an in utero infection (see above) (Couvreur and Desmonts 1988). Statistically it is more likely to be unilateral, and is usually painless. A common presentation consists of blurred vision and/or aching in one eye, during the second decade; however, disease is often discovered incidentally. Initially, an inflammatory exudate clouds the vitreous; when the retina is visualized, fluffy cotton-wool-like patches are present and these later become sharply demarcated to form a choroidoretinal scar (Kwantes 1987). Retinoblastoma is a possible differential diagnosis (Frenkel 1984). Old quiescent lesions may also be noted incidentally on routine examination. Recurrence of activity may occur many years later, and satellite lesions appear in proximity to an old scar. Prolonged smouldering lesions have been described; these may either follow corticosteroid administration which has been inadequately 'covered' by chemotherapy (see below), or complicate a recrudescent *T gondii* infection in an immunosuppressed individual. Retinal oedema, optic neuritis, iridocyclitis and rarely pan-uveitis can ensue; blindness and glaucomas are recognized long-term sequelae. Serum IgG antibody is usually mildly elevated but stable (see below); only complete absence of antibody excludes a diagnosis of toxoplasmal uveitis.

T gondii Infection in the Immunosuppressed Individual

Most cases occur as a result of reactivation of a chronic (latent) infection following a reduction of CMI; this can result from administration of an immunosuppressive agent, Hodgkin's disease, a lymphoma, or from AIDS. Histologically, tachyzoites are present in widespread lesions of the brain and lungs; this may occur whenever CMI is depressed and the tissue cysts become reactivated. A severe febrile illness with prostration, generalized rash and multiple organ involvement (including myocarditis, focal pneumonia and hepatic necrosis) may all be present (Manson-Bahr and Bell 1987). However, the most common presentation results from cerebral involvement (Elkin et al. 1985; Tang et al. 1986). Approximately 30% of toxoplasma-antibody-positive AIDS patients develop a toxoplasmic encephalitis (McCabe and Remington 1988). Encephalitis in fact occurs in 3%–40% of patients with AIDS (Luft and Remington 1988) and may present with headache, convulsions, disorientation and coma as well as numerous focal manifestations (CSF may be xanthochromic, with an elevated protein and mononuclear cell count, and normal glucose). A focal neurological deficit may be present: mild hemiparesis, cerebellar or brain-stem lesions, ataxia, or a cranial nerve lesion (Navia et al. 1986). If untreated, death is likely within a few days (Kwantes 1987; McCabe and Remington 1988) and recovery is a rare event (Hakes and Armstrong 1983). Lesions are often focal (especially in association with AIDS) and the clinical presentation often simulates a cerebral abscess or tumour; they may be multicentric. Viral encephalitis and cerebral tumours should be differentiated (Manson-Bahr and Bell 1987). Other CNS lesions associated with HIV infection (Lantos et al. 1989) should be ruled out. Hydrocephalus, resulting from a blocked Sylvian aqueduct, may be present. Generalized septicaemia and other severe febrile diseases should be excluded. Disseminated organ involvement may occur in AIDS; testicular disease, with necrotic seminiferous tubules has, for example, been reported (Nistal et al. 1986). When detectable serum IgG concentration is usually elevated but stable.

   Primary infection in the immunosuppressed individual follows either from the usual portal of entry (see above) or alternatively (and more frequently) from a leucocyte transfusion or organ (especially cardiac) transplant. Whilst resembling a generalized *T gondii* infection in an immunointact individual, the disease is overall more severe; serum antibody concentration is either rising or stable. Although prolonged survival has been recorded, 70% of patients die within 1 year of diagnosis of a *T gondii* infection in AIDS (Gerberding 1988).

Diagnosis

Diagnostically, parasite identification (usually after inoculation of fresh biopsy-material into a mouse, hamster or cell-culture) is the only definitive method; lymph-node biopsy is virtually but not completely diagnostic. Material for inoculation (tissue-biopsy, placental tissue, ventricular fluid, buffy-coat from a centrifuged blood-specimen (McCabe and Remington 1983), or a post-mortem sample) should be conveyed to the laboratory in saline containing 100 µg penicillin + 100 µg streptomycin/ml; any contact with formalin and/or freezing must be avoided. Mice manifest evidence of a *T gondii* infection 4–6 weeks after inoculation: typical cysts (recognizable in imprints – see below) are present in cerebral tissue, and antibodies in peripheral blood (Kwantes 1987); tachyzoites may be visualized in peritoneal fluid after 4–18 days (Manson-Bahr and Bell 1987). Tissue impression smears (imprints) can be made from CSF, and specimens of lymph-node, muscle, brain, eye, or the products of conception. Tissue should be dried, fixed with methanol, and stained with Giemsa; ovoid organisms (7 × 3 µm) which possess a red nucleus and blue cytoplasm can then be demonstrated (Frenkel 1984). Tissue sections stained with haematoxylin and eosin reveal ovoid or rounded tachyzoites (3 × 4 µm) or bradyzoites (which are similar in size but more closely packed) (McCabe and Remington 1983; Frenkel 1984); parasite-glycogen can be stained using a periodic acid-Schiff technique. Peroxidase–antiperoxidase (McCabe and Remington 1983; Dutton 1984), fluor-escent-antibody or enzyme staining, and electron-microscopical (to delineate the ultrastructural features) techniques may all be applied to facilitate identification. In a preliminary study, transmission electron-microscopy has been shown to be valuable in the rapid demonstration of detailed features of the tachyzoite (Tang et al. 1986). The presence of cell or tissue necrosis, with tachyzoites (or cysts), indicates active infection whilst the presence of cysts alone suggests a chronic infection (except in placental tissue and in the newborn). Fine-needle aspiration is sometimes of value; cytopathological features of acute glandular toxoplasmosis can closely parallel these histopathological changes (Hall 1984), but this pro-cedure is of limited value due to sampling error (Luft and Remington 1988). In practice, diagnosis usually rests on the clinical picture in association with positive *T gondii* serology (Luft and Remington 1988); absence of both IgG and IgM antibodies excludes infection (Kwantes 1987).

Some of the problems encountered in diagnosis have been reviewed (Hakes and Armstrong 1983; McCabe and Remington 1983; Dutton 1984; Hall 1984); it can be especially difficult in HIV-infected individuals (Luft and Remington 1988). An ECG is of value if myocarditis (a potentially lethal complication) is suspected. The indications for brain biopsy in the diagnosis of a *T gondii* infection in AIDS are controversial (Luft and Remington 1988). Presence of an intracra-nial mass lesion(s) on CT-scanning (see below), together with positive serology in an AIDS patient in the UK or USA makes the diagnosis extremely likely on probability grounds; however, when another diagnosis, e.g. tuberculoma, *Cryp-tococcus neoformans* or Kaposi's sarcoma (more likely in African AIDS), is a possibility this procedure is valuable (Löwenberg et al. 1983; Elkin et al. 1985; Ackerman et al. 1986; Tang et al. 1986). Typical CT appearances in a *T gondii* infection consist of multiple areas of nodule or ring-enhancement with a predilection for white matter, the corticomedullary junction or basal ganglia; areas of low density are present surrounding the lesions. Figure 9.2 shows a CT-scan from a 5-week-old child with a congenital *T gondii* infection, and Fig. 9.3 a CT-scan in an AIDS patient with cerebral involvement – before and after treatment (Cook 1987). Nuclear magnetic resonance imaging (NMR) will detect lesions which are not apparent on CT-scanning (Luft and Remington 1988); this technique will presumably be used far more in the future.

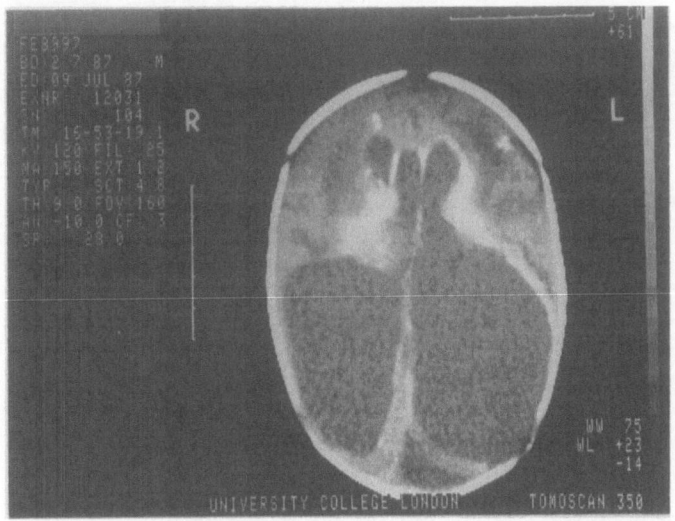

Fig. 9.2. CT-scan of a 5-week-old child showing very extensive intracerebral calcification and gross hydrocephalus with periventricular lucency. The diagnosis was congenital *T gondii* infection, which was confirmed by positive serology.

Serological Diagnosis

Serological events depend upon the type of individual at risk; laboratory details and the significance of the various test results have been carefully documented (Fleck and Kwantes 1980; McCabe and Remington 1983; Couvreur and Desmonts 1988).

Recent Infection in the Immunointact

ELISA or immunofluorescent antibody (IFA) techniques can be used to separate serum IgM from IgG (which increases approximately 2 weeks after infection and peaks within 1–2 months); specific IgM (which usually appears in the first week of illness) remains present for 2–3 months after onset of infection, and when present confirms the suspicion of an acute *T gondii* infection (Kwantes 1987). A rising Sabin–Feldman dye-test (DT)* titre is of value (very high titres (mainly representing *T gondii*-IgG) are attained in the acute glandular form of the disease (Bannister 1982)), but the concentration is frequently at its peak when the patient first consults a physician; a high titre (e.g. >250 iu) may persist for several years but is not diagnostic unless IgM is also present. The DT, complement fixation (CF) test using cuticular antigen, and IFA test measure the same antibody, and

---

*The DT, which remains the reference test, is difficult to carry out, and is performed only by a few specialist laboratories; it is dependent upon lysis of live *T gondii* parasites by the patient's antibody in the presence of complement, and does not separate IgG and IgM. Although almost specific for *T gondii* infection, this is not strictly so; *Hammondia hammondi*, a coccidian related both to *T gondii* and *Sarcocystis* sp exhibits some cross-reaction (Fleck and Kwantes 1980).

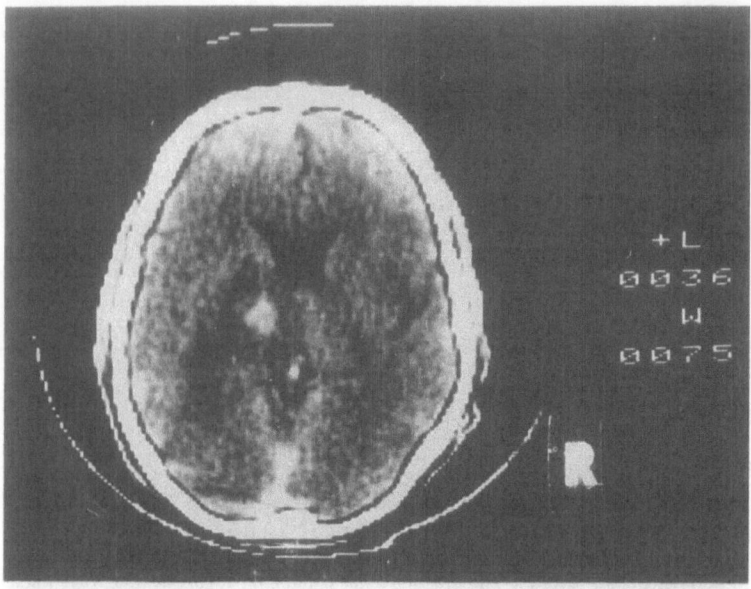

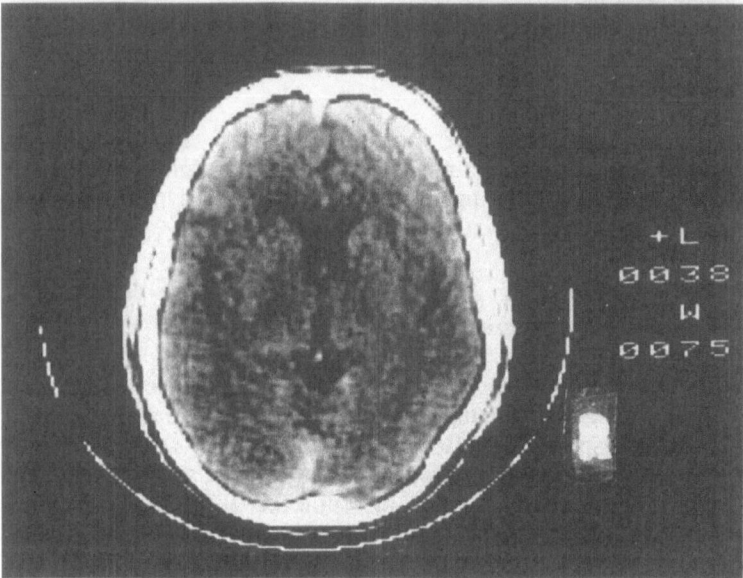

Fig. 9.3a,b. CT-scans in a man suffering from the acquired immune deficiency syndrome and an active intracerebral *T gondii* infection: **a** before, and **b** during chemotherapy (see text) (Cook 1987). Two 'mass lesions' are demonstrated in **a**. Lesions recurred at a later date despite continuing treatment.

maximum titres are achieved several weeks after the onset of infection (Kwantes 1987). Indirect haemagglutination (IHA) and a CF test which utilizes a soluble antigen measure a different antibody however; the titre may take several months to attain a maximum level, and the IHA usually exhibits a markedly later rise than the DT in acute disease (Bannister 1982). In summary, if the DT and IFA titres are elevated, and IHA and CF remain low, a *recent* infection is likely (Kwantes 1987).

Other tests which have been used include (Hall 1984; Manson-Bahr and Bell 1987): latex agglutination, direct agglutination, Indian ink immunoreaction, lymphocyte transformation to *T gondii* antigens (McCabe and Remington 1983), and a skin test (which is dependent on CMI, remains positive for only several months after an acute infection, but is of epidemiological value only (McCabe and Remington 1983; Frenkel 1984; Kwanted 1987)). A battery of serological tests was used in 27 previously healthy individuals who could accurately identify the date of onset of an acute *T gondii* infection (Welch et al. 1980); an IgM-IFA titre of >1 : 160 proved the best indicator of infection acquired during the previous 2–4 months, the DT gave an imprecise prediction of the date of infection, and the CF and HA were less useful.

An IgM-ELISA is now used by all three toxoplasma reference laboratories (Leeds, Swansea and St George's Hospital, Tooting) in England and Wales. Using 1500 clinical specimens, 100% specificity and 97% sensitivity has been claimed in the diagnosis of an acute *T gondii* infection using an IgM-ELISA (using an antibody capture technique) (Wielaard et al. 1983); IgM peaked within one month, and could be demonstrated up to an average of 8 months after onset of infection. *T gondii*-IgM antibody detection by ELISA (using antibody class capture) has been confirmed to be sensitive and specific (it is easily automated) in the diagnosis of acute infection (Payne et al. 1982; Joss et al. 1989). In addition to IgM, IgA antibodies to *T gondii* surface protein have been sought using a double-sandwich ELISA (Loon et al. 1983; Decoster et al. 1988); this seems valuable in the separation of acute from chronic cases of *T gondii* infection, and might have an important role both in pregnancy and in HIV-infected patients (see below).

Chronic Infection

In the UK almost all cases of *T gondii* choroidoretinitis result from infection in utero (Fleck and Kwantes 1980). Confirmation that choroidoretinitis has been caused by a previous *T gondii* infection is, however, often difficult or impossible; DT titres are usually only mildly elevated (e.g. 4–6 iu) (Bannister 1982). However, even a very low IgG antibody titre is confirmatory evidence of a presumptive diagnosis (Dutton 1984; Frenkel 1984). Detection of toxoplasma antibody in aqueous humour has been shown to be a valuable adjunct in the diagnosis of ocular involvement by *T gondii* (McCabe and Remington 1983; Dutton 1984). An Indian ink immunoreaction method has been compared with an IFAT for the diagnosis of ocular *T gondii* infection in Egypt (Safar et al. 1984); it proved specific, simple and rapid. Recrudescent disease may be accompanied by high, low or occasionally by absence of antibody (e.g. in the immuno-suppressed – see below).

Infection During Pregnancy

Ideally, IgM antibody should be sought every 3 weeks during pregnancy; a rising titre is significant (Manson-Bahr and Bell 1987). Seroconversion should be an indication for chemotherapy, and consideration of abortion (see below). [The presence of any IgG in maternal blood at the beginning of pregnancy renders complete foetal protection.] Serological results on antenatal specimens are similar to those already outlined (Joynson and Payne 1988); on the basis of their personal experience these authors concluded that there are 1200 acute maternal *T gondii* infections annually in the UK. However, if a history suggesting *T gondii* infection in pregnancy is elicited, the organism should be sought in placental tissue (by animal inoculation).

Congenital Infection

An elevated antibody titre in the presence of a compatible clinical history and physical signs (see above) is highly suggestive. It is important to distinguish between passive transfer of maternal antibody and actively acquired antibody (which includes IgM) (Manson-Bahr and Bell 1987). If *T gondii* antibody either rises or remains elevated for more than 6 months, diagnosis becomes definite; a 10-fold fall in IgG within 3 months indicates that the infant was not infected (Manson-Bahr and Bell 1987). A positive IgM-ELISA (which is highly sensitive and specific in the diagnosis of congenital *T gondii* infection) (Naot et al. 1981; Desmonts et al. 1988; Chatterton et al. 1989) strongly suggests an in utero *T gondii* infection; however, it is only present in cord blood in 25% of cases, and this finding can result from a placental 'leak' (antibody has a half-life of 3–5 days); a repeat sample from the *infant* should be examined to exclude this possibility (Kwantes 1987). A negative IgM does *not* therefore exclude congenital toxoplasmosis (Naot et al. 1981), and the IgG concentration should be measured serially (see above). The presence of IgG antibody alone at the age of even 8 or 12 months does not necessarily prove infection; this could still result from maternal transfer (McCabe and Remington 1983). An IgM-IFA test is of very limited use (Naot et al. 1981). Measurement of IgA antibody is of value in detecting an acute infection (see above) (Decoster et al. 1988). The value of prenatal diagnosis using foetal blood samples has been reviewed (Desmonts et al. 1985); in addition to IgM detection, blood and amniotic fluid was inoculated into mice, and serial foetal ultrasonography (to detect ventricular enlargement) carried out.

Infection in Immunocompromised Individuals (Including AIDS Sufferers)

Problems involved in the diagnosis of a *T gondii* infection in patients with AIDS have been reviewed (Cook 1987; Gerberding 1988). Ideally, parasite (tachyzoite) identification in stained tissue imprints should be obtained (Datry et al. 1984); it is necessary to identify *T gondii* in CSF, a brain-biopsy (Gerberding 1988), lung-biopsy or bone-marrow aspirate (Kwantes 1987). Failing this, attempts should be made to detect IgM antibody; the result, however, is unpredictable (see above) (Luft and Remington 1988; Heurkens et al. 1989). Whereas IgM antibody is rarely demonstrated in AIDS patients with *T gondii* encephalitis in the USA (Gerberding 1988), it is apparently detectable in 20% in France (Luft and Remington 1988); in the USA, less than one-third have elevated IgG antibody in serum but a much higher percentage in CSF. Detection of IgA antibodies (see above) might prove more valuable in the diagnosis of acute infection in AIDS patients (Decoster et al. 1988). Demonstration of space-occupying lesions using CT-scanning (Roué et al 1984) (see below) suggests a poor prognosis.

T gondii Antigen Detection

Detection of parasite antigens (which promises to be of great value in distinguishing acute from chronic infection) in serum and other body-fluids is not widely carried out (Hall 1984; Gerberding 1988; Heurkens et al. 1989); however, a number of reports have recently been made and when generally available, suitable tests will circumvent reliance on antibody detection (which may be absent in AIDS patients and others who are immunosuppressed (Löwenberg et al. 1983; McCabe and Remington 1983; Hirsch et al. 1984; Jehn et al. 1984; Heurkens et al. 1989), and who are infected with *T gondii* (Frenkel 1984)). An ELISA detected antigenaemia in 15 (65%) out of 23 serum samples from 22 patients who had recently had an acute *T gondii* infection (Araujo and Remington 1980); results in 28 and 55 serum samples from healthy and chronically infected patients respectively were all negative. Detection of *T gondii* antigens using a dot-immunobinding technique (Brooks et al. 1985) has given results which are initially encouraging; antigen could be detected in serum 2 days after infection in mice, and in CSF from four of six children with a congenital infection. Western blot analysis has shown that *T gondii* possesses several major antigens and antigenic components (Sharma et al. 1983; Weiss et al. 1988); this might have a value in distinguishing between tachyzoite and bradyzoite antigens, and probably explains much of the antibody diversity encountered in both acute and chronic infections. Preliminary studies have indicated that antigen detection in amniotic fluid and in CSF from newborn infants suffering from congenital infection is possible (Araujo and Remington 1980; Brooks et al. 1985). A method designed to detect *T gondii* antigen-containing complexes in active toxoplasmosis has been documented (Knapen et al. 1985); although this development should be treated with caution, it offers some hope.

Management

The major indications for chemotherapy are: (i) a *symptomatic* acute infection in an immunocompetent individual (see below); (ii) infection in all immunosuppressed individuals; (iii) where there is evidence of a foetal *T gondii* infection and/ or ocular involvement; and (iv) pregnant women in whom there is good evidence of recently acquired disease (McCabe and Remington 1983; Couvreur and Desmonts 1988). In addition, routine chemoprophylaxis prior to bone-marrow transplant has been suggested if there is evidence of a previous *T gondii* infection (Hirsch et al. 1984; Jehn et al. 1984; Ackerman et al. 1986). The presence of a high IgM antibody titre alone is *not* an indication for chemotherapy (Hall 1984). An acute symptomatic infection consisting of a pyrexial illness, severe malaise, widespread glandular involvement and/or myocardial and CNS involvement certainly warrants chemotherapy (Kwantes 1987); however, minor acute infections do not.

   Although the use of chemotherapy during pregnancy has for long been a matter of considerable controversy (due largely to potentially toxic effects of chemotherapy on the foetus), good evidence now exists that the dangers of *T gondii* infection (one-third of foetuses become infected) outweigh these problems (McCabe and Remington 1983). Good evidence also exists that treatment in utero diminishes the likelihood of congenital defects (McCabe and Remington 1983, 1988; Kasper and Kass 1988; McCabe and Remington 1988); furthermore, early treatment of the infected infant with sulphadiazine + pyrimethamine, which should continue for 6–12 months (Wilson et al. 1980; Kasper and Kass 1988) (whether or not signs are present), almost certainly reduces the incidence of undesirable late sequelae (McCabe and Remington 1983). In foetal and neonatal infection, recurrent choroidoretinitis is common (although the frequency of this complication is also reduced by chemotherapy). When good evidence exists for an initial infection *during* pregnancy (a high IgG titre in early pregnancy indicates a prior infection (see above)) – especially during the first trimester – abortion should be carefully considered; subsequent pregnancies are completely without risk. A chronic asymptomatic *T gondii* infection (in which there is a solitary elevation of IgG antibody) is a benign condition, unless immunosuppression ensues; recrudescence is then a significant possibility.

   Table 9.1 summarizes various chemotherapeutic regimens which have been used to treat a *T gondii* infection. Two chemotherapeutic regimens are now in general use (McCabe and Remington 1983; Manson-Bahr and Bell 1987): sulphadiazine (or occasionally another sulphonamide) + pyrimethamine (these two agents act synergistically (McCabe and Remington 1983; Kwantes 1987)) (Leport et al. 1988), and spiramycin. The former regimen is effective against actively multiplying tachyzoites, but *not* bradyzoites in tissue cysts (Luft and Remington 1988); chronic infections persist in most cases and this is an especial problem with AIDS encephalitis (Kwantes 1987; Manson-Bahr and Bell 1987),

Table 9.1. Some therapeutic regimens which have been used against *Toxoplasma gondii* infection in immunocompromised (including AIDS) patients (Cook 1987)

Chemotherapeutic agent (Tuazon et al. 1987; Wanke et al. 1987; Weller 1987)	Suggested dose regimen (often continued indefinitely)	Side-effects
Sulphadiazine + pyrimethamine	1–2 g ⎫ oral daily for 50 mg, qds ⎭ 4–6 weeks (+ folinic acid)	Bone-marrow depression, fever, rash, phlebitis, hypotension, abnormal liver function
Trimethoprim + sulphamethoxazole ('co-trimoxazole')	30 mg/kg ⎫ oral daily for 150 mg/kg ⎭ minimum of 3 weeks	(See text)
Clindamycin[a,b] (Tuazon and Labriola 1987)	2–4 g oral, daily (2–6 weeks)	Antibiotic-associated colitis
Spiramycin[b] (Leport et al 1986)	500–750 mg qds oral for 4–6 weeks	Gastrointestinal, epigastric pain acute colitis, contact dermatitis

[a]This antibiotic penetrates the blood–brain barrier poorly, and its ability to diffuse into cerebral tissue is unknown.
[b]These agents have been combined with pyrimethamine (25 mg daily) (Wanke et al. 1987).

although transient improvement has been reported (Gerberding 1988). Doses are: sulphadiazine 0.5–2.0 g (children 25–35 mg/kg) four times daily + pyrimethamine 75 mg (children 2 mg/kg) daily for 3 days, followed by 25 mg (children 1.0 mg/kg) daily for 4–6 weeks (Manson-Bahr and Bell 1987). Blood and platelet counts should be made twice-weekly (McCabe and Remington 1983; Kwantes 1987). Toxic side-effects are: bone-marrow depression, severe skin rashes, thrombocytopenia and leucopenia (Hakes and Armstrong 1983; Leport et al. 1988); these are reduced by folinic acid 5–15 mg (children 1 mg) daily (Frenkel 1984; Manson-Behr and Bell 1987).

Pyrimethamine is best avoided during the first trimester of pregnancy (Kwantes 1987) due to fears (almost certainly unwarranted) of teratogenicity (McCabe and Remington 1983; Gerberding 1988); after this, it is perfectly safe and its administration probably reduces the likelihood of a congenital defect (see below). In infants infected in utero, three or four courses of the combined regimen should be given during the first year of life; these can be alternated with spiramycin (see below).

Sulphadiazine + pyrimethamine is also the recommended chemotherapeutic regimen for CNS involvement (encephalitis) in AIDS patients (Leport et al. 1988; Luft and Remington 1988); however, because activity of this combination is limited to the replicating tachyzoite, a recrudescence after withdrawal occurs in approximately 80% of cases (Luft and Remington 1988). Good results have been recorded but life-long therapy is necessary (Leport et al. 1988); 14 (58%) out of 24 infections resolved completely. Sulphadiazine-induced crystalluria accompanied by renal impairment has been documented in an AIDS patient given this regimen (Sahai et al. 1988). A trimethoprim–sulphamethoxazole combination has been used unsuccessfully in cerebral *T gondii* infection after a bone-marrow transplant in a patient with aplastic anaemia (Emerson et al. 1981); however, sulphadiazine + pyrimethamine produced a cure.

The dose-regimen for spiramycin (a macrolide antibiotic)* (Luft and Remington 1988) is 500–750 mg four times (children 50–100 mg twice) daily for 4–6 weeks (Manson-Bahr and Bell 1987). This agent is virtually free of side-effects and has been widely used in France (Freukel 1984; McCabe and Remington 1988); it is not teratogenic and is also safe in the immunodepressed (including AIDS) patient. However, it does not cross the placenta freely and the foetal concentration is therefore low (Frenkel 1984); as a consequence, it probably does *not* reduce the incidence of congenital disease, and in this situation the sulphadiazine + pyrimethamine combination is more efficacious and should always be used (Kwantes 1987).

Peri-ocular clindamycin has been used for ocular involvement (Elliot et al. 1985). In the management of choroidoretinitis, corticosteroids (e.g. prednisolone 50–75 mg daily) may be indicated, but they must not be used without a chemotherapeutic 'cover' (see above) (Frenkel 1984); acute vitreous inflammation usually subsides within 5–10 days, and the dose can then be tapered rapidly. The value of spiramycin in the treatment of ocular lesions (Kwantes 1987) (and AIDS encephalitis (Luft and Remington 1988)) is limited.

Table 9.1 also lists some other chemotherapeutic regimens which have been used in AIDS patients (Cook 1987). Spiramycin (sometimes given in conjunction

---

*Although readily available in most countries, this agent is obtainable in the USA only by special request from the FDA.

with pyrimethamine) (see above) has been used but results overall are not encouraging (Leport et al. 1986). Clindamycin, given initially or as maintenance therapy alone or in combination with pyrimethamine (Rolston and Hoy 1987; Luft and Remington 1988; Rolston 1988), has also been used to good effect in CNS involvement in AIDS; however, clindamycin penetrates the blood–brain barrier poorly, and antibiotic-associated colitis is an occasional sequel (McCabe and Remington 1983; Frenkel 1984). A trimethoprim–sulphamethoxazole combination has not been adequately evaluated (Couvreur and Desmonts 1988). Other agents which have been tried include: roxithromycin (Rolston and Hoy 1987), trimetrexate (a dehydrofolate reductase inhibitor), arprinocid (6-amino-9-(2-chlorofluorobenzyl)-purine), γ-interferon (IFN-γ), and recombinant interleukin-2 (IL-2) (Luft and Remington 1988). The overall value of zidovudine in AIDS-associated infection has not been adequately assessed.

Anti-*T gondii* chemotherapeutic agents have been assessed experimentally (Nguyen and Stadtsbaeder 1985; Harris et al. 1988). 'Co-trimoxazole' has been compared with spiramycin in mice infected in mid-pregnancy; the former agent (which is contraindicated in pregnancy and the neonate in the UK and USA) was superior, and successful delivery and survival of offspring were both significantly greater (Nguyen and Stadtsbaeder 1985). In an in vitro study, pyrimethamine at high dose had a similar inhibiting effect to sulphadiazine + pyrimethamine at low dose, and spiramycin was effective only at high concentration and with prolonged incubation (Harris et al. 1988); clindamycin, methotrexate and difluoromethylornithine (given alone or in combination with sulphadiazine or pyrimethamine) were all ineffective; spirogermanium was effective, but only when a near toxic concentration was used; 5-fluorouracil was as effective – when combined with pyrimethamine – as high-dose pyrimethamine. There is an urgent need for new agents, especially in AIDS encephalitis (Luft and Remington 1988); whether γ-interferon will be useful requires careful study (McCabe and Remington 1988).

Prevention and Public Health Aspects

Prevention of a *T gondii* infection (which is crucially important in the previously uninfected pregnant woman) depends on avoidance of ingestion of oocysts (via contaminated soil), and tissue cysts (in infected undercooked meat) (Frenkel 1984; McCabe and Remington 1983; Couvreur and Desmonts 1988; McCabe and Remington 1988). Approximately 80% of women in the UK and USA have *not* been infected before their first pregnancy (see above); therefore strict hygienic standards and satisfactory cooking habits are extremely important (Frenkel and Dubey 1972). However, advice on elaborate hygienic rituals is unlikely to be widely accepted (Editorial 1989).

Cats become infected as soon as they start catching mice and birds; by 1–2 years old they are usually immune (Manson-Bahr and Bell 1987). Therefore attention to hand-washing after contact with cats – especially kittens (Frenkel and Dubey 1972) – is essential, especially in pregnancy; also contact with soil which should be assumed to be contaminated with cat faeces (oocysts remain viable for up to a year, or more) must be avoided. In a woman who has no anti-*T gondii* IgG in early pregnancy, complete avoidance of cats should in fact be recommended (Manson-Bahr and Bell 1987). Childrens' sandpits should always be covered when not in use, to prevent contamination by cat faeces; this also prevents deposition of dog faeces and the subsequent risk of *Toxocara canis* infection (Cook 1989). Serological testing of cats is of little or no value (Elliot et al. 1985), although widespread immunization has been recommended (Fleck and Kwantas 1980; Koppe et al. 1986). Tissue cysts remain viable in pork, mutton, goat (and other animal meat) for many days at room temperature (they are easily destroyed at 60–66 °C, and less effectively at −20 °C) (McCabe and Remington 1983; Couvreur and Desmonts 1988); pregnant women should therefore avoid all undercooked meat. Hands should be very carefully washed after handling meat in cooking (Frenkel and Dubey 1972); bradyzoites from tissue cysts on the skin are inactivated by soap and water, alcohol, and chemical disinfectants (Frenkel 1984).

Routine systematic screening of every pregnant woman would be necessary to detect all acute infections and to treat accordingly (Fleck and Kwantes 1980; Hall 1983; Couveur and Desmonts 1988; McCabe and Remington 1988); this is legally mandatory in France and Austria (McCabe and Remington 1983, 1988; Koppe et al. 1986), but not in the UK or USA. Alternatively, every woman should perhaps be screened before marriage (or the first attempt to become pregnant) (Koppe et al. 1986). Another recommendation is that a suitable serological test is applied on all pregnant women as soon as possible (certainly by 10–12 weeks gestation) to identify those at risk, i.e. if this has not already been carried out before pregnancy (McCabe and Remington 1983); those with a negative result should then be re-tested at 20–22 weeks, and this would allow sufficient time to either consider possible therapeutic abortion or for specific chemotherapy to be started; a third test would be performed near or at term in order to identify mothers and infants infected late in pregnancy and they could be treated. It is obviously essential that if/when introduced, testing is performed by a laboratory which is entirely reliable (McCabe and Remington 1983, 1988), otherwise needless abortions, in addition to missed cases of foetal infection, will occur.

There is no doubt, therefore, that prenatal diagnosis in the pregnant woman is feasible (Desmonts et al. 1985; Daffos et al. 1988); in addition to serological testing (see below), mouse inoculation with amniotic-fluid samples and foetal ultrasonography are of value. In the former study only one case of congenital *T gondii* infection was detected amongst 209 cases with a negative prenatal diagnosis. Recently, Daffos and his colleagues working in France (Daffos et al. 1988) have reported accurate prenatal identification of foetuses infected with *T gondii* in a large group of 746 women with a maternal infection; tissue culture from foetal blood and amniotic fluid, rather than mouse inoculation was used to establish the diagnosis, and in addition foetal blood was tested for *T gondii*-specific IgM and the foetal brain was also examined by ultrasonography. Out of 39 infections diagnosed in utero 24 were aborted and the remainder continued, these mothers being treated with spiramycin throughout pregnancy; if foetal infection was demonstrated, pyrimethamine + either sulfadoxine or sulphadiazine were added (McCabe and Remington 1983). Of the 15 foetuses born with congenital toxoplasmosis, all remained clinically well during follow-up except 2 who had choroidoretinitis. Ideally, therefore, this procedure should be adopted before a decision to abort is made; however, the linchpin to this approach consists of very careful serological screening to identify those at risk (see above) (McCabe and Remington 1988). Only by careful serial screening during pregnancy (as exists in France), will identification of 'at risk' women in pregnancy be possible in the UK.

The cost of antenatal testing has been an inhibiting factor (Joynson and Payne 1988); in 1984 the currently used blood test cost approximately £4.00, but the use of an IgM-ELISA on antenatal specimens collected for other tests would apparently have reduced this to £1.00 or less. In another assessment, two potential strategies for congenital toxoplasmosis prevention in the UK have been examined (Henderson et al. 1984): (i) a serological surveillance service (as above) followed by subsequent treatment; and (ii) a health education campaign to prevent acquisition of the infection during pregnancy. These authors consider that the latter approach is more likely to save resources, and advise further assessment of its potential effectiveness; however, they stress that there are many unknown factors, e.g. an uncertain overall prevalence, and the largely unexplored incidence of severe manifestations (both mentally and ophthalmologically) in the UK. If the problem in the UK is as common as experience in Scotland suggests (Williams et al. 1981; Chatterton et al 1989) (not all would agree (Fleck and Kwantes 1980)), the cost of setting up preventive programmes might well be justified (Wilson et al. 1980). In the USA, millions of dollars are needed each year to care for victims of toxoplasmosis (McCabe and Remington 1988). Government funding might be necessary for a major preventive strategy.

Although most infections in immunosuppressed individuals result from recrudescence of existing lesions, the wisdom of AIDS patients keeping feline pets (bearing in mind that *T gondii* encephalitis is invariably fatal) should perhaps be questioned.

The possibility of vaccine production is being addressed (Boothroyd et al. 1988); the possible use of *Salmonella* sp as a carrier of recombinant antigens is undergoing exploration.

Conclusions

T gondii infection produces potentially serious, and often lethal, consequences to the foetus and immunosuppressed individual (including those with AIDS). There seems little chance of eliminating the infection from the domestic cat population of the UK. More data are required on overall prevalence, and incidence of foetal abnormalities resulting from an in utero *T gondii* infection. The major problem in diagnosis centres on distinguishing a recent from a chronic infection (where tissue cysts and bradyzoites predominate), and this is especially difficult in AIDS. Serial screening of pregnant women who have not previously been infected (already mandatory in several other countries) should probably be introduced to the UK; continued production of infants with severe disabilities (which may not manifest for some years) is now completely unacceptable. As soon as an in utero infection is diagnosed a decision regarding effective chemotherapy (now known to be at least partially effective) or, alternatively, abortion must be made. Diagnostic methods have improved and *T gondii* antigen detection techniques offer advantages over older ones, especially in the immunosuppressed individual. Chemotherapy remains unsatisfactory; the regimens which offer the best (but by no means excellent) results are accompanied by significant side-effects, and newer agents are urgently required – this is especially so in AIDS patients, in whom *T gondii* infection is one of the most common 'opportunistic' infections.

References

Ackerman Z, Or R, Maayan S (1986) Cerebral toxoplasmosis complicating bone marrow transplantation. Israel J Med Sci 22:582–586

Ahmed HJ, Mohammed HH, Yusuf MW, Ahmed SF, Huldt G (1988) Human toxoplasmosis in Somalia. Prevalence of *Toxoplasma* antibodies in a village in the lower Scebelli region and in Mogadishu. Trans R Soc Trop Med Hyg 82:330–332

Araujo FG, Remington JS (1980) Antigenemia in recently acquired acute toxoplasmosis. J Infect Dis 141:144–150

Bannister B (1982) Toxoplasmosis 1976–80: review of laboratory reports to the Communicable Disease Surveillance Centre. J Infect 5:301–306

Benenson MW, Takafuji ET, Lemon SM, Greenup RL, Sulzer AJ (1982) Oocyst-transmitted toxoplasmosis associated with ingestion of contaminated water. N Engl J Med 307:666–669

Boothroyd JC, Nagel SD, Burg JL, Perelman D (1988) Molecular approaches to the study of *Toxoplasma gondii*. In: Leech JH, Sande MA, Root RK (eds) Parasitic infections. Churchill Livingstone, New York and Edinburgh, pp 259–269

Brooks RG, Sharma SD, Remington JS (1985) Detection of *Toxoplasma gondii* antigens by a dot-immunobinding technique. J Clin Microbiol 21:113–116

Chatterton JMW, Skinner LJ, Joss AWL, Ho-Yen DO (1989) Diagnosis of congenital toxoplasmosis in Scotland. J Infect 18:249–255

Cook GC (1987) Opportunistic parasitic infections associated with the acquired immune deficiency syndrome (AIDS): parasitology, clinical presentation, diagnosis and management. Q J Med 65:967–983

Cook GC (1989) Canine associated zoonoses: an unacceptable hazard to human health. Q J Med 70:5–26

Cook GC (1990) *Toxoplasma gondii* infection: a potential danger to the unborn fetus and AIDS sufferer. Q J Med 74:3–19

Couvreur J, Desmonts G (1988) Toxoplasmosis. In: MacLeod CL (ed) Parasitic infections in pregnancy and the newborn. Oxford University Press, Oxford, pp 112–142

Daffos F, Forestier F, Capella-Pavlovsky M, Thulliez P, Aufrant C, Valenti D, Cox WL (1988) Prenatal management of 746 pregnancies at risk for congenital toxoplasmosis. N Engl J Med 318:271–275

Darde ML, Bouteille B, Pestre-Alexandre M (1988) Isoenzymic characterization of seven strains of *Toxoplasma gondii* by isoelectrofocusing in polyacrylamide gels. Am J Trop Med Hyg 39:551–558

Datry A, Lecso G, Rozenbaum W, Danis M, Gentilini M (1984) Cerebral toxoplasmosis in AIDS: a simple laboratory technique for diagnosis. Trans R Soc Trop Med Hyg 78:679–680

Decoster A, Darcy F, Caron A, Carpron A (1988) IgA antibodies against P30 as markers of congenital and acute toxoplasmosis. Lancet ii:1104–1107

Desmonts G, Daffos F, Forestier F, Capella-Pavlovsky M, Thulliez P, Chartier M (1985) Prenatal diagnosis of congenital toxoplasmosis. Lancet i:500–504

Dubey JP, Beattie CP (1988) Toxoplasmosis in animals and man. CRC Press, Boca Raton, p 220

Dutton GN (1984) The diagnosis of toxoplasmosis. Br Med J 289:1078

Editorial (1989) Topical zoonoses. J Infect 18:105–110

Elkin CM, Leon E, Grenell SL, Leeds NE (1985) Intracranial lesions in the acquired immunodeficiency syndrome: radiological (computed tomographic) features. JAMA 253:393–396

Elliot DL, Tolle SW, Goldberg L, Miller JB (1985) Pet-associated illness. N Engl J Med 313:985–995

Emerson RG, Jardine DS, Milvenan ES, D'Souza BJ, Elfenbein GJ, Santos GW, Saral R (1981) Toxoplasmosis: a treatable neurologic disease in the immunologically compromised patient. Pediatrics 67:653–655

Fisher MA, Levy J, Helfrich M, August CS, Starr SE, Luft BJ (1987) Detection of *Toxoplasma gondii* in the spinal fluid of a bone marrow transplant recipient. Pediatr Infect Dis 6:81–83

Fleck DG, Kwantes W (1980) The laboratory diagnosis of toxoplasmosis. Public Health Laboratory Service monograph 13. Her Majesty's Stationery Office, London, p 20

Frenkel JK (1984) Toxoplasmosis. In: Strickland GT (ed) Hunter's tropical medicine, 6th edn. Saunders, Philadelphia, pp 593–605

Frenkel JK, Dubey JP (1972) Toxoplasmosis and its prevention in cats and man. J Infect Dis 126:664–673

Frenkel JK, Ruiz A (1980) Human toxoplasmosis and cat contact in Costa Rica. Am J Trop Med Hyg 29:1167–1180

Frenkel JK, Ruiz A (1981) Endemicity of toxoplasmosis in Costa Rica: transmission between cats, soil, intermediate hosts and humans. Am J Epidemiol 113:254–269

Gerberding JL (1988) Diagnosis and management of cerebral toxoplasmosis in patients with acquired immunodeficiency syndrome. In: Leech JH, Sande MA, Root RK (eds) Parasitic infections. Churchill Livingstone, New York and Edinburgh, pp 271–284

Hakes TB, Armstrong D (1983) Toxoplasmosis: problems in diagnosis and treatment. Cancer 52:1535–1540

Hall SM (1983) Congenital toxoplasmosis in England, Wales, and Northern Ireland: some epidemiological problems. Br Med J 287:453–455

Hall SM. The diagnosis of toxoplasmosis (1984) Br Med J 289:570–571

Harris C, Salgo MP, Tanowitz HB, Wittner M (1988) *In vitro* assessment of antimicrobial agents against *Toxoplasma gondii*. J Infect Dis 157:14–22

Henderson JB, Beattie CP, Hale EG, Wright T (1984) The evaluation of new services: possibilities for preventing congenital toxoplasmosis. Int J Epidemiol 13:65–72

Heurkens AHM, Koelma IA, Planque MM de, Polderman AM, Meer JWM van der (1989) Failure to diagnose fatal disseminated toxoplasmosis in a bone marrow transplant recipient: the possible significance of declining antibody titres. J Infect 18:283–288

Hirsch R, Burke BA, Kersey JH (1984) Toxoplasmosis in bone marrow transplant recipients. J Pediatr 105:426–428

Hutchison WM, Dunachie JF, Work K (1968) The faecal transmission of *Toxoplasma gondii*. Acta Pathol Microbiol Scand 74:462–464

Jehn U, Fink M, Gundlach P, Schwab WD, Bise K, Deckstein WD, Wilske B (1984) Lethal cardiac and cerebral toxoplasmosis in a patient with acute myeloid leukemia after successful allogeneic bone marrow transplantation. Transplantation 38:430–433

Joss AWL, Skinner LJ, Moir IL, Chatterton JMW, Williams H, Ho-Yen DO (1989) Biotin-labelled antigen screening test for toxoplasma IgM antibody. J Clin Pathol 42:206–209

Joynson DHM, Payne R (1988) Screening for toxoplasma in pregnancy. Lancet ii:795–796

Kasper DL, Kass EH (1988) Infectious disease rounds: toxoplasmosis in a premature infant. Rev Infect Dis 10:624–626

Knapen F van, Panggabean SO, Leusden J van (1985) Demonstration of *Toxoplasma* antigen containing complexes in active toxoplasmosis. J Clin Microbiol 22:645–650

Koppe JG, Loewer-Sieger DH, Roever-Bonnet H de (1986) Results of 20-year follow-up of congenital toxoplasmosis. Lancet i:254–256

Kwantes W (1987) Toxoplasmosis. In: Weatherall DJ, Ledingham JGG, Warrell DA (eds) Oxford textbook of medicine, 2nd edn. Oxford University Press, Oxford, 5.506–5.509

Lantos PL, McLaughlin JE, Scholtz CL, Berry CL, Tighe JR (1989) Neuropathology of the brain in HIV infection. Lancet i:309–311

Leport C, Vilde JL, Kathama C, Regnier B, Matheron S, Saimot AG (1986) Failure of spiramycin to prevent neurotoxoplasmosis in immunosuppressed patients. JAMA 255:2290

Leport C, Raffi F, Matheron S, KatlamaC, Regnier B, Saimot AG, Marche C, Vedrenne C, Vilde JL (1988) Treatment of central nervous system toxoplasmosis with pyrimethamine/sulfadiazine combination in 35 patients with the acquired immunodeficiency syndrome: efficacy of long-term continuous therapy. Am J Med 84:94–100

Loon AM van, Logt JTM van der, Heessen FWA, Veen J van der (1983) Enzyme-linked immunosorbent assay that uses labeled antigen for detection of immunoglobulin M and A antibodies in toxoplasmosis: comparison with indirect immunofluorescence and double-sandwich enzyme-linked immunosorbent assay. J Clin Microbiol 17:997–1004

Löwenberg B, Gijn J van, Prins E, Polderman AM (1983) Fatal cerebral toxoplasmosis in a bone marrow transplant recipient with leukemia. Transplantation 35:30–34

Luft BJ, Remington JS (1988) Toxoplasmic encephalitis. J. Infect Dis 157:1–6

Manson-Bahr PEC, Bell DR (eds) (1987) Toxoplasmosis. In: Manson's tropical diseases, 19th edn. Baillière Tindall, London, pp 207–212

McCabe RE, Remington JS (1983) The diagnosis and treatment of toxoplasmosis. Eur J Clin Microbiol 2:95–104

McCabe R, Remington JS (1988) Toxoplasmosis: the time has come. N Engl J Med 318:313–315

Naot Y, Desmonts G, Remington JS (1981) IgM enzyme-linked immunosorbent assay test for the diagnosis of congenital *Toxoplasma* infection. J Pediatr 98:32–36

Navia BA, Petito CK, Gold JW, Cho ES, Jordan BD, Price RW (1986) Cerebral toxoplasmosis complicating the acquired immune deficiency syndrome: clinical and neuropathological findings in 27 patients. Ann Neurol 19:224–238

Nguyen BT, Stadtsbaeder S (1985) Comparative effects of cotrimoxazole (trimethoprim-sulphamethoxazole) and spiramycin in pregnant mice infected with *Toxoplasma gondii* (Beverley strain). Br J Pharmacol 85:713–716

Nicolle C, Manceaux L (1909) Sur un protozoaire nouveau du Gondi. Arch Inst Pasteur (Tunis) 4:97–103

Nistal M, Santana A, Paniaqua R, Palacios J (1986) Testicular toxoplasmosis in two men with the acquired immunodeficiency syndrome (AIDS). Arch Pathol Lab Med 110:744–746

Paradisi F, Bartoloni A, Aquilini D, Roselli M, Nunez LE, Manzone G, De Majo E, Parri F (1989) Serological survey of toxoplasmosis in the Santa Cruz region of Bolivia. Trans R Soc Trop Med Hyg 83:213–214

Payne R, Isaac M, Francis JM (1982) Enzyme-linked immunosorbent assay (ELISA) using antibody class capture for the detection of antitoxoplasma IgM. J Clin Pathol 35:892–896

Peach W, Fowler J, Hay J (1989) Incidence of *Toxoplasma* infection in a population of European starlings *Sturnus vulgaris* from Central England. Ann Trop Med Parasitol 83:173–177

Pinkerton H, Weinman D (1940) Toxoplasma infection in man. Arch Pathol 30:374–392

Rolston KVI (1988) Clindamycin in cerebral toxoplasmosis. Am J Med 85:284

Rolston KVI, Hoy J (1987) Role of clindamycin in the treatment of central nervous system toxoplasmosis. Am J Med 83:551–554

Roué R, Debord T, Denamur E, Ferry M, Dormont D, Barre-Sinoussi F, Rouzioux C (1984) Diagnosis of toxoplasma encephalitis in absence of neurological signs by early computerised tomographic scanning in patients with AIDS. Lancet ii:1472

Ruiz A, Frenkel JK (1977) Isolation of *Toxoplasma* from cat feces deposited in false attics of homes in Costa Rica. J Parasitol 63:931–932

Ruiz A, Frenkel JK (1980a) *Toxoplasma gondii* in Costa Rican cats. Am J Trop Med Hyg 29:1150–1160

Ruiz A, Frenkel JK (1980b) Intermediate and transport hosts of *Toxoplasma gondii* in Costa Rica. Am J Trop Med Hyg 29:1161–1166

Sabin AB, Feldman HA (1948) Dyes as microchemical indicators of a new immunity phenomenon affecting a protozoon parasite (*Toxoplasma*). Science 108:660–663

Safar EH, Azab ME, Osman ZM (1984) Diagnosis of ocular and glandular toxoplasmosis using the Indian ink immunoreaction. Trans R Soc Trop Med Hyg 78:169–172

Saffer LD, Krug SAL, Schwartzman JD (1989) The role of phospholipase in host cell penetration by *Toxoplasma gondii*. Am J Trop Med Hyg 40:145–149

Sahai J, Heimberger T, Collins K, Kaplowitz L, Polk R (1988) Sulfadiazine-induced crystalluria in a patient with the acquired immunodeficiency syndrome: a reminder. Am J Med 84:791–792

Sharma SD, Mullenax J, Araujo FG, Erlich HA, Remington JS (1983) Western blot analysis of the antigens of *Toxoplasma gondii* recognised by human IgM and IgG antibodies. J Immunol 131:977–983

Tang TT, Harb JM, Dunne WM, Wells RG, Meyer GA, Chusid MJ, Casper JT, Camitta BM (1986) Cerebral toxoplasmosis in an immunocompromised host: a precise and rapid diagnosis by electron microscopy. Am J Clin Pathol 85:104–110

Teutsch SM, Juranek DD, Sulzer A, Dubey JP, Sikes RK (1979) Epidemic toxoplasmosis associated with infected cats. N Engl J Med 300:695–699

Tuazon CU, Labriola AM (1987) Management of infectious and immunological complications of acquired immunodeficiency syndrome (AIDS): current and future prospects. Drugs 33:66–84

Wanke C, Tuazon CU, Kovacs A, Dina T, Davis DO, Barton N, Katz D, Lunde M, Levy C, Conley FK, Lane HC, Fauci AS, Masur H (1987) *Toxoplasma* encephalitis in patients with acquired immune deficiency syndrome: diagnosis and response to therapy. Am J Trop Med Hyg 36:509–516

Weiss LM, Udem SA, Tanowitz H, Wittner M (1988) Western blot analysis of the antibody response of patients with AIDS and toxoplasma encephalitis: antigenic diversity among *Toxoplasma* strains. J Infect Dis 157:7–13

Welch PC, Masur H, Jones TC, Remington JS (1980) Serologic diagnosis of acute lymphadenopathic toxoplasmosis. J Infect Dis 142:256–264

Weller IVD (1987) Treatment of infections and antiviral agents. Br Med J 295:200–203

Wielaard F, Gruijthuijsen H van, Duermeyer W, Joss AWL, Skinner L, Williams H, Elven EH van (1983) Diagnosis of acute toxoplasmosis by an enzyme immunoassay for specific immunoglobulin M antibodies. J Clin Microbiol 17:981–987

Williams KAB, Scott JM, Macfarlane DE, Williamson JMW, Elias-Jones TF, Williams H (1981) Congenital toxoplasmosis: a prospective survey in the West of Scotland. J Infect 3:219–229

Wilson CB, Remington JS, Stagno S, Reynolds DW (1980) Development of adverse sequelae in children born with subclinical congenital *Toxoplasma* infection. Pediatrics 66:767–774

Wolf A, Cowen D, Paige B (1939) Human toxoplasmosis: occurrence in infants as an encephalomyelitis. Verification by transmission to animals. Science 89:226–227

Young R (1989) Postmen dogged by rise in canine attacks. The Times, London, 29 August, p 3

Chapter 10

Neurocysticercosis: Clinical Features and Advances in Diagnosis and Management

Pigs whose meat is tender have bladders which are like hailstones in the region of the thigh, neck and loin. If they are few in number, the meat is leaner; if there are many, the meat becomes soft and filled with serous fluid.

Aristotle (384–322 BC),
History of Animals

Introduction

Cysticercosis, which is probably the most common parasitic cause of neurological disease in man (Del Brutto and Sotelo 1988) (*Plasmodium falciparum* is the only serious contender), consists of infection by the larval stage (*Cysticercus cellulosae*) (McGreevy and Nelson 1984; Cook 1990) of the pig tapeworm *Taenia solium* (Cook 1988a). The disease was described in pigs by Aristophanes and Aristotle in the third century BC, and Paranoli is credited with the first human account (which involved the corpus callosum) in 1550 (Nieto 1982). The term *cysticercus* was first used by Laennec. One of the largest series of cases was documented in British soldiers and their families in India (Dixon and Lipscomb 1961); 92% of 450 affected individuals described by these authors had a history of epilepsy.

Although accurate information on prevalence rates is rarely available, the disease is known to be endemic in all continents with the exception of Australasia (Manson-Bahr and Bell 1987); however, even there cases are now being identified in immigrants. Exceptionally high rates exist in Latin America – from Mexico to Chile. In Mexico City 1.4%–3.6% of autopsies in the general population provide evidence of cysticercosis (McGreevy and Nelson 1984); the disease accounts for approximately 10% of neurological admissions, as well as up to one-third of craniotomies for intracranial space-occupying lesions. Important foci exist in the USSR, China, India, Pakistan, the Philippines and Indonesia

(Muller et al. 1987) (see below), and the disease occurs sporadically throughout Africa. Although now rare in northern Europe, it remains a problem in the Iberian peninsula and the Slavic countries. In North America, the disease was until recently fairly unusual; however, during the last decade it has become a significant problem in immigrant populations (Earnest et al 1987), and series of 127 and 238 cases of neurocysticercosis have recently been recorded at Los Angeles (McCormick et al. 1982; Scharf 1988). The disease is apparently being diagnosed with increased frequency in children at Los Angeles (Mitchell and Crawford 1988). Cysticercosis is overall unusual in Jews and Muslims because pork consumption in these ethnic groups is generally low; however, this fact does not prevent ingestion of *T solium* eggs in contaminated food or water. This fact, and not ingestion of uncooked pork, is the cause of human cysticercosis.

The highest prevalence rates therefore exist in communities where there is a close contact between man and pigs, and most importantly where hygienic standards and practices are low. Pork is of course also often eaten raw or is undercooked. Affected communities are often rural ones (Muller et al. 1987). Faecal contamination of foodstuffs is the usual source of infection; however, flies have been shown to play a part in the spread of *T solium* eggs. Cases caused by aberrant sexual practices and witch doctors have also been recorded. In Irian Jaya, an 'epidemic' of epilepsy which resulted in villagers suffering from extensive burns after falling into their domestic fires, had its origin in a gift of infected pigs from Bali. Recent examination of a random sample of 242 Ekari people in Irian Jaya revealed that 42 had palpable cysticercal nodules (Muller et al. 1987); 8 of them gave a history of fits and 6 of burns.

Parasitology and Pathogenesis

Man is the sole *definitive* host for adult *T solium* and is therefore the only source of eggs (McGreevy and Nelson 1984). Following ingestion of viable cysticerci in contaminated meat from the *intermediate* host (the pig) – 'measly pork' – the scolex (or head) (Šlais 1982) when digested out of the cyst attaches to the small-intestinal wall. Here, it grows into a mature tapeworm in 5–12 weeks and may live in the human small-intestine for up to 25 years; it is unusual (but not impossible) for more than one adult to be present simultaneously. The scolex anchors itself by means of four muscular suckers and a double row of hooklets which are present on the rostellum; the remainder of the worm (the strobila), which ultimately consists of up to 1000 proglottides or segments, varies from 2 to 10 metres in length, and may extend into the ileum. Gravid segments break off from the worm's distal end and may be swept out intact in faeces; alternatively, gravid segments disintegrate in the colon with the liberation of thick-walled eggs (31–43 μm in diameter) which after elimination in faeces may remain viable in soil for several weeks. The cycle is completed when eggs (via human faeces) are ingested by pigs with the eventual production of cysticerci in various organs, especially skeletal muscle. If human cannibalism both existed and was widely practised, this could theoretically play a significant role in the life-cycle. Treatment of *T solium* infection is with praziquantel, niclosamide, dichlorophen or mepacrine

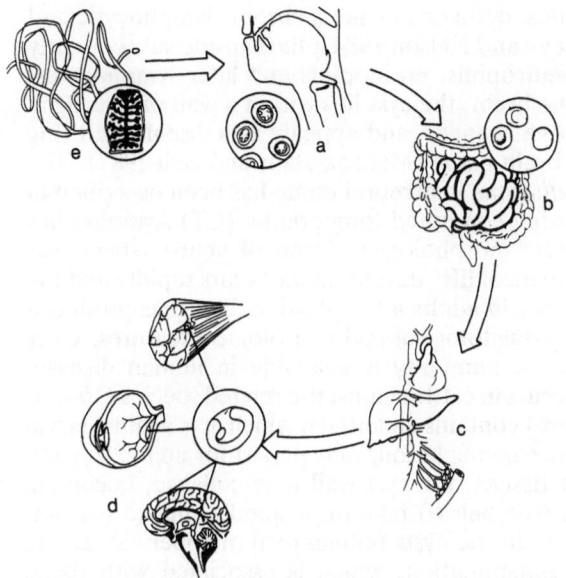

Fig. 10.1. Life-cycle of *Taenia solium* leading to cysticercosis. (a) Eggs (contained in food contaminated with human faeces) are ingested and swallowed by man (the definitive host); (b) eggs hatch in the small-intestine and the oncosphere emerges in the presence of bile-salts; (c) after penetration of the small-intestinal wall, oncospheres undergo haematogenous spread to all parts of the body, where they undergo development and growth, and transform to cysticerci; (d) cysticerci (approximately 10 mm at the widest point) lodge in many tissues, e.g. subcutaneous tissue, but more importantly muscle bundles, the eye and brain (neurocysticercosis); (e) adult *T solium* in the human small-intestinal lumen (this has originated from consumption of 'measly pork' containing cysticerci – in most cases by another human); this is the source of viable eggs (present within gravid proglottides). After indiscriminate defaecation the proglottides degenerate with liberation of free eggs which can contaminate foodstuff.

(McGreevy and Nelson 1984; Manson-Bahr and Bell 1987); some physicians follow chemotherapy with a laxative some 2 to 4 hours later to expel any residual *T solium* eggs.

Human cysticercosis arises when man becomes an incidental *intermediate* host (McGreevy and Nelson 1984). Figure 10.1 summarizes the life-cycle leading to cysticercosis. Eggs are ingested in food and water contaminated by human faeces. They begin to hatch in the stomach (the egg-wall is dissolved by gastric secretions) and the process is completed in the duodenum. Here, oncospheres emerge, penetrate the intestinal mucosa, and enter local lymphatics and mesenteric vessels. From here they are transmitted to many organs: central nervous system, skeletal muscles, heart, eye and oral cavity, etc., in addition to subcutaneous tissues. Within 2 to 3 months, the oncospheres lose their hooks and develop into fluid-filled 'bladder-worms' or cysticerci. External autoinfection can also give rise to cysticercosis, i.e. an individual harbouring an adult *T solium* may via his/her faeces produce a self-infection by the faecal–oral route. Although in theory internal autoinfection could result from a reversal of peristalsis, so that gravid proglottides would enter the stomach from the small-intestine (with subsequent hatching of eggs), this has never been proved and if it does occur is undoubtedly a rare event (Manson-Bahr and Bell 1987).

As they mature in various tissues, cysticerci evoke a chronic lymphocytic and granulomatous reaction (McGreevy and Nelson 1984); the capsule subsequently fibroses and is surrounded by neutrophils, eosinophils and later lymphocytes, plasma cells and giant cells. In the brain, the cyst lies within a wall of neuroglia which later undergoes degenerative changes, and appears as a discoloured ring which is walled off from normal brain tissue (Manson-Bahr and Bell 1987). The morphology of the scolex of *C cellulosae* in cerebral tissue has been described in detail (Šlais 1982). A study utilizing computed tomography (CT) scanning has produced evidence of two different morphological forms of neurocysticercosis (Flisser et al. 1988); in the early years of life, development occurs rapidly and the cysts have a similar appearance, but in adults a long-lasting disease is produced which is associated with diverse parasitological and neurological features. Only very limited evidence of protective immunity is available in human disease, despite some evidence that this occurs in cattle against the related species *C bovis*. The activated embryo (oncosphere) contains an antigen which acts against larval cysts in the tissues. These space-occupying lesions may persist for up to 20 years. In muscles and some other soft tissues, the cyst-wall may collapse, becoming flattened, and after calcification (see below) take on a spindle-shaped (or oat-shaped) form. However, in the brain the cysts remain oval or spherical. Dying cysts are surrounded by acute inflammation, which is associated with tissue damage. When dead, they either resolve or remain in situ and subsequently calcify (this may occur after 3 years, but takes much longer in the brain). As calcification occurs, symptoms usually subside and may disappear completely (see below).

Clinical Aspects

Presentation of disease is usually from 2 months to 30 years after infection (mean 5 years (Wiederholt and Grisolia 1982; Grisolia and Wiederholt 1982)); most individuals at presentation are aged 20–50 years. The initial symptom is usually awareness of small subcutaneous nodules or intramuscular swellings; a myositis may also be present; Fig. 10.2 shows a patient who had had many subcutaneous nodules removed by a highly motivated surgeon on the supposition that they were caused by an *Onchocerca volvulus* infection; in addition to the fact that he had not lived in a rural area which was endemic for that infection, histology showed that they actually resulted from *C cellulosae* infection. Every organ may be affected by this parasitosis; symptoms depend on the number, age and location of cysts. If neurological involvement does not occur, cysticercosis remains a benign disease. One estimate is that the brain is involved in 60%, and the eye in 3% of infections (Grisolia and Wiederholt 1982; Wiederholt and Grisolia 1982; McGreevy and Nelson 1984). Any part of the central nervous system can be involved; symptoms result in approximately 50% of cases. Fits, increased intracranial pressure and stroke are the commonest manifestations (Grisolia and Wiederholt 1982; McCormick et al. 1982; Wiederholt and Grisolia 1982; Case records of the Massachusetts General Hospital 1986; Earnest et al. 1987). Ten out of 11 cases recently documented in Indian children presented with features of raised intracranial pressure (Kalra et al. 1987).

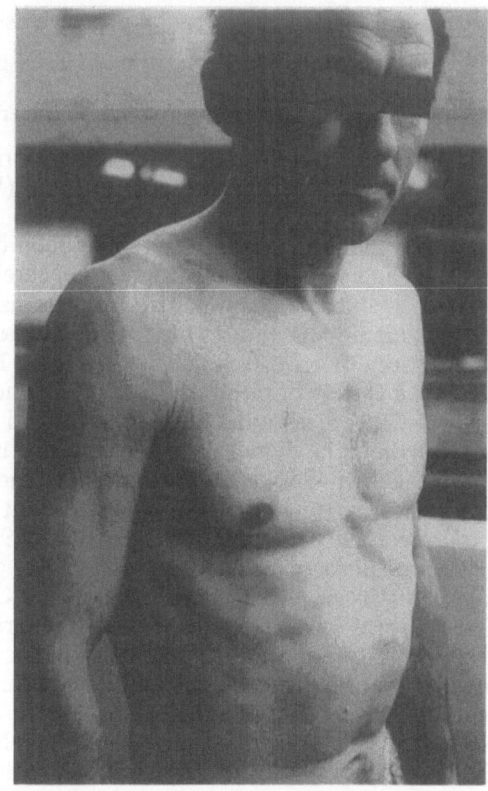

Fig. 10.2. A 48-year-old man who had had 84 subcutaneous swellings removed surgically on the supposition that they were caused by an *Onchocerca volvulus* infection (Chap. 12); serology for cysticercosis (CFT) was positive at 1:160, and histology and examination of one of them showed conclusive evidence of cysticercosis. He had previously worked for 22 years in Sudan and Uganda.

The possibility of neurocysticercosis should be considered in anyone suffering from fits who has resided in an endemic area (Manson-Bahr and Bell 1987). Clinical presentations in two large series of cases have recently been recorded at Los Angeles (McCormick et al. 1982; Scharf 1988). Although the classical presentation may be a mixed one (multiple cysts are present in over 50% of patients), clinical neurocysticercosis can be divided roughly into four main groups (Zenteni-Alanis 1982; McGreevy and Nelson 1984; Manson-Bahr and Bell 1987; Del Brutto and Sotelo 1988):

1. Parenchymal cysts. The subarachnoid space is involved in a high percentage of cases (Lotz et al. 1988). This is the most common state of affairs, and the cysts cause fits, acute or progressive focal abnormalities and raised intracranial pressure. Epilepsy is usually caused by fresh, live cysts, and may be either focal (Jacksonian) or general.

2. Meningeal cysts (subarachnoid involvement). These are often in the basal meninges and occur in approximately 50% of affected patients (often in conjunction with parenchymal cysts). There may be intense inflammation with obstructive hydrocephalus, arterial thromboses and stroke.

3. Ventricular cysts. These may be free-floating, or attached, and are most common in the fourth ventricle. They are found in approximately 15% of affected patients. They become symptomatic when they block the aqueduct of Sylvius,

and can cause raised intracranial pressure associated with severe headaches and vomiting.

4. Spinal-cord cysts. These are found in only 3% of cases, and cause arachnoiditis with transverse myelitis, or alternatively signs of a local mass lesion.

In addition, a rare widely disseminated form which consists of vast numbers of small cysts, has been reported from India (Wadia et al. 1988); this apparently carries a poor prognosis.

Clinical manifestations which have been described in another series of cases (Grisolia and Wiederholt 1982) include: cerebral infarction, ocular involvement, dementia, spinal arachnoiditis, thrombosis of superficial cortical vessels by chronic meningitis (and which give rise to 'cerebrovascular events'), and a hemisensory deficit. Korsakoff's psychosis, Parkinson's disease, motor neurone disease, a variety of pituitary fossa syndromes and isolated cranial nerve palsies have also been documented (Grisolia and Wiederholt 1982); cerebellar syndromes, diplopia, dementia, schizophrenia, manic-depressive disease, dysarthria and the Brown–Séquard syndrome are others (Dixon and Lipscomb 1961). In children an acute encephalitis may account for the initial clinical presentation (Rodriguez-Carbajal and Boleagu-Durán 1982; Earnest et al. 1987).

A particularly severe and aggressive type of disease is a racemose meningobasal form (Brown and Voge 1982; Rabiela-Cervantes et al 1982; Itabashi 1983; Case records of the Massachusetts General Hospital 1986); groups of cysts arborize into extensive grape-like clusters around the basal cisterns with the production of hydrocephalus and dementia. Ocular cysticerci float freely in the anterior and vitreous chambers, or adhere to subretinal tissue (McGreevy and Nelson 1984). The latter may cause papilloedema (Grisolia and Wiederholt 1982), haemorrhage and vasculitis of the disc. In the vitreous chamber, larvae may cause clouding, choroidoretinitis and retinal detachment. The lachrymal glands and eyelids may also be affected.

Idiopathic epilepsy, multiple intracranial space-occupying lesions, chronic meningitis, and other causes of raised intracranial pressure can be mimicked. Differential diagnoses also include: tuberculosis (especially tuberculomas), coccidioidomycosis, cryptococcosis, neurosyphilis, sarcoidosis, and primary and secondary malignancies involving the central nervous system (Grisolia and Wiederholt 1982; McGreevy and Nelson 1984). In certain tropical locations, the following should also be considered (Chap. 8): hydatidosis, angiostrongyliasis ('eosinophilic meningitis'), gnathostomiasis, paragonimiasis, schistosomiasis, filariasis, ascariasis and ancyclostomiasis (Grisolia and Wiederholt 1982; McCormick et al. 1982; Case records of the Massachusetts General Hospital 1986). The most common causes of death are status epilepticus and complications resulting from intracranial hypertension.

Diagnosis

History of exposure in an endemic area, even 30 years or more previously, is important. In an endemic area, neurocysticercosis is the most common cause of epilepsy in young adults. Family and friends, as well as the patient, occasionally have a current infection with *T solium*; faecal examination may then reveal eggs. The entire body should be palpated for subcutaneous and intramuscular nodules; a high 'index of suspicion' in an individual known to have been at risk is also very important (Cook 1988a). Definitive diagnosis depends on histological examination of a cysticercal cyst, which if subcutaneous can be excised under local anaesthesia. A fluid-filled opaque bladder 1 to 70 mm in diameter contains a single, solid, white sphere (the scolex) (Šlais 1982). A translucent membrane with a central 'milk spot' is characteristic; if alive, the parasite may evaginate its head and neck, or it may be induced to do so by immersion in hot saline (Manson-Bahr and Bell 1987).

In children, a skull-radiograph often shows sutural diastasis (Kalra et al. 1987). However, the 'hallmark' of neurocysticercosis radiologically consists of multiple elliptiform intracranial calcifications; a central calcified scolex surrounded by a calcified cyst wall is pathognomonic (Grisolia and Wiederholt 1982; McGreevy and Nelson 1984). Calcification does not, however, usually occur until at least 3 years after infection and often very much later. In one study, intracranial calcification was found in 36% of cases within 10 years of the presumed date of infection (Dixon and Lipscomb 1961); however, 97% already had calcification in skeletal muscles. Figure 10.3 shows multiple intracranial calcifications in the brain of an individual with neurocysticercosis, and Fig. 10.4 in the thigh muscles of a man heavily infected with cysticercosis. CT-scanning may reveal non-calcified cysts, and this is the most valuable radiological procedure (Grisolia and Wiederholt 1982; McCormick et al 1982; Earnest et al. 1987; Braconier and Christensson 1988; Dellen and McKeown 1988; Flisser et al. 1988; Sotelo et al. 1988; Woo et al. 1988; Agapejev et al. 1989). It is also of value in the widely disseminated form of the disease (Wadia et al. 1988). When present in the ventricles contrast-enhancement is usually necessary because cyst and cerebro-

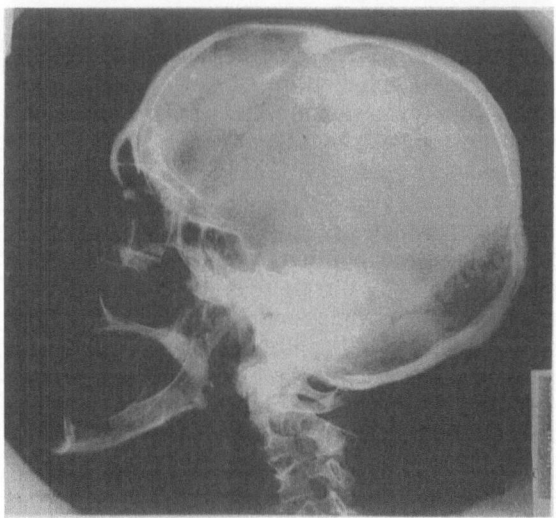

Fig. 10.3. Skull-radiograph of a man suffering from neurocysticercosis. Multiple areas of calcification are shown.

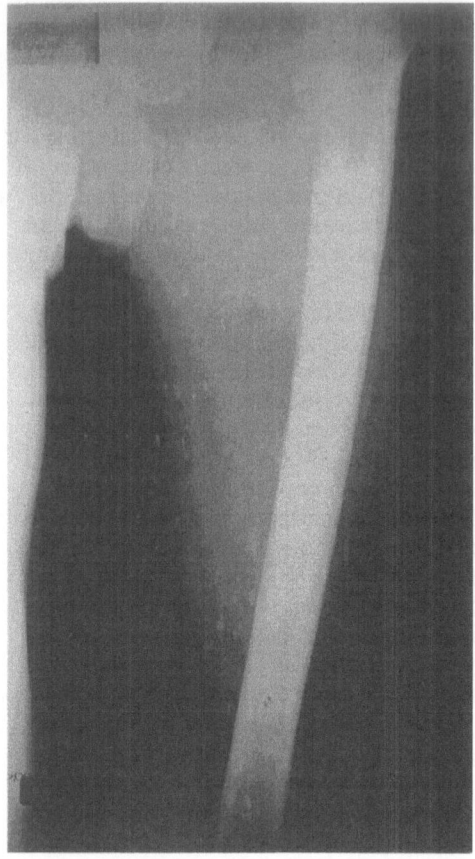

Fig. 10.4. Radiograph of the thigh of a man with cysticercosis involving the deep muscles. The calcifications are spindle-shaped, in contrast to the rounded or oval ones in the brain.

spinal fluid absorption values are similar (McGreevy and Nelson 1984). Angiography, isotope scanning, pneumoencephalography, ventriculography, electroencephalography and myelography occasionally yield abnormal results but these techniques have largely been replaced by CT-scanning (Grisolia and Wiederholt 1982; Rodríguez-Carbajal and Boleaga-Durán 1982). CT patterns in parenchymal disease can be summarized as: (i) small calcifications or granulomas; (ii) rounded areas of low density which are not enhanced by contrast medium; (iii) hypodense or isodense lesions surrounded by oedema and ring-like or nodular enhancement after administration of contrast medium; and (iv) diffuse brain swelling, associated with small lateral ventricles and multiple nodular ring-like areas of enhancement following contrast medium administration (Del Brutto and Sotelo 1988); the first of these various manifestations usually represents 'burnt-out' disease. A recent report from South Africa, documents a close correlation between appearances on nuclear magnetic resonance (NMR) imaging and histopathological features (Lotz et al. 1988); this technique proved highly effective, and the high degree of resolution allowed visualization of larval protoscoleces. The superiority of NMR for the localization of some intraventricular and subarachnoid cysts was also demonstrated in a study at Réunion (Bouilliant-Linet et al. 1988).

Although an eosinophilia, with or without an overall leucocytosis (Grisolia and Wiederholt 1982; McCormick et al. 1982; Earnest et al. 1987) is sometimes present, this is of little or no value diagnostically. The finding of *T solium* eggs in a faecal specimen is overall an unusual finding (McCormick et al. 1982). Cerebrospinal fluid pressure is occasionally elevated in neurocysticercosis (Grisolia and Wiederholt 1982). A pleocytosis of 5 to 500 cells or more, with either a lymphocyte or eosinophil predominance can occur but this is inconstant (Grisolia and Wiederholt 1982; McCormick et al. 1982; McGreevy and Nelson 1984; Earnest et al. 1987). Protein changes are non-specific; total protein and IgG may sometimes be elevated (Grisolia and Wiederholt 1982; McGreevy and Nelson 1984). A very low glucose concentration apparently carries a bad prognosis (McCormick et al. 1982; Earnest et al. 1987). Surgical biopsy is sometimes necessary for a definitive diagnosis (Grisolia and Wiederholt 1982).

Serology: Recent Advances

Immunodiagnosis has recently improved; although formerly unreliable (Espinoza et al 1982; Manson-Bahr and Bell 1987) it is becoming increasingly sensitive and specific (Cook 1988a). Widely divergent sensitivity of serodiagnostic tests has, however, been reported in different studies; these are due not only to the techniques used but also the characteristics of the patient populations and cyst viability (Schantz et al. 1988). Cross-reactions with hydatidosis, *Coenurus cerebralis*, and other tapeworms occasionally prove troublesome. Antigens from *C cellulosae*, *C bovis*, and adult tapeworms (*T solium* and *T saginata*) have all been used. Limited evidence suggests that antigen derived from cysticercal fluid possesses far greater reactivity than that from the cyst-wall (Baily et al. 1988). An indirect haemagglutination test has proved useful, but negative results certainly do not rule out active infection (Powell et al. 1966; Botero and Castano 1982; Grisolia and Wiederholt 1982; Wiederholt and Grisolia 1982).

An ELISA with sensitivity which varied between 61% and 79% was documented in 1982 (Diwan et al. 1982; Espinoza et al. 1982); however, cross-reaction with hydatid and schistosomal infections (and possibly angiostrongyliasis also) proved troublesome. A good deal of work has recently been carried out using an ELISA incorporating *C cellulosae* (and in some cases *T solium*) antigen, on both serum and CSF specimens, with generally good results. Whilst a group in Mexico considered in 1986 that serological tests for neurocysticercosis still lacked reliability (Rosas et al. 1986), this conclusion can no longer be widely upheld.

When antigen from *C cellulosae* fluid is available, the ELISA now produces results which are both sensitive and specific (Baily et al. 1988). Experiences of serum and CSF testing using and ELISA designed to detect IgG antibodies against *C cellulosae* and *T solium* antigens have been reported from Colombia (Ramírez and Pradilla 1987), Mexico (Corona et al. 1986; Espinoza et al. 1986; Téllez-Girón et al. 1987), and Durban, South Africa (Pammenter et al. 1987). In the Colombia report 89% and 93% sensitivity and specificity rates respectively, for detection of serum IgG antibodies against cysticercal antigen, were documented. In Mexico, comparable figures (87% and 90%) were reported for serum testing, with an 87% sensitivity and 100% specificity for CSF specimens (Corona et al. 1986); a significantly higher rate of sensitivity using both serum and CSF testing was reported in those whose disease ran a 'malignant' course ($P < 0.01$). In another study from Mexico, 85% and 90% sensitivity rates in serum and CSF, respectively, were recorded with specificity approaching 100% (Espinoza et al. 1986); humoral responses did not correlate significantly with the clinical and laboratory findings; IgM, IgA and IgE were detected less frequently. The dot ELISA-linked and the standard ELISA (for detection of *C cellulosae* antigen) have been compared using CSF specimens from 48 cases of neurocysticercosis; although both gave 100% specificity, sensitivity rates were only 59% and 77% respectively (Téllez-Girón et al. 1987). Examination of both serum and CSF from the same individual has been advocated (Pammenter et al. 1987); when both specimens were analysed, 87% of 212 patients with neurocysticercosis could be diagnosed serologically, but when using CSF alone this rate fell to 67%. Using an ELISA incorporating any one of three monoclonal antibodies generated from mice immunized with *C cellulosae* scolex protein antigen, 100% positivity was reported on serum samples in a study from São Paulo, Brazil (Nascimento et al. 1987). Hybridoma-derived reagents for use with larval cestodes might also prove valuable in the future (Manson-Bahr and Bell 1987).

Management: Chemotherapy or Surgery?

Until 1979 the only form of treatment for this disease was surgical (Botero and Castaño 1982). Since then chemotherapy has produced generally encouraging results and these have been reviewed (Cook 1988a,b). Experimental work using electron-microscopy demonstrated that praziquantel (prazinoisoquinolone) can destroy the tegument along the whole pseudostrobila and the scolex of the related species *C fasciolaris* (Thomas et al. 1982); furthermore using ^{14}C-praziquantel, penetration of the cyst-wall and death of the cysticercus was apparent. Assessment of the efficacy of chemotherapy can be evaluated in vivo by CT-scanning (McCormick et al. 1982) in conjunction with serial measurement of serum antibody titres against cysticercal antigen (Botero and Castaño 1982; Groll 1982; Markwalder et al. 1984). Early clinical trials using this agent in cysticercosis were carried out in Mexico, Colombia, Chile, Brazil and South Korea (Groll 1982); dosage varied from 5–10 to 75 mg/kg daily, with an overall total dose ranging from 45–60 to 1050 mg/kg. Satisfactory results were reported in 172 out of 192 cases of neurocysticercosis. In a study in Colombia, 31 cases of neurocysticercosis (14 had previously undergone surgery) were treated with praziquantel combined with prednisolone (Botero and Castaño 1982); only one patient died, and this contrasted with a 50%–80% fatality rate in a group of 'historical' controls observed at the same institution. In another early assessment, 20 out of 40 cases of the disease treated at São Paulo received dexamethasone in addition to praziquantel (Spina-França et al. 1982); the authors concluded that by reducing inflammatory phenomena 'the administration of corticosteroids alongside praziquantel is highly indicated'. Whether the addition of a corticosteroid is beneficial was, however, unclear from these early studies (see below).

   Several subsequent reports involved either single or very small numbers of cases (deGhetaldi et al. 1983; Markwalder et al. 1984; Case records of the Massachusetts General Hospital 1986; Norman and Kapadia 1986; Binstock et al. 1987; Pascoe et al. 1987; Schwartz et al. 1987; Braconier and Christensson 1988;

Baily and Levy 1989) and, although most results have been encouraging overall, they are difficult to evaluate accurately. Praziquantel is not without side-effects, however. The most frequent problem has been the *CSF reaction syndrome*; this is characterized by fever, headache, meningismus, and exacerbation of many of the neurological symptoms of the disease. It is considered to be caused by an inflammatory reaction to dead and dying larvae, possibly analogous to the Jarisch–Herxheimer reaction (Case records of the Massachusetts General Hospital 1986). Simultaneous administration of corticosteroids has produced encouraging results in prevention and/or attenuation of this reaction (Spina-França 1982; deGhetaldi et al. 1983; Dellen and McKeown 1988; Norman and Kapadia 1986) (see below).

The first large series of cases to be treated with praziquantel *without* a corticosteroid 'cover' was published as recently as 1984 from Mexico (Sotelo et al. 1984a). Twenty-six patients were treated with 50 mg praziquantel/kg daily for 15 days; after 3 months all had improved clinically and 13 were asymptomatic. Furthermore, the total number of cysts, which was 152 at the beginning of treatment, had reduced to 51 with a reduction in mean diameter by 72%; CT-scans showed improvement in 25 cases, and total remission of cysts in nine. An inflammatory reaction (see above) was common however (and involved 92%); both protein and cell concentrations in CSF increased during treatment. In 17 untreated 'historical' controls followed for a mean of 9 months, CT-scans showed either no change or worsening of disease. A further large group of 141 patients with neurocysticercosis treated with praziquantel 50 mg/kg daily (approximately half of them also received prednisolone 30 mg daily) has been recorded (Robles et al. 1987); 75 of them were subsequently considered cured (they were asymptomatic after 5 years and their cysts or nodules had either disappeared or had calcified), while 35 showed both clinical and radiological improvement. However, intraventricular cysts in 5 of them had to be removed surgically (being unaffected by praziquantel), and 31 were unchanged or had actually worsened. Failure of intraventricular cysts to improve was considered to be due to an inadequate concentration of praziquantel in the CSF.

An attempt has recently been made from experience obtained in treating 40 patients to delineate the indications for use of praziquantel (50 mg/kg daily for 15 and, in severe cases, 30 days) in neurocysticercosis (Vasconcelos et al. 1987); these authors concluded that the groups which should be treated with this chemotherapeutic agent are those with: (i) active cerebral cysticercosis (with cysts in the brain parenchyma or subarachnoid space); (ii) cysts in brain parenchyma, subarachnoid space and the ventricular system; and (iii) miliary cysticercosis (in which many cysts will be too small to be detected by CT-scanning). Those with cysts solely within the ventricular system should probably always be treated surgically, and *not* with praziquantel alone; group (ii) patients might also require surgery later.

Although still a controversial matter, nearly all physicians now strongly favour the addition of a corticosteroid 'cover' to reduce the incidence of the CSF reaction syndrome (Ciferri 1984; deGhetaldi et al. 1984; Sotelo et al. 1984b; Case records of the Massachusetts General Hospital 1986; Worthington and Horowitz 1987); either dexamethasone or prednisolone should be given before and during praziquantel treatment. Recommended dosage is 30–40 mg prednisolone, or 12–16 dexamethasone daily (Ciferri 1984; Sotelo et al. 1984b; Worthington and Horowitz 1987). Del Brutto and Sotelo (1988), however, consider that dexamethasone should only be given when intracranial hypertension develops during therapy; these authors cite evidence that simultaneous administration of a corticosteroid significantly reduces the plasma praziquantel concentration. Another group of physicians considers that praziquantel administration without corticosteroids becomes increasingly hazardous as neurocysticercosis becomes progressively severe (and advanced) (deGhetaldi et al. 1984). In widely disseminated disease praziquantel + corticosteroids were given to 3 patients in India; this regimen proved valueless, however, and they all died (Wadia et al. 1988).

Recently, albendazole (15 mg/kg body-weight daily for 1 month) has been used in seven patients with neurocysticercosis (two had previously shown partial response to praziquantel) (Escobedo et al. 1987); when treatment was begun, 157 cysts were delineated by CT-scanning and at 3 months after treatment the number was 22, i.e. an 86% reduction. In the two patients who had previously received praziquantel, there was a 100% and 77% response respectively to albendazole. This early evidence is impressive but much larger numbers are obviously required before a valid conclusion can be drawn. In a recent prospective, controlled randomized study, albendazole has been compared with praziquantel in 20 patients while a further five were used as controls (Sotelo et al. 1988); after 3 months, 76% and 73% cyst-remission rates in those treated with a single course of albendazole and praziquantel respectively was demonstrated using CT-scanning. However, an exacerbation of neurological lesions similar to those after praziquantel has been documented, and simultaneous corticosteroid administration is then necessary (Del Brutto and Sotelo 1988). Albendazole (15 mg/kg daily for 21 days, followed after a 7-day interval by 20–30 mg/kg daily for 30 days) has been combined with dextrochloropheniramine (a potent anti-histamine with good CNS penetration) (18 mg daily for at least 4–6 months) in a clinical trial at São Paulo, Brazil (Agapejev et al. 1989); this combination produced promising results but it is unclear whether it has any advantages over albendazole when given alone. Limited use of flubendazole (another benzimidazole compound) has also been documented (Earnest et al. 1987). A further potentially useful chemotherapeutic agent is metriphonate (Trujillo-Valdés et al. 1982); 93 patients suffering from neurocysticercosis were given 7.5 mg/kg body-weight daily for 5 consecutive days. Assessment by CT-scanning and immunological response indicated a satisfactory outcome at between 6 months and 10 years in approximately 80%. Here too, further evidence from large (preferably controlled) studies is required.

In certain situations, especially when CSF pressure is significantly raised, surgery is, however, still the major line of treatment (Grisolia and Wiederholt 1982; Escobedo et al. 1982; McCormick et al 1982; Wiederholt and Grisolia 1982; McGreevy and Nelson 1984; Earnest et al. 1987; Robles et al. 1987; Del Brutto and Sotelo 1988); this applies to several groups. Cases in which intracranial hypertension is associated with intraventricular cysts and hydrocephalus, and in which cysticerci are localized to the chiasma with an inflammatory reaction and adhesive arachnoiditis, fall into this category (Escobedo et al. 1982). Removal of intraventricular (especially when freely mobile) or spinal cysts may also be required (Earnest et al. 1987). Surgery also continues to be important in the treatment of cysts which do not respond to chemotherapy (Robles et al. 1987; Vasconcelos et al. 1987). Ventricular, ventriculoperitoneal or other types of shunting are occasionally required (Wiederholt and Grisolia 1982). Treatment with high-dose corticosteroids is probably indicated before chemotherapy in patients with spinal cord involvement.

One report, from Los Angeles, suggests that in children intraparenchymal cysts are usually 'benign' and do not require active chemotherapy (Mitchell and Crawford 1988). The racemose meningobasal form still carries a poor prognosis; it can be complicated by right internal carotid artery occlusion (Bia and Barry 1986). Sudden death may occur when obstructive hydrocephalus develops rapidly.

Control

Prophylaxis (and control) centres on improved public health measures. Man is the sole definitive host; therefore health education is of paramount importance (McGreevy and Nelson 1984); indiscriminate human defaecation must be strongly discouraged and sewage should be treated to kill *T solium* eggs. Husbandry practices must also be improved so that pigs do not wander widely and consume human faeces. The source of human infection with adult *T solium* is infected pork; cysticerci in meat can be killed by freezing at -20 °C for 12 hours, or by cooking at 50 °C. Careful inspection of pork is obviously of value. Whenever a *T solium* infection is diagnosed in man, it should be treated with the appropriate anti-parasite agent(s) (see above); furthermore, family members and close contacts should be investigated for the presence of infection, and treated accordingly.

In Mexico, antibodies which might be protective are present in 50% of affected individuals (Flisser et al. 1979). This suggests that human vaccination might theoretically be possible in high-risk areas. Therefore, in areas with a high prevalence of neurocysticercosis, and where rearing of pigs is still uncontrolled in rural areas and human defaecation remains indiscriminate, this possibility is worthy of serious consideration (Larralde et al. 1982).

Conclusions

Neurocysticercosis remains a major world-wide health problem and accounts for numerous neurological presentations and hospital admissions. An especially high 'index of suspicion' for this disease is required when dealing with neurological problems in individuals who have lived in or visited areas where the disease is common. Where and when *C cellulosae* (preferably fluid) antigen is available, serological testing (using an ELISA) is now both sensitive and specific in the diagnosis of active neurocysticercosis. Treatment has been revolutionized by the advent of effective chemotherapy; praziquantel (50 mg/kg daily for 14–15 days) has been shown to be of overall value (placebo-controlled trials would not now be ethically justified), but albendazole and metriphonate have not been adequately evaluated. When epilepsy persists after a full course of chemotherapy, a second course given up to 6 months after the first often achieves success. There can now be no doubt that a corticosteroid 'cover' should be added to any chemotherapeutic regimen for active neurocysticercosis. Nevertheless, surgery is still indicated in certain situations, especially when the ventricular system is involved, and intracranial hypertension is present. Prognosis has therefore improved substantially since the introduction of chemotherapy; long-term anti-epileptic agents are now rarely necessary. Complications of surgical (including shunting) procedures, such as meningitis are now unusual (Wiederholt and Grisolia 1982), but disease involving the ventricular system must always be viewed seriously (Escobedo et al. 1982; McCormick et al. 1982; Earnest et al. 1987). Extirpation of basilar cysticerci (McCormick et al. 1982) still carries a significant mortality rate.

References

Agapejev S, Meira DA, Barraviera B, Machado JM, Pereira PCM, Mendes RP, Kamegasawa A, Ueda AK (1989) Neurocysticercosis: treatment with albendazole and dextrochloropheniramine. Trans R Soc Trop Med Hyg 83:377–383

Baily GG, Levy LF (1989) Racemose cysticercosis treated with praziquantel. Trans R Soc Trop Med Hyg 83:95–96

Baily GG, Mason PR, Trijssenar FEJ, Lyons NF (1988) Serological diagnosis of neurocysticercosis: evaluation of ELISA tests using cyst fluid and other components of *Taenia solium* cysticerci as antigens. Trans R Soc Trop Med Hyg 82:295–299

Bia FJ, Barry M (1986) Parasitic infections of the central nervous system. Neurol Clin 4:171–206

Binstock PD, Azimi PH, Williams RA (1987) Cerebral cysticercosis in a 22-month-old infant. Am J Clin Pathol 88:655–658

Botero D, Castaño S (1982) Treatment of cysticercosis with praziquantel in Colombia. Am J Trop Med Hyg 31:811–821

Bouilliant-Linet E, Brugières P, Coubes P, Gaston A, Laporte P, Marsault C (1988) Cysticercose cérébrale: intérêt diagnostique de la scanographie. A propos de 117 observations. J Radiol 69:405–412

Braconier JH, Christensson B (1988) Cerebral cysticercosis successfully treated with praziquantel. Scand J Infect Dis 20:105–108

Brown WJ, Voge M (1982) Neuropathology of parasitic infections. Oxford University Press, Oxford, p 240

Case records of the Massachusetts General Hospital (1986) Case 11, 1986: cerebral cysticercosis. N Engl J Med 314:767–774

Ciferri F (1984) Praziquantel for cysticercosis of the brain parechyma. N Engl J Med 311:733

Cook GC (1988a) Neurocysticercosis: parasitology, clinical presentation, diagnosis, and recent advances in management. Q J Med 68:575–583

Cook GC (1988b) Chemotherapy of parasitic infections. Curr Opin Infect Dis 1:423–438

Cook GC (1990) Protozoan and helminthic infections of the central nervous system. In: Kass EH, Weller TH, Wolff SM, Tyrrell DAJ (eds) Handbook of infectious diseases. B.C. Decker, Toronto (in press)

Corona T, Pascoe D, González-Barranco D, Abad P, Landa L, Español B (1986) Anticysticercous antibodies in serum and cerebrospinal fluid in patients with cerebral cysticercosis. J Neurol Neurosurg Psychiatr 49:1044–1049

deGhetaldi LD, Norman RM, Douville AW (1983) Cerebral cysticercosis treated biphasically with dexamethasone and praziquantel. Ann Intern Med 99:179–181

deGhetaldi LD, Norman RM, Douville AW (1984) Praziquantel for cysticercosis of the brain parenchyma. N Engl J Med 311:732–733

Del Brutto OH, Sotelo J (1988) Neurocysticercosis: an update. Rev Infect Dis 10:1075–1087

Dellen JR van, McKeown CP (1988) Praziquantel (pyrazinoisoquinolone) in active cerebral cysticercosis. Neurosurgery 22:92–96

Diwan AR, Coker-Vann M, Brown P, Subianto DB, Yolken R, Desowitz R, Escobar A, Gibbs CJ, Gajdusek C (1982) Enzyme-linked immunosorbent assay (ELISA) for the detection of antibody to cysticerci of *Taenia solium*. Am J Trop Med Hyg 31:364–369

Dixon HBF, Lipscomb FM (1961) Cysticercosis: an analysis and follow-up of 450 cases. Medical Research Council, London, p 58 (Special report series 299)

Earnest MP, Reller LB, Filley CM, Grek AJ (1987) Neurocysticercosis in the United States: 35 cases and a review. Rev Infect Dis 9:961–979

Escobedo F, González-Mariscal G, Revuelta R, Ruben M (1982) Surgical treatment of cerebral cysticercosis. In: Flisser A, Willms K, Laclette JP, Larralde C, Ridaura C, Beltran F (eds) Cysticercosis: present state of knowledge and perspectives. Academic Press, New York, pp 201–205

Escobedo F, Penagos P, Rodriguez J, Sotelo J (1987) Albendazole therapy for neurocysticercosis. Arch Intern Med 147:738–741

Espinoza B, Flisser A, Plancarte A, Larralde C (1982) Immunodiagnosis of human cysticercosis: ELISA and immunoelectrophoresis. In: Flisser A, Willms K, Laclette JP, Larralde C, Ridaura C, Beltran F (eds) Cysticercosis: present state of knowledge and perspectives. Academic Press, New York, pp 163–178

Espinoza B, Ruiz-Palacios G, Tovar A, Sandoval MA, Plancarte A, Flisser A (1986) Characterization by enzyme-linked immunosorbent assay of the humoral immune response in patients with neurocysticercosis and its application in immunodiagnosis. J Clin Microbiol 24:536–541

Flisser A, Pérez-Montfort R, Larralde C (1979) The immunology of human and animal cysticercosis: a review. Bull WHO 57:839–856

Flisser A, Madrazo I, Gonzalez D, Sandoval M, Rodriguez-Carbajal J, De-Dios J (1988) Comparative analysis of human and porcine neurocysticercosis by computed tomography. Trans R Soc Trop Med Hyg 82:739–742

Grisolia JS, Wiederholt WC (1982) CNS cysticercosis. Arch Neurol 39:540–544

Groll EW (1982) Chemotherapy of human cysticercosis with praziquantel. In: Flisser A, Willms K, Laclette JP, Larralde C, Ridaura C, Beltran F (eds) Cysticercosis: present state of knowledge and perspectives. Academic Press, New York, pp 207–218

Itabashi HH (1983) Pathology of CNS cysticercosis. Bull Clin Neurosci 48:6–17

Kalra V, Paul VK, Marwah RK, Kochhar GS, Bhargava S (1987) Neurocysticercosis in childhood. Trans R Soc Trop Med Hyg 81:371–373

Larralde C, Flisser A, Pérez-Montfort R (1982) Vaccination against cysticercosis: perspectives on the immunological prevention of human disease. In: Flisser A, Willms K, Laclette JP, Larralde C, Ridaura C, Beltran F (eds) Cysticercosis: present state of knowledge and perspectives. Academic Press, New York, pp 675–684

Lotz J, Hewlett R, Alheit B, Bowen R (1988) Neurocysticercosis: correlative pathomorphology and MR imaging. Neuroradiology 30:34–41

Manson-Bahr PEC, Bell DR (eds) (1987) In: Manson's tropical diseases, 19th edn. Baillière Tindall, London, pp 527–529, 536–540

Markwalder K, Hess K, Valavanis A, Witassek F (1984) Cerebral Cysticercosis: treatment with praziquantel. Report of two cases. Am J Trop Med Hyg 33:273–280

McCormick GF, Zee C-S, Heiden J (1982) Cysticercosis cerebri: review of 127 cases. Arch Neurol 39:534–539

McGreevy PB, Nelson GS (1984) Cysticercosis. In: Strickland GT (ed) Hunter's tropical medicine, 6th edn. Saunders, Philadelphia, pp 783–786

Mitchell WG, Crawford TO (1988) Intraparenchymal cerebral cysticercosis in children: diagnosis and treatment. Pediatrics 82:76–82

Muller R, Lillywhite J, Bending JJ, Catford JC (1987) Human cysticercosis and intestinal parasitism amongst the Ekari people of Irian Jaya. J Trop Med Hyg 90:291–296

Nascimento E, Tavares CA, Lopes JD (1987) Immunodiagnosis of human cysticercosis (Taenia solium) with antigens purified by monoclonal antibodies. J Clin Microbiol 25:1181–1185

Nieto D (1982) Historical notes on cysticercosis. In: Flisser A, Willms K, Laclette JP, Larralde C, Ridaura C, Beltran F (eds) Cysticercosis: present state of knowledge and perspectives. Academic Press, New York, pp 1–7

Norman RM, Kapadia C (1986) Cerebral cysticercosis: treatment with praziquantel. Pediatrics 78:291–294

Pammenter MF, Rossouw EJ, Epstein SR (1987) Diagnosis of neurocysticercosis by enzyme-linked immunosorbent assay. S Afr Med J 71:512–514

Pascoe M, Lyall I, Saines N, Nolan C (1987) Cerebral cysticercosis: a case report with particular reference to recent advances in diagnosis and treatment. Aust NZ J Med 17:55–57

Powell SJ, Proctor EM, Wilmot AJ, MacLeod IN (1966) Cysticercosis and epilepsy in Africans: a clinical and serological study. Ann Trop Med Parasitol 60:152–158

Rabiela-Cervantes MT, Rivas-Hernández A, Rodríguez-Ibarra J, Castillo-Medina S, Cancino F de M

(1982) Anatomopathological aspects of human brain cysticercosis. In: Flisser A, Willms K, Laclette JP, Larralde C, Ridaura C, Beltran F (eds) Cysticercosis: present state of knowledge and perspectives. Academic Press, New York, pp 179–200

Ramírez G, Pradilla G (1987) Use of enzyme-linked immunosorbent assay in the diagnosis of cysticercosis. Arch Neurol 44:898

Robles C, Sedano AM, Vergas-Tentori N, Galindo-Virgen S (1987) Long-term results of praziquantel therapy in neurocysticercosis. J Neurosurg 66:359–363

Rodríguez-Carbajal J, Boleagu-Durán B (1982) Neuroradiology of human cysticercosis. In: Flisser A, Willms K, Laclette JP, Larralde C, Ridaura C, Beltran F (eds) Cysticercosis: present state of knowledge and perspectives. Academic Press, New York, pp 139–162

Rosas N, Sotelo J, Nieto D (1986) ELISA in the diagnosis of neurocysticercosis. Arch Neurol 43:353–356

Schantz PM, Tsang VCW, Maddison SE (1988) Serodiagnosis of neurocysticercosis. Rev Infect Dis 10:1231–1233

Scharf D (1988) Neurocysticercosis: Two hundred thirty-eight cases from a California hospital. Arch Neurol 45:777–780

Schwartz A, Aulich A, Hammer B (1987) CT-verlaufsbeobachtungen bei neurocysticerkose unter praziquanteltherapie. Radiologe 27:237–242

Šlais J (1982) Morphology of the scolex of *Cysticercus cellulosae* in brain cysticercosis. In: Flisser A, Willms K, Laclette JP, Larralde C, Ridaura C, Beltran F (eds) Cysticercosis: present state of knowledge and perspectives. Academic Press, New York, pp 235–259

Sotelo J, Escobedo F, Rodriguez-Carbajal J, Torres B, Rubio-Donnadieu F (1984a) Therapy of parenchymal brain cysticercosis with praziquantel. N Engl J Med 310:1001–1007

Sotelo J, Escobedo F, Rodriguez-Carbajal J, Torres B, Rubio-Donnadieu F (1984b) Praziquantel for cysticercosis of the brain parenchyma. N Engl J Med 311:734

Sotelo J, Escobedo F, Penagos P (1988) Albendazole vs praziquantel for therapy for neurocysticercosis: a controlled trial. Arch Neurol 45:532–534

Spina-França A, Nobrega JPS, Livramento JA, Machado LR (1982) Administration of praziquantel in neurocysticercosis. Tropenmed Parasitol 33:1–4

Téllez-Girón E, Ramos MC, Dufour L, Alvarez P, Montante M (1987) Detection of *Cysticercus cellulosae* antigens in cerebrospinal fluid by dot enzyme-linked immunosorbent assay (dot-ELISA) and standard ELISA. Am J Trop Med Hyg 37:169–173

Thomas H, Andrews P, Mehlhorn H (1982) Results on the effect of praziquantel in experimental cysticercosis. Am J Trop Med Hyg 31:803–810

Trujillo-Valdés VM, González-Barranco D, Sandoval-Islas ME, Villanueva-Díaz G, Orozco-Bohne R (1982) Chemotherapy of human cysticercosis using metrifonate. In: Flisser A, Willms K, Laclette JP, Larralde C, Ridaura C, Beltran F (eds) Cysticercosis: present state of knowledge and perspectives. Academic Press, New York, pp 219–226

Vasconcelos D, Cruz-Segura H, Mateos-Gomez H, Alanis GZ (1987) Selective indications for the use of praziquantel in the treatment of brain cysticercosis. J Neurol Neurosurg Psychiatr 50:383–388

Wadia N, Desai S, Bhatt M (1988) Disseminated cysticercosis: new observations, including CT scan findings and experience with treatment by praziquantel. Brain 111:597–614

Wiederholt WC, Grisolia JS (1982) Cysticercosis: an old scourge revisited. Arch Neurol 39:533

Woo E, Yu YL, Huang CY (1988) Cerebral infarct precipitated by praziquantel in neurocysticercosis – a cautionary note. Trop Geogr Med 40:143–146

Worthington M, Horowitz H (1987) Case 11, 1986: cysticercosis. N Engl J Med 316:693–694

Zenteno-Alanis GH (1982) A classification of human cysticercosis. In: Flisser A, Willms K, Laclette JP, Larralde C, Ridaura C, Beltran F (eds) Cysticercosis: present state of knowledge and perspectives. Academic Press, New York, pp 107–126

Chapter 11

Parasitic Zoonoses with a Canine Reservoir: An Unacceptable Human Health Hazard

It cannot be helped that dogs bark
and vomit their foul stomachs,
. . . but care can be taken that
they do not bite or inoculate their mad humours.

William Harvey (1578–1657),
On the circulation of the blood, [second essay to Jean Riolan]

Introduction

Human parasitoses (and other infections) which possess a reservoir in the canine population (Cook 1989) have received extensive coverage in the medical literature of the USA; in the UK awareness of this group of diseases seems less acute. In this chapter, I attempt to summarize those parasitic infections which maintain a zoonotic presence in 'man's best friend'. Dog populations of the UK and USA have been estimated at 6 and 55 million respectively (Baxter 1984a; Elliot et al. 1985). Problems are not, however, confined to the Western world; for example, in Nigeria dogs are also an important source of human disease (Okoh 1983).

Dog owners are frequently oblivious both to the variety and possible sequelae of these zoonoses and their consequences, both to themselves and also their children (Egerton 1982; Baxter and Leck 1984; Hubbert 1984; Warner 1984; Roth and Gleckman 1985; Kirkwood 1987). While toxocariasis and hydatidosis come immediately to mind, many other potential hazards result from numerous other parasites (and ectoparasites), bacteria, viruses, and mycoses (Cook 1989). Bites (which are of minor importance in the context of parasitoses), are a common and often neglected paediatric problem (infection takes place via infected saliva) and constitute the most dramatic means of transmission (Lauer and White 1982), but conveyance via faecal contamination of fingers, fomites, food and water is in practice far more common. The dog heartworm (*Dirofilaria immitis*) utilizes a mosquito vector. Certain rickettsial infections, e.g. plague and Rocky Mountain spotted fever, can be transmitted by ectoparasites (ticks).

Table 11.1 summarizes many parasitic infections known to be transmitted between dogs and man, and also those common to both species, and which might therefore have a significant canine reservoir. Many of these infections, which can produce significant morbidity and occasionally mortality, can present in unusual ways; only when a case history includes careful reference to household pets, with details of their species, will some of them be even considered in the differential diagnosis. The infected dog may remain completely healthy while remaining a potential source of human infection.

Table 11.1. Some canine-associated parasitic infections to which man is vulnerable (Elliot et al. 1985; Okoh 1983; Egerton 1982; Baxter and Leck 1984; Hubbert 1984; Warner 1984; Roth and Gleckman 1985; Kirkwood 1987)

Causative organism	Dog to man transmission established		Present in both species but dog to man transmission not established
	World-wide significance	Limited geographical areas only	
Protozoa	*Entamoeba histolytica* *Coccidiosis* *Pneumocystis carinii*[a]	South American trypanosomiasis Visceral leishmaniasis	*Giardia lamblia* *Toxoplasma gondii*
Nematodes	*Toxocara canis* Visceral and ocular larva migrans *Trichuris vulpis*	*Capillaria hepatica* *Gnathostoma spinigerum* *Dioctophyma renale* *Dracunculus medinensis* *Dirofilaria immitis* *Brugia pahangi* *Ancylostoma caninum,* *A ceylanicum*, and *A braziliense* Cutaneous larva migrans	*Strongyloides stercoralis* *Trichinella spiralis* *Thelazia callipaeda* (oriental eye worm)
Trematodes		*Clonorchis sinensis* *Opisthorchis viverrini* *Echinostoma* sp *Heterophyes heterophyes* *Metagonimus yokogawai* *Paragonimus* sp	*Schistosoma mansoni,* *S japonicum*
Cestodes	*Echinococcus granulosus* *Dipylidium caninum* *Taenia* (*multiceps*) sp		*Diphyllobothrium latum*
Arachnids	Scabies dermatitis	Tick/ Trombiculid dermatitis	
Insects Ectoparasites	Flea-bite dermatitis *Sarcoptes scabiei* var *canis* (canine scabies) *Ctenocephalides canis* (canine flea) *Cheyletiella* sp (canine mite)	*Tunga penetrans*	

[a] This organism, which is now considered by some to be a fungus, is traditionally classified as a protozoan parasite (*The Lancet* 1988; ii: 522) (Chap. 2).

Protozoan Parasites

The dog is one of several mammals which can maintain a reservoir of *Entamoeba histolytica* (Chap. 6); however it undoubtedly plays a minor role in transmission compared with direct man-to-man spread (Wolfe 1984). A very wide range of animals, which includes dogs, can harbour various small-intestinal coccidia including *Cryptosporidium* sp (Case records of the Massachusetts General Hospital 1985) (Chap. 4), and *Giardia lamblia* (Sykes and Fox 1989) (Chap. 3); while oocyst excretion from the former is probably important in some human cases, infection via faecal cysts has so far not been established in the case of *G lamblia* although a strong possibility exists (Thompson 1983; Baxter 1984a; Warner 1984). Dogs are not infrequently infected with *Toxoplasma gondii* (Chap. 9); cats are, however, a far more important reservoir (Elliot et al. 1985) and the practical importance of canine transmission is unclear. In Nigeria, a 58% infection rate was demonstrated serologically in pet dogs (Okoh 1983); toxoplasma meningoencephalitis in a mongrel dog has been demonstrated there. In some South American countries, dogs constitute an important reservoir of *Trypanosoma cruzi* infection (Chap. 12); living close to man they have an important capacity in infecting domiciliated reduviid bugs (Marsden 1984). Dogs form a very important reservoir for visceral leishmaniasis in the Mediterranean littoral, South America and China (Chulay and Manson-Bahr 1984); the cutaneous forms of the disease also affect dogs.

Nematode Infections

Toxocariasis (Visceral and Ocular Larva Migrans)

The nematode *Toxocara canis* occurs world-wide, and constitutes one of the two most important canine helminthic zoonoses (Egerton 1982; Okoh 1983; Baxter and Leck 1984; Warner 1984; Elliot et al. 1985; Roth and Gleckman 1985; Kirkwood 1987). Man is an abnormal ('dead-end') host. Epidemiology and pathogenesis in relation to this organism have both been extensively reviewed (Glickman and Schantz 1981). One estimate for prevalence in England and Wales, based on serological tests, is 16 000 new infections annually (Baxter and Leck 1984); this includes many subclinical cases. For the 10-year period 1975–1984, 107 clinical cases were reported (Kirkwood 1987); accurate figures are impossible to obtain, however, because, with the exception of New York City, this is not a notifiable disease (Gunby 1979). Infection occurs world-wide and many epidemiological surveys have recorded prevalence rates in tropical and subtropical countries (Abo-Shehada 1989). Although *T canis* has been known to be a parasite of dogs since 1782, human infection (with larvae) was not described until 1952 (Beaver et al. 1952); in 1921, however, Fülleborn had recognized the potential for infectivity of *Toxocara* sp in man (Glickman and Schantz 1981).

Parasitology and Pathogenesis

Figure 11.1 shows the life-cycle of *T canis*. Dogs become infected both directly from contaminated soil and also when larvae (which are passed transplacentally) are conveyed in bitches' milk; the faeces and vomit of an infected pup are also infectious (Editorial 1989). By the time adult life is reached, few dogs continue to pass eggs. Adult *T canis* lives in the dog small-intestine (infection usually occurs in utero or perinatally (Gillespie 1987)); human infection occurs after ingestion of embryonated ova (85 × 75 μm) which hatch into larvae (350 × 20 μm) in the lumen of the proximal small-intestine.

Figure 11.2 shows a larva of *T canis*. After penetration of the intestinal mucosa, larvae enter the portal circulation and/or lymphatics, and are transmitted to the liver; here they are either halted or pass into the lungs, subsequently into the systemic circulation, and thence to any other organ (*visceral larva migrans*). They give rise to eosinophil-containing granuloma (1–2 mm in diameter) formation. Most human infections presumably occur after accidental ingestion of embryo-

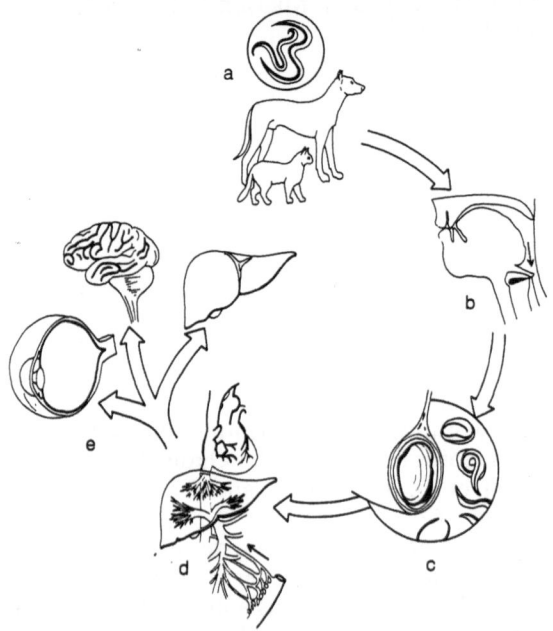

Fig. 11.1. Life-cycle of *Toxocara canis* (and *T cati*). (a) Adults of *T canis* (and *T cati*) live in the small-intestine of dogs (and cats) – in which the life-cycle is similar to that of *Ascaris lumbricoides* in man (Fig. 3.3); (b) an embryonated egg is ingested and swallowed in contaminated food, or after playing with an infected dog (or cat); (c) larva hatches in the small-intestine; (d) after penetration of the small-intestinal wall and entry to the portal venous system larvae are widely distributed in human tissues; (e) most important organs affected are the eye (*ocular larva migrans*), brain, and liver (*visceral larva migrans*). Man is thus a 'dead-end' host.

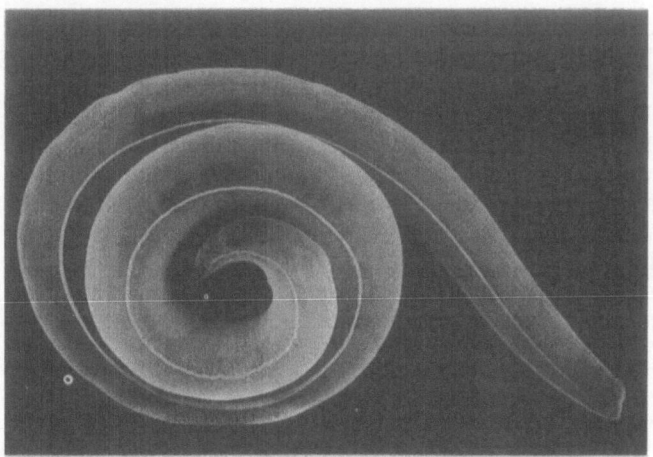

Fig. 11.2. Scanning electron-micrograph of larva of *T canis* (× 880).

nated ova from soil (maturation takes 2–3 weeks) which has been contaminated by canine faeces, or in children by the sucking of contaminated fingers; pica and recent contact with puppies have been clearly associated with a high prevalence rate of infection (Glickman and Schantz 1981). In one study a high incidence of positive serological tests (16%) was demonstrated in dog breeders compared with a sample from the general public (3%) (Baxter and Leck 1984).

The possibility has been raised that *T canis* (and possibly other nematodes also) can by mechanical means introduce pathogenic viruses (including poliomyelitis and Japanese B encephalitis) to the brain (Brown and Voge 1982); however, evidence for this is based largely on circumstantial evidence.

Clinical Aspects

Clinically, although all organs may be affected, ophthalmic involvement (*ocular larva migrans*), which seems to comprise a distinct clinical syndrome, is the most important manifestation (Glickman and Schantz 1981; Gillespie 1987). Varying degrees of unilateral visual loss associated with retinal lesions (including choroidoretinitis) may occur. Presentation is usually with reduced vision or squint, an underlying retinitis, or less commonly uveitis and/or endophthalmitis. These are usually the sole clinical manifestations on examination; an important differential diagnosis is retinoblastoma.

Initially, an acute infection with fever, cough and malaise may be present; this represents the clinical expression of the host's immune response to the migrating larvae (Gillespie 1987). Hepatomegaly, transient pneumonitis (with chronic cough and wheeze), encephalitis (and fits) and lymphadenopathy may occasionally be present. A recent report from Dublin has sought to expand the existing clinical spectrum of the acute disease (Taylor et al. 1988); the most common features were shown to be: abdominal pain, hepatomegaly, anorexia, nausea, vomiting, lethargy, sleep and behaviour disturbances, pneumonia, cough, wheeze, pharyngitis, cervical adenitis, headache, limb pains, and fever. These authors consider that 'covert toxocariasis' is a relatively common infection, of which visceral and ocular larva migrans are but two manifestations. An acute visceral larva migrans syndrome is unusual in children less than 5 years old (Editorial 1989). Rarely, myocardial and CNS involvement (Russegger and Schmutzhard 1989) (Chap. 8) have occasionally resulted in fatalities (Schantz and Glickman 1978). Hepatic capillariasis (caused by *Capillaria hepatica*) can also give rise to visceral larva migrans. A similar clinical presentation can be produced by migrating *Ascaris lumbricoides*, *Strongyloides stercoralis*, and filariae in tropical pulmonary eosinophilia, although in the latter pulmonary symptoms are more pronounced. Other 'wandering' larvae include: *Gnathostoma spinigerum* and *Paragonimus westermani* (Chap. 8), sparganum, and the pentastomids.

Diagnosis

An eosinophilia is often present initially, but is frequently absent by the time ocular involvement is established (Schantz and Glickman 1978; Elliot et al. 1985; Taylor et al. 1988). Serum IgG, and to a lesser extent IgM and IgE may be raised (Schantz and Glickman 1978; Gillespie 1987). A positive ELISA (>32) gives a high degree of sensitivity and specificity (Glickman and Schantz 1981; Gillespie 1987; Taylor et al. 1988). Toxocara antigen may also be detected in an aspirate of vitreous humour (Editorial 1989); this is of value when histological examination is either negative or not feasible. A needle liver-biopsy specimen may show numerous cell-mediated granulomas (surrounding *T canis* larvae) which contain a centre of closely packed eosinophils and histiocytes; these are surrounded by larger histiocytes with pale vesicular nuclei which are sometimes arranged in a palisade-like pattern; atypical multinucleate giant-cells and remnants of second-stage larvae may be identifiable. The serum alkaline phosphatase is frequently elevated. A generalized, transient, peribronchial infiltrate may be demonstrable on chest radiography. Myocardial involvement occasionally produces ECG changes.

Management

No form of chemotherapy is completely successful, and/or adequately evaluated in man (Wiseman et al. 1971; Gillespie 1987; Taylor et al. 1988). Diethylcarbamazine (DEC) 3 mg/kg body weight tds for 21 days, and thiabendazole 50 mg/kg body weight (given as 3 divided doses) daily for at least 5 days have been widely used and both regimens undoubtedly possess larvicidal properties; a corticosteroid 'cover' should be given when ocular involvement is present. Successful results have been claimed from the Federal Republic of Germany in a limited study using fenbendazole (100–500 mg given as 2 divided doses daily for 10 days) (Düwel 1983). Mebendazole (1 g tds for 21 days) has also produced a cure (Bekhti 1984). Experimentally, several other agents have been shown to be larvicidal: albendazole, oxfenbendazole, levamisole and ivermectin (Gillespie 1987; Taylor et al. 1988). In a small clinical study carried out in Switzerland, albendazole proved superior to thiabendazole (Stürchler et al. 1989); the authors recommend a regimen of ≥10 mg/kg daily on 5 consecutive days. Treatment with various chemotherapeutic agents kills larvae in experimental animals which have been infected during the previous 7 days; however, after they have entered the muscles and brain chemotherapy is ineffective, and larvae may in fact reactivate (Abo-Shehada and Herbert 1984).

Other Non-Vector-Borne Nematode Infections

Capillaria hepatica occasionally causes human visceral larva migrans (see above) (Manson-Bahr and Bell 1987); however, this is very much less common than with *T canis*, and ocular involvement is not a major problem. Several nematodes which infect man can reside in canine tissues; amongst these are: *Gnathostoma spinigerum*, *Trichinella spiralis* (in Arctic regions only), *Thelazia callipaeda* (the oriental eye worm), *Dioctophyma renale* (a cause of urinary tract infection) and *Dracunculus medinensis* (the guinea worm) (Baxter and Leck 1984; Manson-Bahr and Bell 1987); however, these parasites all have a localized geographical distribution and in most cases limited clinical relevance.

Although suggested by some available evidence, opinion is divided as to whether *Strongyloides stercoralis* can inhabit the small-intestine of dogs (Baxter and Leck 1984). The dog whipworm (*Trichuris vulpis*) can cause human infection but the importance of this is unclear (Kenney and Eveland 1978; Okoh 1983); a prevalence of up to 52% in stray dogs in the USA has been recorded. Two dog hookworms: *Ancylostoma ceylanicum* and *A caninum* can infect the gastrointestinal tract of man; the former especially, can produce symptoms – principally blood loss and subsequent anaemia in children – and is therefore a significant health hazard (Areekul 1979; Okoh 1983). In Zaria, northern Nigeria, one study showed a 66% prevalence rate for *A caninum* in stray dogs (Okoh 1983).

Another dog hookworm *Ancylostoma braziliense*, is widespread in many parts of the tropics (especially the Caribbean); faecal contamination of holiday beaches in tourist resorts (Areekul 1979; Okoh 1983; Warner 1984; Manson-Bahr and Bell 1987) followed by skin contact, usually the feet, gives rise to *cutaneous larva migrans* (Fig. 11.3). This consists of a pruritic, erythematous, serpiginous eruption; diagnosis is a clinical one and although the infection is self-limiting, usually lasting a few weeks, topical thiabendazole and oral albendazole are of proven value in management. *A caninum* can also cause cutaneous larva migrans (Areekul 1979). A further canine hookworm *Uncinaria stenocephala* which has been observed in British dogs, has also been implicated in cutaneous larva migrans (Baxter and Leck 1984).

Mosquito-Borne Nematodes

Although *Dirofilaria immitis* (often referred to as the canine heartworm) infection occurs in a wide variety of mammals, dogs represent the most important host reservoir (Merrill et al. 1980; Ciferri 1982; Grieve et al. 1983; Neafie and Meyers 1984; Elliot et al. 1985). This infection has been reported from eastern, southern and western USA, southern Europe, Australia, Japan, India, China and South America. It seems to be rare in Africa; the reason for this is unclear.

Adult worms live in a coiled mass in the right ventricle; their microfilariae

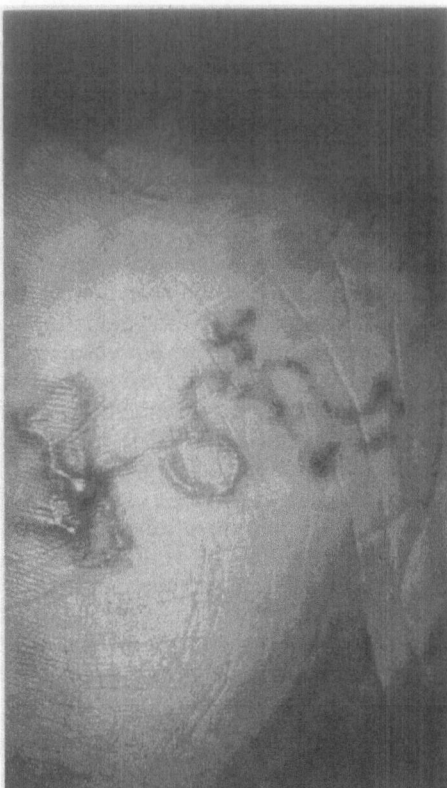

Fig. 11.3. *Larva migrans* rash on the sole of the foot of a young man who had recently returned from a Caribbean holiday. Infection was presumably acquired by walking barefoot on a beach contaminated with dog faeces, probably containing *Ancylostoma braziliense* larvae. He was successfully treated with oral albendazole (400 mg daily for 3 days).

circulate in peripheral blood. An infected dog, in whom the diagnosis can be made by detection of microfilariae in peripheral blood, is usually asymptomatic but a severe infection can cause exercise intolerance, haemoptyses, and subsequently evidence of right ventricular outflow obstruction (Elliot et al. 1985). Transmission to man (a 'dead-end' host) is by many species of mosquito. Partial development of the helminths occurs in the right ventricle, from which they are swept into small pulmonary arteries. A minority of infected individuals are immunosuppressed (Ciferri 1982). Only the immature *D immitis* (100–350 μm in length) has been demonstrated in human lungs; neither mature worms nor microfilariae have been visualized. The consequent lesions are usually limited to the lung periphery; a single, coiled (usually necrotic and occasionally calcified) worm can be detected in the lumen of an artery within a necrotic area, and this is surrounded by a zone of granulomatous infiltration and fibrosis. Clinically, chest discomfort, cough, haemoptyses, fever, chills and malaise may be present, although diagnosis is usually made by detection of a well circumscribed 'coin-lesion' (1–3 cm diameter) during routine chest radiography (Ciferri 1982); in this report, 95% of 59 cases studied possessed a single nodule, whilst the remainder had two in separate lobes. The lesions are often removed surgically (at thoracotomy) because the differential diagnoses include primary and secondary neoplasia (Merrill et al. 1980). An ELISA, which has a high degree of specificity and sensitivity has been documented (Grieve et al. 1983). Peripheral blood eosinophilia is unusual (Elliot et al. 1985). DEC, ivermectin, and dithiazanine have been used but although promising results have been reported their role in treatment is unclear (Grieve et al. 1983). The possibility of effective canine vaccination has been raised; using a rat model, killing of microfilariae has been demonstrated (Tamashiro et al. 1989).

Subcutaneous dirofilariasis is usually caused by *D repens*, which is also mosquito-spread and also has a reservoir in dogs (Neafie and Meyers 1984). Reports have been made in the USA, Africa, Europe and South America. Lesions can occur in any part of the body, but especially the conjunctiva, eyelid, scrotum, breast, arm and leg; they develop over several weeks into tender, painful, erythematous, and occasionally migratory subcutaneous nodules. Chronic lesions are granulomatous and contain epithelioid cells, foreign-body giant cells, histiocytes, and eosinophils. Diagnosis is by identifying *D repens* in a biopsy-specimen; excision is the sole effective treatment.

Dogs in Malaysia have been shown to be infected with *Brugia pahangi* (Mak et al. 1980) (in addition to *D immitis*); experimental infection in man has produced all of the symptoms and signs of tropical pulmonary eosinophilia (TPE, occult filariasis) (Chap. 12); it is therefore possible that dogs might have a relevance in the pathogenesis of this disease (Beaver 1970).

Trematode Infections

Several trematode helminths which are pathogenic to man, can also infect dogs, usually via the consumption of infected freshwater fish; however, the importance of this reservoir is probably of limited significance. Dogs are known to be infected, albeit in tropical countries only (Baxter and Leck 1984; Manson-Bahr and Bell 1987), with: *Clonorchis sinensis* and *Opisthorchis viverrini* (Chap. 3), *Echinostoma* sp, *Heterophyes heterophyes*, *Metagonimus yokogawai* and *Paragonimus* sp. They can also be infected with *Schistosoma mansoni* (Chap. 7), but only in exceptional circumstances, and are unlikely to play a major role in transmission (Karoum and Amin 1985); in a study in Sudan, although 27% of 55 stray dogs were shown at post-mortem to be infected, no evidence of viable ova was detectable on faecal examination. *S japonicum* can also infect dogs, but their role in the transmission of human disease seems of little or no importance.

Cestode Infections

Hydatidosis

Although frequently considered a *tropical* parasitic infection, this is not the case, and *Echinococcus granulosus* infection occurs wherever the parasite (which is usually confined to rural areas) exists and man lives in close proximity to sheep and dogs (McGreevy and Nelson 1984). Although the dog (and other canids) always constitute the definitive host(s) (Elliot et al. 1985) numerous other carnivorous mammals in addition to the sheep can act as important intermediate hosts; these include the goat, pig, cow and camel (Saad and Magzoub 1988). There are, however, strain differences and whereas in the UK the horse can be involved, it is very unlikely that this strain could infect man (McGreevy and Nelson 1984). The infection is distributed in foci throughout the world; in addition to Africa, Asia and South America, Wales, western England and much of the Middle-east are affected (Daly et al. 1984; Elliot et al. 1985; Editorial 1987; Pandey et al. 1988; Watson-Jones and Macpherson 1988, Macpherson et al. 1989). Between 1975 and 1984, 103 laboratory reports were made in England and Wales, with 42 registered deaths (Kirkwood 1987); one estimate is that about 100 new infections occur in England and Wales annually (Baxter and Leck 1984).

Parasitology and Pathogenesis

This tapeworm (which is one of the smallest cestodes) consists of 2–5 segments (3 to 8 mm in length) and attaches to the dog small-intestinal mucosa. Figure 11.4 summarizes the life-cycle of *E granulosus*. Very high prevalence rates may exist in dogs in some localities; for example, in one recent epidemiological study in southern Morocco, 51% of stray and 43% of urban dogs were infected (Pandey et al. 1988). Up to 70 000 worms have been recovered from a dog fed a single

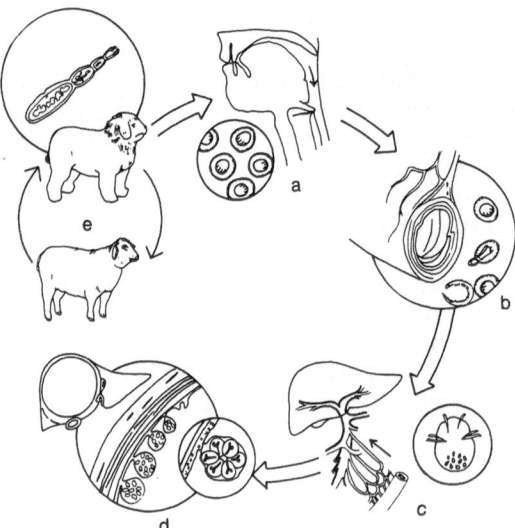

Fig. 11.4. Life-cycle of *Echinococcus granulosus*. (a) Embryonated eggs (from food contaminated with dog faeces) are ingested by man (and sheep) and swallowed; (b) the eggs hatch in the upper small-intestine; (c) oncosphere emerges and by using its hooklets penetrates the small-intestinal wall and enters the portal circulation; (d) the liver is the most usual resting place, although other organs can also be involved; maturation takes several months and an 'hydatid cyst' which contains an outer (acellular) membrane and a germinal layer from which protoscoleces are produced is formed; (e) the definitive host (usually the dog) is infected by consuming an hydatid cyst (usually present in an infected sheep carcass); each protoscolex can produce an adult worm within the canine intestine.

hydatid cyst (McGreevy and Nelson 1984). Human infection is acquired from ingestion of dog faeces (resulting from frequent and intimate contact with dogs, and poor personal hygiene); the eggs hatch in the small-intestine and liberated oncospheres penetrate the mucosa; they are then transported via mesenteric blood and lymphatics to the liver, lungs and other organs. Figure 11.5 shows a protoscolex of *E granulosus* viewed from within a human hydatid cyst. Dogs become infected by ingesting a hydatid cyst present in infected uncooked offal from a sheep, goat or other infected herbivore (McGreevy and Nelson 1984; Elliot et al. 1985). The related species *E multilocularis* produces an altogether more serious disease because it maintains a proliferative stage in man and masses of small cysts, which occasionally metastasize, are produced (Bia and Barry 1986).

Clinical Aspects

Clinically, the majority of human infections are asymptomatic and are discovered either during routine investigation (e.g. chest radiography) (Roth and Gleckman 1985) or at post-mortem examination. However, a significant number result in morbidity with occasional mortality. The liver is most often involved (60%), followed by the lungs (25%) and other organs; 80% of cysts are solitary. Examples of cardiac (Noah et al. 1988) and cerebral involvement (Chap. 8) (Abdulla et al. 1988) have recently been recorded in the Middle-east. Most presentations occur in young adults; however, cerebral and ocular cysts sometimes produce symptoms in children. Presenting symptoms depend on the site of the cyst(s); traumatic rupture, associated either with trauma or surgery, can

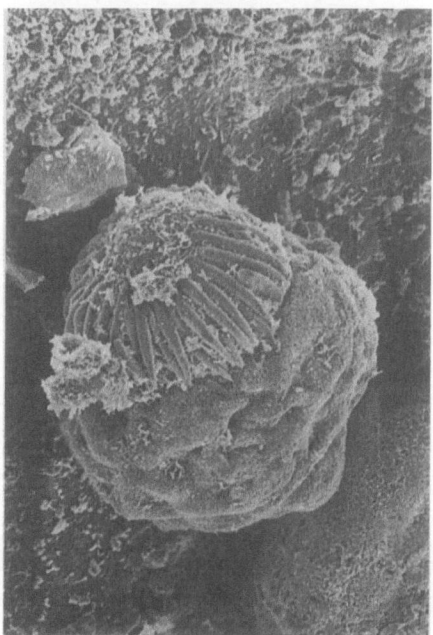

Fig. 11.5. Scanning electron-micrograph of a protoscolex of *E granulosus* (× 700).

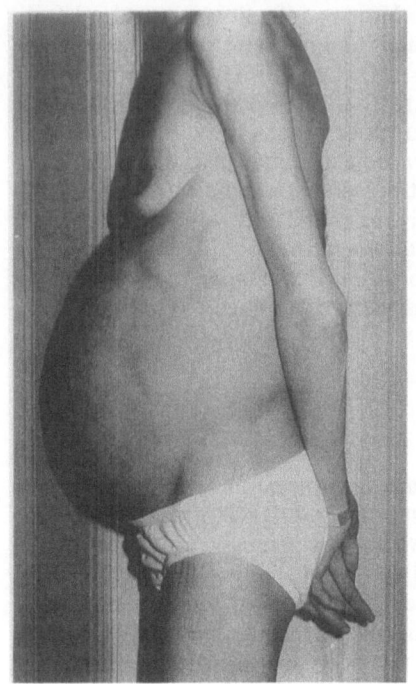

a

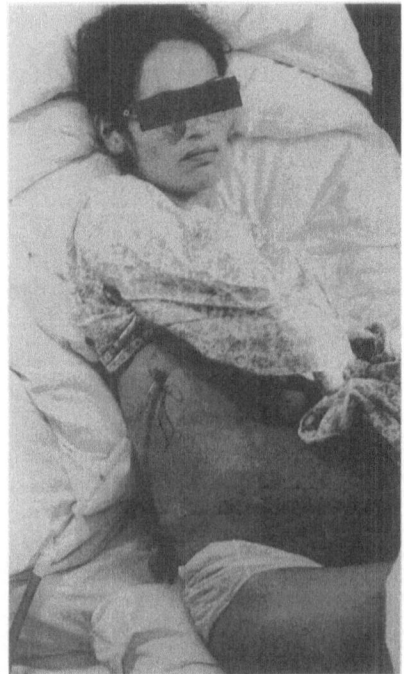

b

Fig. 11.6a,b. A 25-year-old Turkish woman. **a** Generalized abdominal distension caused by multiple hydatid-cysts within the peritoneal cavity. **b** She also had a massive right pleural effusion. A drainage tube was inserted into the chest and intact daughter cysts emerged. Serum IgG was 26.1 g/l, ELISA for hydatidosis positive, and hydatid CFT 1:256. Treatment with albendazole + praziquantel (see text) produced a remarkably good response.

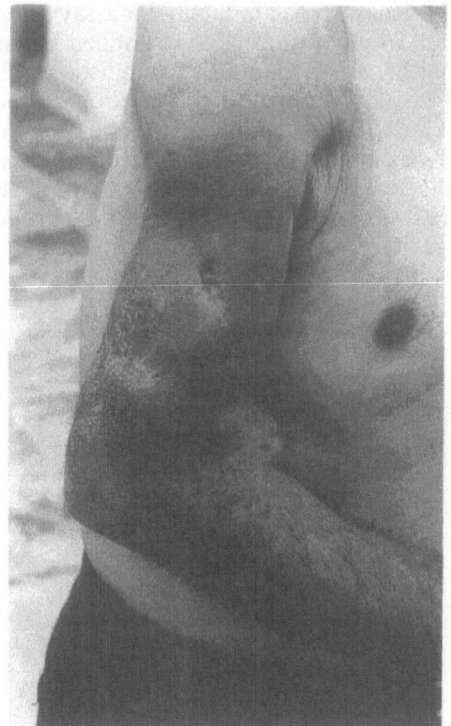
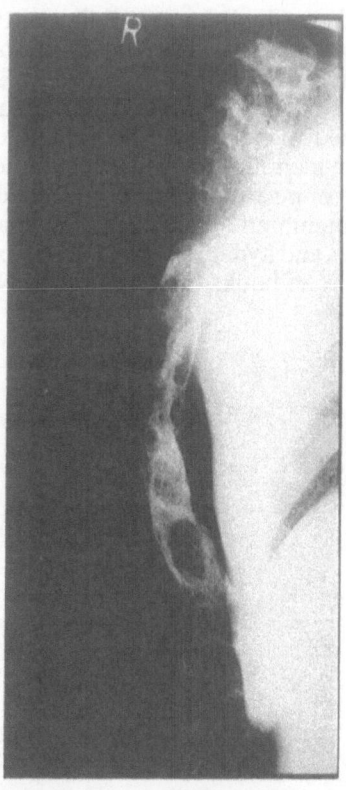

a

b

Fig. 11.7. a A 45-year-old Kuwaiti man who presented with a pathological fracture of the right humerus. **b** Radiograph of the right humerus showing multiple hydatid-cysts. Swabs from the sinuses failed to produce scoleces of *E granulosus*, but hydatid CFT was positive at 1:128.

produce peritonitis and seeding of protoscoleces throughout the peritoneal cavity, pneumothorax and/or an empyema; an anaphalactoid reaction which consists of pruritus, urticaria, oedema, dyspnoea, asthma, vomiting, diarrhoea, colicky pain, shock and death is a rare occurrence. The disease should be suspected in any individual with a space-occupying lesion who has lived in an area where the disease is common. Figure 11.6 shows a Turkish woman with generalized abdominal hydatidosis, and Fig. 11.7 a Kuwaiti man with bone involvement which caused a pathological fracture.

Diagnosis

Localization of the cyst is by radiography, ultrasonography, and/or CT-scanning. However, these techniques are not always as accurate as some investigators have claimed (Hira et al. 1988), and they occasionally suggest an erroneous diagnosis. Figure 11.8 shows ultrasound and CT-scans of hepatic hydatidosis. Eosinophilia is inconstant (Roth and Gleckman 1985). Serological tests have until recently been unreliable, and have lacked specificity and sensitivity (McGreevy and Nelson 1984); however, the ELISA has recently proved valuable, especially when antibody against 'Arc-5' (a genus-specific antigen isolated from unilocular hydatid cyst fluid) is used (Editorial 1987). Recently, an immunoblot assay using an *E granulosus* antigen of 8 kDa molecular weight (unrelated to antigen 5) has given 100% specificity in the daignosis of hepatic hydatidosis (Maddison et al. 1989). Furthermore, cyst-fluid obtained by ultrasound-guided aspiration can be subjected to cytological verification or an ELISA technique (Hira et al. 1988). Parasite identification can be confirmed by examining a cyst(s) removed either at surgery or post-mortem. A single fluid-filled cavity is surrounded by a translucent white membrane which contains opaque dots; these represent scoleces, brood capsules and hydatid 'sand'; the scolex has four spherical suckers, a rostellum and two rows of hooks (McGreevy and Nelson 1984).

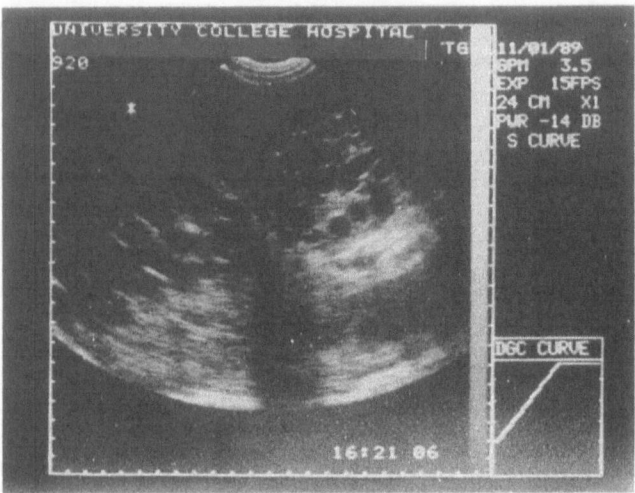

a

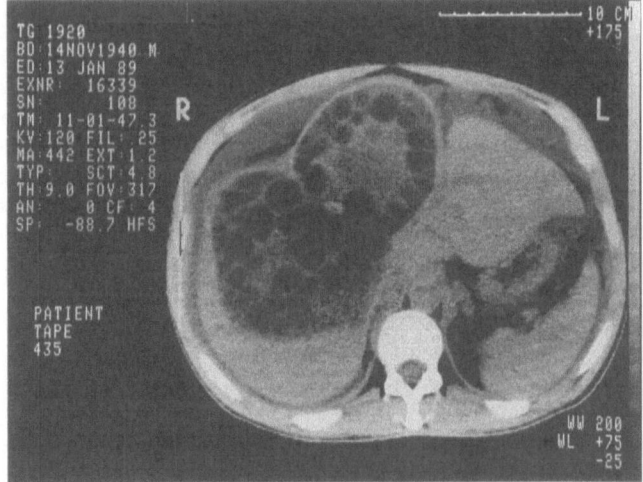

b

Fig. 11.8a,b. Liver hydatid-cysts in a 49-year-old Greek Cypriot man. **a** Ultrasound; **b** CT-scan. Ascitic fluid on admission contained 83 g/l protein; peripheral blood eosinophil count was 0.42×10^9/l, and serum IgG 48.1 g/l. Hydatid ELISA was positive, and CFT 1:1024. He was treated with albendazole + praziquantel; the response was good, but surgery was required at a later date.

Management

Treatment was formerly always surgical, usually after prior injection of the cyst with hypertonic saline, silver nitrate or 0.1% cetrimide; caution was obviously required when dealing with intracranial hydatid disease. The benzimidazole group of compounds has been widely used over the last decade and is still undergoing evaluation (McGreevy and Nelson 1984; Elliot et al. 1985; Editorial 1987). Problems involved in assessing the efficacy of chemotherapy are several: (i) assessment of cyst-viability is not always accurate before chemotherapy is commenced; (ii) major difficulties arise in comparing small series of cases in which different organs are involved; and (iii) assessment of cure is usually difficult. Mebendazole was the first chemotherapeutic agent to be used (Rausch et al. 1986), but the most effective compound to date is undoubtedly albendazole (which is very well absorbed from the small-intestine) (Saimot et al. 1983; Wilson et al. 1987; Horton 1989); there is now excellent evidence which indicates that provided an adequate concentration of this agent (albendazole sulphoxide is the principal metabolite) is attained within the cyst it is scolicidal (Saimot et al. 1983; Morris et al. 1987a; Wilson et al. 1987). Albendazole is also effective as a chemotherapeutic agent in inoperable cases and for prophylaxis prior to surgery (Horton 1989). One regimen which has proved successful is 10–15 mg/kg daily (given as three divided doses) in four one-month courses separated by 14–15-day intervals (Todorov et al. 1988). Horton (1989) has recently reviewed the outcome of a large series of infected patients who were given albendazole chemotherapy over an approximately 5-year period. Two hundred and fifty-three infected patients (there was a total of 269 hepatic cysts, 86 pulmonary, 50 peritoneal, 28 bone, and 23 cysts at other sites) were treated (most received 800 mg albendazole daily in cycles of 28 days, separated by 14 days, for a mean duration of 2.5 (range 1–12) cycles); 72 (28%) were considered cured, 129 (51%) improved, 46 (18%) unchanged and 6 (2%) worse off. In that assessment, 47 patients underwent surgery *after* treatment and in only 5 (11%) were cysts still viable. In 4 (14%) out of 29 cases not treated surgically who were followed-up for 24 months, recurrence of infection was documented. Experience with *E multilocularis* infection was limited, but of 35 who were treated, 2 were cured, 4 improved, the disease had stabilized in 25, and 4 had worsened. Side-effects of albendazole were uncommon in that study: approximately 20% had abnormalities in biochemical tests of liver function; some of those infected with *E multilocularis* developed a leucopenia.

When surgical intervention is necessary, albendazole should be administered pre-operatively; an experimental study using gerbils has demonstrated that a delay in chemotherapy until 15 days *after* peritoneal inoculation of protoscoleces prevents this protective advantageous effect (Morris and Taylor 1988). Viability following chemotherapy can be assessed by the ELISA (Zhanqing et al. 1988), specific IgG, and CT-scanning; complete cyst calcification usually signifies a successful outcome.

Praziquantel (either alone as in combination with albendazole) has undergone extensive study in rats and gerbils infected with *E multilocularis* (Richards et al. 1989; Taylor et al. 1989); it is an active protoscolicidal agent but less active than albendazole in the inhibition of cyst growth. Recently praziquantel has been subjected to clinical trial but its efficacy is currently impossible to evaluate; there is no doubt however, that this compound when present at an adequate concentration is a very active protoscolicidal agent (Morris et al. 1987b).

However, a recent in vitro study has indicated that praziquantel is probably inferior in this respect to albendazole sulphoxide (Taylor et al. 1989). There is currently an urgent need for large multicentre trials to assess accurately the role of albendazole (Davis et al. 1986) and praziquantel. Combination regimens using albendazole + praziquantel seem effective when either of these agents used alone has failed (G. C. Cook unpublished observation). Some cases will probably always require surgery, but only after prior albendazole and/or praziquantel treatment.

Other Cestode Infections

A further common tapeworm of dogs throughout the world is *Dipylidium caninum* (Okoh 1983; Baxter and Leck 1984; Warner 1984; Elliot et al. 1985); man is an occasional and accidental host to the adult parasite (10–70 cm in length and 6–8 mm in breadth). In one study, 31% of a sample of pet dogs examined in Britain was shown to be infected (Baxter and Leck 1984). Human infection occurs after ingesting adult fleas (obligate intermediate hosts) which contain cysticercoids, or after being licked around the mouth by a dog which has recently nipped an infected flea (Baxter and Leck 1984). Infection is most common in infants and children (Margolis 1983; Baxter and Leck 1984; Hubbert 1984). Although usually asymptomatic, abdominal pain, diarrhoea, irritability, pruritus ani and urticaria have been attributed to its presence. Characteristic proglottides can be detected in faecal samples. Praziquantel and niclosamide are effective in management.

Coenuriasis, which is caused by human infection with the larval stage of *Taenia (multiceps)* sp, is a further zoonotic disease involving dogs, which form the definitive host (Manson-Bahr and Bell 1987). The eggs develop into coenuri in subcutaneous tissue and the CNS (Chap. 8); the cyst is usually solitary (2–6 cm in diameter). Presentation is similar to that of neurocysticercosis (Cook 1988); the only form of management currently effective is surgical removal, although high-dose praziquantel is undergoing investigation.

The freshwater fish tapeworm *Diphyllobothrium latum* (and related species) occasionally infect the dog (via infected fish) (Baxter and Leck 1984) – which then acts as a reservoir of infection; treatment is with praziquantel or niclosamide. Related species which also infect dogs can occasionally be demonstrated in man (Goldsmith and Markell 1984).

Ectoparasites

The dog flea *Ctenocephalides canis* (Table 11.1) can infect man, and is a significant problem in warm humid climates (Warner 1984); the frequency of human infection is poorly quantified (Baxter and Leck 1984). Children can occasionally be infected with canine scabies *Sarcoptes scabiei* var *canis* (Warner 1984), although most human disease is caused by the human scabies mite *S scabiei* var *hominis*. Canine scabies mites do not normally burrow into human skin, but produce eruptions which can be papular, vesicular or urticarial (Baxter and Leck 1984). Another mite *Cheyletiella* sp, which is mildly pathogenic to dogs, can cause human dermatitis and other *local* manifestations (Egerton 1982); this infection is especially common in long-haired breeds (Baxter and Leck 1984). Puppies and old debilitated dogs seem particularly at risk for ectoparasitic infections, but here also, the true prevalence is unknown.

Some ectoparasites can be responsible for canine-induced allergy. Allergic reactions to animal danders have been estimated to be important in 6% of individuals treated by 'allergists' in the USA (Elliot et al. 1985); dogs are implicated in some of them. [Children in particular can develop asthma, rhinitis, urticaria and even diarrhoea when exposed to dog fur or scurf (Kirkwood 1987).]

Ectoparasite-Associated Infections

The major zoonoses which are dependent upon vectors for their transmission, are: plague, tularaemia and Rocky Mountain spotted fever (Elliot et al. 1985). Although the causative organism in Lyme disease, *Borrelia burgdorferi* (which relies upon ixodid ticks for transmission), exists in dogs their role, if any, in the spread of this disease has not been clearly established (Elliot et al. 1985).

Yersinia pestis infection (plague), which throughout history has caused devastating epidemics and pandemics (often with a high mortality rate), is enzoonotic in many rodent species (especially *Rattus rattus* and *R norvegicus*); it is dependent on insect vectors (rodent fleas) for transmission. Dogs, which together with other carnivores (including man) can be infected, suffer a brief, self-limited disease (Mann et al. 1984; Elliot et al. 1985); theoretically at least, they constitute an important reservoir (Butler 1984).

Cats, which become infected with *Francisella tularensis*, a Gram-negative coccobacillus, while hunting and feeding on infected animals, can transmit tularaemia to man via their contaminated teeth and claws (Evans et al. 1981; Hubbert 1984); although dogs disseminate the tick vectors, they do not, however, directly transmit the infective organism (Elliot et al. 1985). The disease has been well documented in Japan, the USSR, and North and South America (Sanford 1984).

A reservoir for Rocky Mountain spotted fever, a rickettsial disease (caused by *Rickettsia rickettsii*), is present in many wild rodents and rabbits; dogs act as transient hosts for one of the tick vectors *Dermacentor variabilis*. They are also susceptible to infection which can either be asymptomatic, or result in fever, abdominal pain and haematological abnormalities (Elliot et al. 1985; Roth and Gleckman 1985). The infection (Durack 1988) can therefore be transmitted to individuals handling tick-infected dogs (Roth and Gleckman 1985). Highest prevalence rates exist in the southern Atlantic and south central states of the USA.

Prevention

Throughout the world, the environment, especially in urban areas, is heavily polluted with canine excrement. In the UK, one estimate is that mean daily faecal and urinary output per dog is 100–250 g, and 0.25–1.25 litres respectively (Baxter 1984b); this adds up for a canine population of over 5 million, to a deposition of approximately 1 million kg of faeces, and 4.5 million litres of urine. This is equivalent to the faecal output of nearly 10 million, and urinary output of 3 million humans, and most of this takes place into the outdoor environment; these estimates incidentally exclude the output of stray dogs! A similar estimate from Rome suggests that in that city 19 250 kg of dog faeces, and 82 600 litres of urine are deposited daily (Fantasia and Filetici 1986).

Uncontrolled, ownerless, and poorly supervised dogs should be rigidly controlled (Gunby 1979; Baxter 1984b). Contamination of soil by dogs in urban areas should be avoided; ova of *T canis* can survive in soil for several months (Elliot et al. 1985) and probably years. Dog excreta should be removed from all public places, and owners should regularly carry out rigorous anthelmintic treatment of their pets. Dogs should not be permitted in public parks and childrens' play areas (a good case can be made for their legal exclusion) (Schantz and Glickman 1978). An out-of-court 'four figure' settlement has recently taken place as compensation to a 7-year-old child who, as a result of a *T canis* infection, lost the vision of one eye (*The Independent* 1988); the disease was presumed to have been contracted whilst playing in an urban public park in Blackpool.

Improved health education, especially of children, is also important. Newly acquired weaned puppies and nursing bitches constitute the largest reservoir of *T canis* infection; therefore newly acquired pups should receive an anthelmintic agent, e.g. low doses of piperazine at a 2-week interval before entering the household (Elliot et al. 1985). Limited evidence indicates that fenbendazole might be a safe and effective agent for use in puppies and pregnant bitches (Düwel 1983). However, de-worming is never 100% effective!

In the control of hydatid disease, mass chemotherapy of dogs with praziquantel is effective when widely used (McGreevy and Nelson 1984; Elliot et al. 1985; Kirkwood 1987); ideally this should be repeated at monthly intervals. Infection of dogs must also be prevented; all offal which is likely to be infected should be disposed of, and access to viscera of sheep (and other intermediate hosts) which contains hydatid cysts (Editorial 1987) disallowed.

Several agents, including diethylcarbamazine (DEC), ivermectin, thiacetarsamide, dithiazanine and levamisole, have been used in the treatment of canine *D immitis* infections; however, none of these is without side-effects, some of which are serious (Merrill et al. 1980; Grieve et al. 1983); adverse reactions to DEC can apparently be diminished with lodoxamide ethyl (Desowitz et al. 1982). The possibility of development of a vaccine exists (Grieve et al. 1983; Tamashiro et al. 1989). Ectoparasite-associated diseases are dependent for their transmission on tick-infected dogs (Elliot et al. 1985); the importance of these vectors is clear from a study in Nigeria (Dipeou and Akinboade 1982). Flea shampoos, powders and sprays, and tick and flea collars have only limited value (Elliot et al. 1985).

If domestic dogs must be kept indoors, it is of paramount importance that they should not be cuddled and, worst of all, kissed; such practices are obviously potentially harmful, especially to infants and children.

Conclusions

A wide range of parasites which are pathogenic to man can infect dogs. The domestic dog might be 'man's best friend' but he/she is also a significant health hazard, and the range of parasitic infections transmitted by this species is very considerable (Baxter and Leck 1984; Editorial 1987). In the UK, the most common canine-associated zoonosis is toxocariasis; hydatidosis is of lesser importance numerically. In developing Third World countries, the range is much broader and includes several exotic infections. There is presently little, if any, evidence that the canine-associated zoonoses (excluding *P carinii* – Table 11.1) have an increased incidence in AIDS patients; it is, however, important to maintain careful surveillance because the advisability of HIV-infected individuals keeping pet dogs must be in question.

Patient education, frequent veterinary examination of household pets, and thorough handwashing after canine contact will reduce the incidence of dog-related infections (Baxter 1984). A high 'index of suspicion' is required if these conditions, some of which are potentially lethal, are to be diagnosed early. In the context of parasitic disease, the question: 'do you or your children have contact with dogs or puppies?' might not be as important statistically as 'have you travelled abroad?', but it is certainly well worth asking especially when dealing with a PUO or when a communicable disease is suspected and the cause is not immediately obvious.

Closer co-operation between physicians (and the medical profession in general) and veterinarians might well prove beneficial in the context of this important group of diseases.

References

Abo-Shehada MN (1989) Prevalence of *Toxocara* ova in some schools and public grounds in northern and central Jordan. Ann Trop Med Parasitol 83:73–75

Abo-Schehada MN, Herbert IV (1984) Anthelmintic effect of levamisole, ivermectin, albendazole and fenbendazole on larval *Toxocara canis* infection in mice. Res Vet Sci 36:87–91

Abdulla K, Tapoo AK, Agha HSA (1988) Ruptured cerebral hydatid cyst: a case report. J Trop Med Hyg 91:302–305

Areekul S (1979) Zoonotic potential of hookworms from dogs and cats in Thailand. J Med Assoc Thai 62:399–402

Baxter DN (1984a) The deleterious effects of dogs on human health: dog-associated injuries. Community Med 6:29–36

Baxter DN (1984b) The deleterious effects of dogs on human health. III. Miscellaneous problems and a control programme. Community Med 6:198–203

Baxter DN, Leck I (1984) The deleterious effects of dogs on human health. II. Canine zoonoses. Community Med 6:185–197

Beaver PC (1970) Filariasis without microfilaremia. Am J Trop Med Hyg 19:181–189

Beaver PC, Snyder CH, Carrera GM, Dent JH, Lafferty JW (1952) Chronic eosinophilia due to visceral larva migrans: report of three cases. Pediatrics 9:7–19

Bekhti A (1984) Mebendazole in toxocariasis. Ann Intern Med 100:463

Bia FJ, Barry M (1986) Parasitic infections of the central nervous system. Neurol Clin 4:171–206

Brown WJ, Voge M (1982) Neuropathology of parasitic infections. Oxford University Press, Oxford, p. 240.

Butler T (1984) Plague. In: Strickland GT (ed) Hunter's tropical medicine, 6th edn. Saunders, Philadelphia, pp 340–349

Case Records of the Massachusetts General Hospital (1985) Case 39, 1985: infectious diarrhea due to *Cryptosporidium*. N Engl J Med 313:805–815

Chulay JD, Manson-Bahr PEC (1984) Visceral leishmaniasis (Kala-azar). In: Strickland GT (ed) Hunter's tropical medicine, 6th edn. Saunders, Philadelphia, pp 578–585
Ciferri F (1982) Human pulmonary dirofilariasis in the United States: a critical review. Am J Trop Med Hyg 31:302–308
Cook GC (1988) Neurocysticercosis: parasitology, clinical presentation, diagnosis, and recent advances in management. Q J Med 68:575–583
Cook GC (1989) Canine-associated zoonoses: an unacceptable hazard to human health. Q J Med 70:5–26
Daly JJ, McDaniel RC, Husted GS, Harmon H (1984) Unilocular hydatid cyst disease in the Mid-South. JAMA 251:932–933
Davis A, Pawlowski ZS, Dixon H (1986) Multicentre clinical trials of benzimidazolecarbamates in human echinococcosis. Bull WHO 64:383–388
Desowitz RS, Palumbo NE, Perri SF, Sylvester MS (1982) Inhibition of the adverse reaction to diethylcarbamazine in Dirofilaria immitis-infected dogs by lodoxamide ethyl. Am J Trop Med Hyg 31:309–312
Dipeou OO, Akinboade OA (1982) Scavenging dogs and the spread of tick infestation in Nigeria. Int J Zoonoses 9:90–96
Durack DT (1988) Rus in urbe: spotted fever comes to town. N Engl J Med 318:1388–1390
Düwel D (1983) Toxocariasis in human and veterinary medicine – and how to prevent it. Helminthologia 20:277–286
Editorial (1987) Man, dogs, and hydatid disease. Lancet i:21–22
Editorial (1989) Topical zoonoses. J Infect 18:105–110
Egerton JR (1982) Pets and zoonoses. Med J Aust 2:311
Elliot DL, Tolle SW, Goldberg L, Miller JB (1985) Pet-associated illness. N Engl J Med 313:985–995
Evans ME, McGee ZA, Hunter PT, Schaffner W (1981) Tularemia and the tomcat. JAMA 246:1343
Fantasia M, Filetici E (1986) Are dog stools an hazard of spreading Salmonella? Eur J Epidemiol 2:318–319
Gillespie SH (1987) Human toxocariasis. J Appl Bacteriol 63:473–479
Glickman LT, Schantz PM (1981) Epidemiology and pathogenesis of zoonotic toxocariasis. Epidemiol Rev 3:230–250
Goldsmith R, Markell EK (1984) Diphyllobothriasis. In: Strickland GT (ed) Hunter's tropical medicine, 6th edn. Saunders, Philadelphia, pp 761–763
Grieve RB, Lok JB, Glickman LT (1983) Epidemiology of canine heartworm infection. Epidemiol Rev 5:220–246
Gunby P (1979) Rising number of man's best friends ups human toxocariasis incidence. JAMA 242:1343–1344
Hira PR, Behbehani K, Shweiki H, Abu-Nema T, Soni CR (1988) Hydatid liver disease: problems in diagnosis in the Middle East endemic area. Ann Trop Med Parasitol 82:357–361
Horton RJ (1989) Chemotherapy of Echinococcus infection in man with albendazole. Trans R Soc Trop Med Hyg 83:97–102
Hubbert WT (1984) 'Caution: pets may be hazardous to your health'. JAMA 251:934–935
Independent (1988) Payment of girl blinded by [virus] in dog excrement. The Independent, 11 August, p 4
Karoum KO, Amin MA (1985) Domestic and wild animals naturally infected with Schistosoma mansoni in the Gezira Irrigation Scheme, Sudan. J Trop Med Hyg 88:83–89.
Kenney M, Eveland LK (1978) Infection of man with Trichuris vulpis, the whipworm of dogs. Am J Clin Pathol 69:199
Kirkwood JK (1987) Animals at home – pets as pests: a review. J R Soc Med 80:97–100
Lauer EA, White WC (1982) Dog bites: a neglected problem in accident prevention. Am J Dis Child 136:202–204
Macpherson CNL, Spoerry A, Zeyhle E, Romig T, Gorfe M (1989) Pastoralists and hydatid disease: an ultrasound scanning prevalence survey in East Africa. Trans R Soc Trop Med Hyg 83:243–247
Maddison SE, Slemenda SB, Schantz PM, Fried JA, Wilson M, Tsang VCW (1989) A specific diagnostic antigen of Echinococcus granulosus with an apparent molecular weight of 8KDA. Am J Trop Med Hyg 40:377–383
Mak JW, Yen PKF, Lim KC, Ramiah N (1980) Zoonotic implications of cats and dogs in filarial transmission in Peninsular Malaysia. Trop Geogr Med 32:259–264
Mann JM, Hull HF, Schmid GP, Droke WE (1984) Plague and the peripheral smear. JAMA 251:953
Manson-Bahr PEC, Bell DR (eds) (1987) Manson's tropical diseases, 19th edn. Baillière Tindall, London, p 1557
Margolis B (1983) Dog tapeworm infestation in an infant. Am J Dis Child 137:702

Marsden PD (1984) American trypanosomiasis. In: Strickland GT (ed) Hunters' tropical medicine, 6th edn. Saunders, Philadelphia, pp 565–573

McGreevy PB, Nelson GS (1984) Cystic hydatid disease. In: Strickland GT (ed) Hunters' tropical medicine, 6th edn. Saunders, Philadelphia, pp 774–778

Merrill JR, Otis J, Logan WD, Davis MB (1980) The dog heartworm (*Dirofilaria immitis*) in man: an epidemic pending or in progress? JAMA 243:1066–1068

Morris DL, Taylor DH (1988) Optimal timing of post-operative albendazole prophylaxis in *E granulosus*. Ann Trop Med Parasitol 82:65–66

Morris DL, Chinnery JB, Georgiou G, Stamatakis G, Golematis B (1987a) Penetration of albendazole sulphoxide into hydatid cysts. Gut 28:75–80

Morris DL, Taylor D, Daniels D, Richards KS (1987b) Determination of minimum effective concentration of praziquantel in *in vitro* cultures of protoscoleces of *Echinococcus granulosus*. Trans R Soc Trop Med Hyg 81:494–497

Neafie RC, Meyers WM (1984) Dirofilariasis. In: Strickland GT (ed) Hunter's tropical medicine, 6th edn. Saunders, Philadelphia, pp 685–686

Noah MS, Hawas N el Din, Joharjy I, Abdel-Hafez M (1988) Primary cardiac echinococcosis: report of two cases with review of the literature. Ann Trop Med Parasitol 82:67–72

Okoh AEJ (1983) Canine diseases of public health significance in Nigeria. Int J Zoonoses 10:33–39

Pandey VS, Ouhelli H, Moumen A (1988) Epidemiology of hydatidosis/echinococcosis in Quarzazate, the pre-Saharian region of Morocco. Ann Trop Med Parasitol 82:461–470

Rausch RL, Wilson JF, McMahon BJ, O'Gorman MA (1986) Consequences of continuous mebendazole therapy in alveolar hydatid disease – with a summary of a ten-year clinical trial. Ann Trop Med Parasitol 80:403–419

Richards KS, Morris DL, Taylor DH (1989) *Echinococcus multilocularis*: ultrastructural effect of *in vivo* albendazole and praziquantel therapy, singly and in combination. Ann Trop Med Parasitol 83:479–484

Roth RM, Gleckman RA (1985) Human infections derived from dogs. Postgrad Med 77:169–180

Russegger L, Schmutzhard E (1989) Spinal toxocaral abscess. Lancet ii:398

Saad MB, Magzoub M (1988) Experimental transmission of hydatid infection from camels and cattle to dogs. Ann Trop Med Parasitol 82:363–365

Saimot AG, Meulemans A, Cremieux AC, Giovanangeli MD, Hay JM, Delaitre B, Coulaud JP (1983) Albendazole as a potential treatment for human hydatidosis. Lancet ii:652–656

Sanford JP (1984) Tularemia. In: Strickland GT (ed) Hunter's tropical medicine, 6th edn. Saunders, Philadelphia, pp 339–340

Schantz PM, Glickman LT (1978) Toxocaral visceral larva migrans. N Engl J Med 298:436–439

Stürchler D, Schubarth P, Gualzata M, Gottstein B, Oettli A (1989) Thiabendazole *vs*. albendazole in treatment of toxocariasis: a clinical trial. Ann Trop Med Parasitol 83:473–478

Sykes TJ, Fox MT (1989) Patterns of infection with *Giardia* in dogs in London. Trans R Soc Trop Med Hyg 83:239–240

Tamashiro WK, Ibrahim MS, Moraga DA, Scott AL (1989) *Dirofilaria immitis*: studies on anti-microfilarial immunity in Lewis rats. Am J Trop Med Hyg 40:368–376

Taylor DH, Morris DL, Richards KS (1989) *Echinococcus granulosus*: in vitro maintenance of whole cysts and the assessment of the effects of albendazole sulphoxide and praziquantel on the germinal layer. Trans R Soc Trop Med Hyg 83:535–538

Taylor DH, Morris DL, Reffin D, Richards KS (1989) Comparison of albendazole, mebendazole and praziquantel chemotherapy of echinococcus multilocularis in a gerbil model. Gut 30:1401–1405

Taylor MRH, Keane CT, O'Connor P, Mulvihill E, Holland C (1988) The expanded spectrum of toxocaral disease. Lancet i:692–695

Thompson RG (1983) Giardia 'species'. Lancet i:1327

Todorov T, Vutova K, Petkov D, Balkanski G (1988) Albendazole treatment of multiple cerebral hydatid cysts: case report. Trans R Soc Trop Med Hyg 82:150–152

Warner RD (1984) Occurrence and impact of zoonoses in pet dogs and cats at US air force bases. Am J Publ Health 74:1239–1243

Watson-Jones DL, Macpherson CNL (1988) Hydatid disease in the Turkana district of Kenya. VI. Man: dog contact and its role in the transmission and control of hydatidosis amongst the Turkana. Ann Trop Med Parasitol 82:343–356

Wilson JF, Rausch RL, McMahon BJ, Schantz PM, Trujillo DE, O'Gorman MA (1987) Albendazole therapy in alveolar hydatid disease: a report of favorable results in two patients after short-term therapy. Am J Trop Med Hyg 37:162–168

Wiseman RA, Woodruff AW, Pettitt LE (1971) The treatment of toxocaral infection: some experimental and clinical observations. Trans R Soc Trop Med Hyg 65:591–598

Wolfe MS (1984) Amebiasis In: Strickland GT (ed) Hunter's tropical medicine, 6th ed. Saunders, Philadelphia, pp 477–495
Zhanqing S, Xinhua F, Zhongxi Q, Ruilin L, Chunrong Y (1988) Application of biotin–avidin system, determination of circulating immune complexes, and evaluation of antibody response in different hydatidosis patients. Am J Trop Med Hyg 39:93–96

Chapter 12

The 'Exotic' Systemic Parasitoses: Limited Geographical Distribution; Rarely Encountered in the UK

Every physician almost hath his favourite disease.

Henry Fielding (1707–1754),
Tom Jones

Introduction

The majority of the protozoan and helminthic infections which have been covered in the previous chapters are either indigenous to the United Kingdom, or are introduced (not infrequently) by travellers and members of the minor ethnic groups (often after visits to their relations in Africa, Asia or the Caribbean). In this chapter the emphasis is on two groups of protozoan infections – trypanosomiasis and leishmaniasis – and a helminthic one – filariasis. These are rarely encountered in the UK and when they are, they are usually referred to one of the specialist centres; therefore the average physican has little or no experience of their diagnosis and chemotherapy. As with so many of the infections outlined in this monograph, serological diagnosis has improved remarkably during the last decade or so. However, chemotherapy has lagged behind that which is now available for many of the other parasitoses; older, toxic preparations are still widely in use (Cook 1988). The reason(s) for this is that little or no financial reward results from the development of chemotherapeutic agents for these diseases, which are localized geographically to tropical countries – mostly in Africa or India. In consequence the pharmaceutical industry tends not to invest in research in this neglected area (Garattini 1988; Scott 1988). Despite this, there have been some advances and these have been reviewed recently (Cook 1990).

The Trypanosomiases

Two major disease entities are grouped under this heading: African (caused by *Trypanosoma brucei* sp) and South American (which results from a *T cruzi* infection) trypanosomiasis. They are clinically very dissimilar and the sole reason for their close proximity in the minds of many physicians is that the causative organisms are taxonomically related and belong to the same genus.

African Trypanosomiasis

The major importance of this infection lies in the fact that untreated it can produce irreversible damage to the central nervous system which nearly always results ultimately in death; therefore, this account should be read in conjunction with that of CNS involvement by *T brucei* sp in Chap. 8.

Parasitological, pathological and general clinical aspects of this disease, which is caused by either *T b rhodesiense* or *T b gambiense*, have been reviewed (Brown and Voge 1982; Molyneux et al. 1984; Spencer 1984). *T b rhodesiense* has a geographical distribution which involves East and Central Africa, whilst *T b gambiense* is a West African disease with a distribution which takes in some central parts of the continent. Whereas man is the only relevant reservoir for *T b gambiense*, *T b rhodesiense* is a zoonotic disease and man is an incidental host; bushbuck, hartebeest, other forms of antelope, and to a lesser extent cattle, lion and hyena constitute important animal reservoirs. One estimate is that about 35 million people are at risk from this disease, but that there are only 6000–10 000 clinical cases annually. *T b rhodesiense* infection is now increasingly recognized in British and American tourists to the game-parks of East and Central Africa (Duggan and Hutchinson 1966) and it is an occupational hazard for gamewardens and fishermen. Congenital infection (Traub et al. 1978), and transmission by blood transfusion are rare events. Following a bite by the tsetse fly *Glossina* sp, the early acute phase of the disease (usually far more severe in the case of *T b rhodesiense*) – which has little, if any, impact on the CNS – is characterized by an intermittent fever, rash (which is irregular, circinate and evanescent), transitory oedema, and evidence of haemolymphatic involvement. A primary lesion (trypanosomal chancre) may develop 5–15 days after infection at the site of the bite.

Trypanosomes were first demonstrated in cattle, which suffered from a disease known locally as nagana, by Sir David Bruce (1895). The presence of trypanosomes in human blood was documented by Dutton (1902); he recognized the organisms in the blood of a European patient who had lived in Gambia and named the organism *T gambiense*. Castellani (1903) first demonstrated trypanosomes in the CSF (of a Ugandan patient), and Robertson (1913) gave a detailed account of trypanosomes in the vector *Glossina* sp (the tsetse fly) in 1913. Meanwhile, Stephens and Fantham (1910) had discovered the morphologically identical parasite *T rhodesiense* which was associated with a more acute infection. The latter disease can be epidemic and has accounted for high mortality rates in East and Central Africa; it has also been a major obstacle to cattle production in Africa.

Parasitology and Pathogenesis

Figure 12.1 summarizes the life-cycle of *T b rhodesiense*, and Fig. 12.2 shows a trophozoite of *T brucei* sp. The pathogenesis of the disease has still not been completely unravelled; complex immunological events include: immune complex deposition in target organs, hypocomplementaemia (with an increase in immuno-conglutinin), an activated kinin system, and autoantibody production directed against antigenic components of brain, erythrocytes and myocardium. A polyclonal hypergammaglobulinaemia with a marked increase in immunoglobulin M (IgM) is a striking and constant feature; however, only a small proportion of this IgM represents specific antitrypanosome antibody. The trypanosome survives in the human host by periodically changing its surface antigenic (glycoprotein) coat thereby preventing the development of an immune response (Turner 1980; Molyneux et al. 1984). Once established, immunosuppression develops and there is an impairment of both cellular and humoral immune responses (Hudson and Terry 1979; Nantulya et al. 1982; Hayes and Cox 1984; Oka et al. 1984).

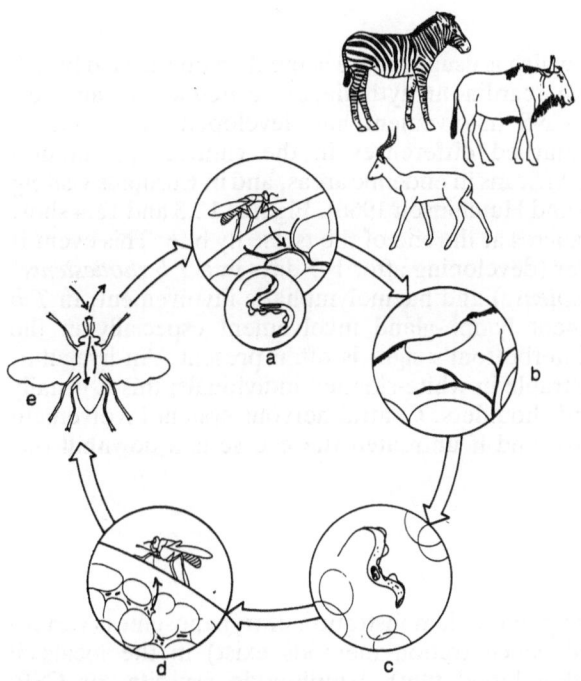

Fig. 12.1. Life-cycle of *Trypanosoma brucei rhodesiense*. (a) Infection occurs when a metacyclic trypomastigote (15–20 µm in length) is injected by a tsetse fly bite (several East and Central African mammals act as reservoir hosts); (b) a primary chancre at the site of infection results from replication by binary fission; (c) the replication-cycle continues in the blood-stream and lymphatics (the CSF may also be invaded); (d) a tsetse fly is infected whilst sucking blood from an infected individual; (e) a trypomastigote transforms to a procyclic trypomastigote in the insect's mid-gut lumen and migrates to the salivary gland (the life-cycle can then be completed).

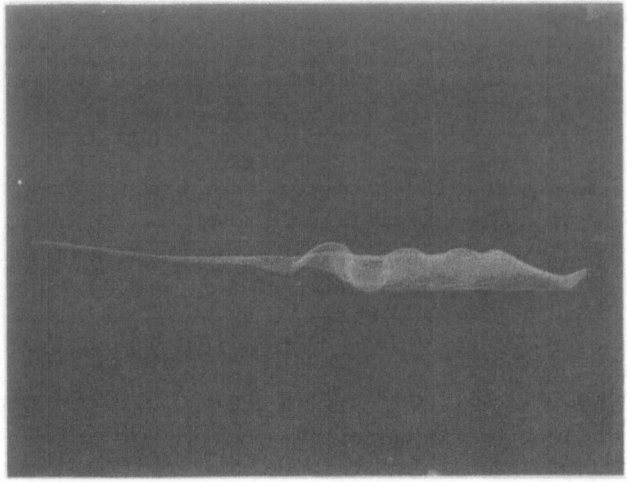

Fig. 12.2. Scanning electron-micrograph showing a trophozoite of *Trypanosoma brucei* sp (× 3500).

Clinical Aspects

In a *T b rhodesiense* infection, which is usually more acute than one caused by *T b gambiense*, death resulting from a cardiac arrhythmia, associated with a pancarditis, may occur even before CNS involvement has developed. It should be appreciated that there are marked differences in the clinical presentation between the disease involving Africans in endemic areas, and in Europids visiting or working in Africa (Duggan and Hutchinson 1966). Figures 12.3 and 12.4 show examples of trypanosomal chancres at the site of the tsetse fly bite. This event is followed by parasitaemia, fever (developing after 1–7 days in a *T b rhodesiense*, or months later with *T b gambiense*) and haemolymphatic involvement; in *T b gambiense* infections, prominent lymph-gland involvement especially in the posterior cervical region (Winterbottom's sign) is often present. An irregular, circinate rash may be demonstrable in white-skinned individuals; this is usually most marked on the trunk and shoulders. Central nervous system involvement occurs subsequently (Chap. 8), and if untreated the course is a downhill one leading to death.

Diagnosis

Diagnosis depends ultimately upon the demonstration of trypanosomes (various filtration, centrifugation, and concentration methods exist) in the localized chancre, blood (thick and thin blood film), lymph-node aspirate, or CSF; serological tests (including an ELISA) are of limited value (Molyneux et al. 1984). Various animal inoculation and culture techniques are now available. Whilst there is usually evidence of anaemia (predominantly haemolytic), thrombocytopenia, coagulation abnormalities, abnormal liver function tests, hypocomplementaemia, an increase in plasma kinins, and DIC also occur; none of these features is, however, diagnostic. Serum IgM concentration is increased in

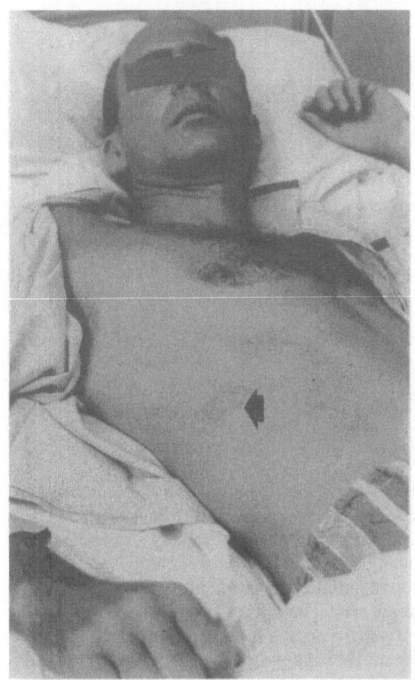

a

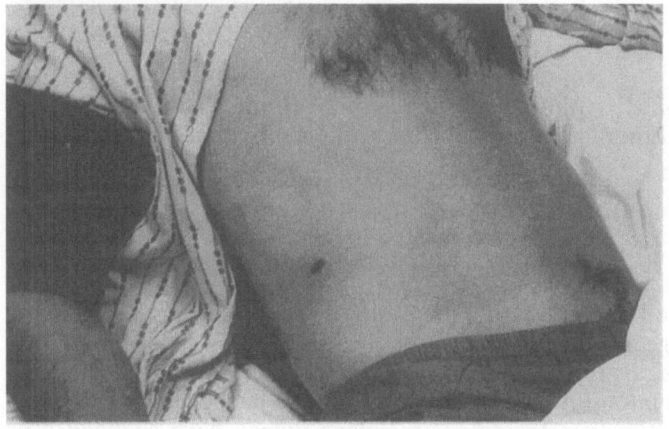

b

Fig. 12.3.a,b A 46-year-old man who presented with a febrile illness following a safari holiday in Kenya and Malawi. A trypanosomal chancre is shown **a** at admission to hospital, and **b** 3 days later. He also had significant lymphadenopathy in the right axilla, and a faint erythematous rash on his trunk. His spleen was enlarged to 2 cm below the left costal margin. A peripheral blood-film contained numerous *T b rhodesiense* trophozoites. CSF showed a mild elevation of protein only. He responded satisfactorily to intravenous suramin and melarsoprol (see text).

both serum and CSF; when CNS involvement is present (Chap. 8), CSF pressure may be raised, contain >25 mg/dl protein, and possess a cell count >5 leucocytes per mm^3; Mott (morular) cells may rarely be present (Molyneux et al. 1984). Differential diagnoses include: malaria, Kala-azar, tuberculosis, brucellosis, viral

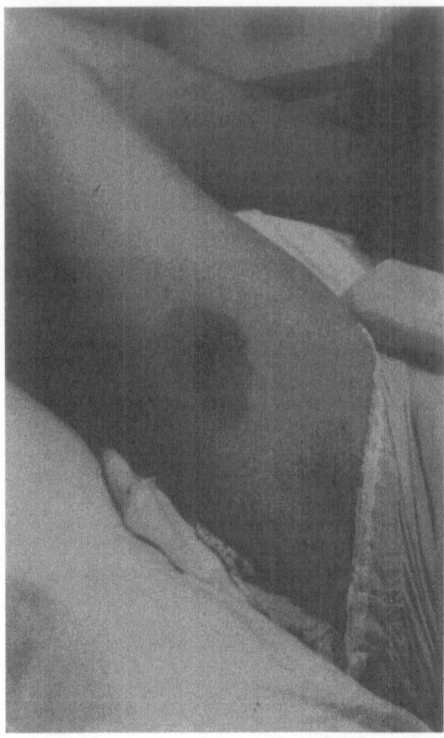

Fig. 12.4. A 29-year-old Irish woman who developed a febrile illness 5 days after returning from a safari holiday in the Lwangwa valley, eastern Zambia. A trypansomal chancre is shown on her right upper arm. Peripheral blood contained 400 *T b rhodesiense* trophozoites per µl. Chemotherapy with suramin was carried out satisfactorily. She also developed tropical pyomyositis which required a prolonged course of antibiotics (Weinberg et al. 1989).

encephalitis, tick typhus, syphilis, lymphomas, CNS tumours, psychoses, and meningitis caused by other infections which provoke a mononuclear response in the CSF.

Management

Chemotherapy is based on the use of two classes of agents: those used (i) in the early (pre-CNS) stage of the disease, and (ii) when CNS involvement has occurred (Molyneux et al. 1984; Spencer 1984). Of the older agents, suramin and the pentamidines fall into group (i) (see below), and melarsoprol ('Mel B') and nitrofurazone into group (ii). Treatment regimens (which have changed little over the last 40 years (Pepin et al. 1989a)) are also outlined in Chap. 8 (Manson-Bahr and Bell 1987a). Recently α-difluoromethylornithine has been subjected to clinical trial, especially in *T b gambiense* infections (Chap. 8).

At an early stage of the disease, suramin and the pentamidines are alternative drugs; however, neither is generally considered to penetrate the blood–brain barrier to a significant extent (although there is limited evidence to the contrary (Raseroka and Ormerod 1985)). Therefore, if CNS involvement is absent, one of these agents – preferably suramin (total dose 5–7 g) should be administered; a slow intravenous infusion (the 10% aqueous solution must be used within 30 minutes of reconstitution) of 20 mg/kg (maximum dose 1.0 g), which should be preceded by a test dose of 200 mg, is given on days 1, 3, 7, 14 and 21. Suramin is, however, a toxic compound; an idiosyncratic reaction is encountered only rarely, but renal damage (the unchanged and unmetabolized compound is deposited in the renal tubules) is important; urine should therefore be examined before each injection, and whilst mild proteinuria is frequently detected this is not an indication for suspending treatment (an increasing presence of casts and/or red blood cells should, however, be taken seriously). Other side-effects include: exfoliative dermatitis, bone-marrow depression, haemolytic anaemia, jaundice, hepatitis, adrenal insufficiency and diarrhoea. When CNS involvement is present, melarsoprol ('Mel B') is indicated (Chap. 8); this should not, however, be the first line of attack in the *absence* of CNS involvement. Some experimental evidence indicates that CNS involvement occurs in all *T b rhodesiense* infections, the parasite persisting in the choroid plexuses (see above); one management strategy is to *always* give melarsoprol after the suramin course. Limited experimental evidence suggests that if a trypanocidal compound is given at a non-curative dosage, invasion of cerebral tissue resulting in a severe encephalitis may result (Schmidt and Bafort 1985); it is therefore important that a full therapeutic regimen is always used.

Recently, α-difluoromethylornithine (eflornithine, DFMO) – an ornithine decarboxylase inhibitor – has been subjected to clinical trial in *T b gambiense* infections (McCann et al. 1987; Cook 1990); even in late-stage disease (with CNS involvement) results have so far been encouraging. In one study, all of 21 patients who completed a course of treatment showed complete clearance of CNS trypanosomes, with a return of CSF to normal, and no evidence of relapse during a 6–30 month follow-up period (Chap. 8). However, this agent has not been formally compared with melarsoprol as a first-line treatment (Pepin et al. 1989a). In *T b gambiense* infections, nifurtimox (which has been commercially available for the treatment of acute Chagas' disease for 15 years) has undergone clinical trial in Zaire with encouraging results (Pepin et al. 1989b); this agent is only indicated, however, in arseno-resistant cases and the optimal dose-regimen has not yet been established.

The efficacy of nitrothiazole compounds has been tested in experimental studies (Jennings 1987). A suramin+metronidazole combination has been successfully tested in mice (Raseroka and Ormerod 1986).

While the untreated disease is invariably fatal, acute cases – especially those in Europids who have visited East and Central African game-parks – usually respond rapidly, and long-term sequelae are most unusual. In the presence of severe CNS involvement and/or a CSF protein concentration of >40 mg/dl when treatment is begun the prognosis is usually bad (Chap. 8). Serial CSF examination is necessary during follow-up and a relapse is readily recognized by an elevation in the cell count; this is followed by a rise in IgM concentration despite the fact that the patient may be asymptomatic. A further treatment course is indicated if a recrudescence is suspected.

South American Trypanosomiasis (Chagas' Disease)

This disease, which is caused by *T cruzi*, is a major health problem in South and Central America; one estimate is that 20 million people are infected (Manson-Bahr and Bell 1987b). The infection is conveyed by reduviid bugs which inhabit the roofs of mud houses in rural areas. Congenital transmission of infection can occur and the foetus may either be born prematurely or even macerated or dead (Bittencourt 1976; Brown and Voge 1982); intracranial calcification has been described in a child who survived but had congenital disease (Pehrson et al. 1982). Transmission by maternal milk has also been demonstrated (Marsden 1984). It can also be acquired by blood transfusion.

Human infection with *T cruzi* consists of an acute phase during which a parasitaemia is present (and lasts a few weeks), and a chronic one which is usually life-long; only a small percentage of those affected develop symptoms. Overall a great deal of morbidity and mortality occurs (Köberle 1974). The major clinical manifestations are: cardiac complications in both phases, and the mega-syndromes (see below) in the later phase of the disease. Chronic infection should not be equated with Chagas' disease (Neva 1988); only a minority of infected individuals develop the disease which Chagas described.

The disease was first accurately documented by Carlos Chagas (1909). The pathogenesis of the mega-syndromes (which result from parasympathetic denervation) was worked out later by Köberle (1974). Cases are only rarely seen in the UK; those which are encountered are usually very longstanding chronic cases, usually with one of the mega-syndromes.

Parasitology and Pathogenesis

T cruzi is a polymorphic trypanosome which multiplies in the hindgut of its vector – the reduviid bug, which lives in the roofs of houses in much of South America. Over 100 naturally infected wild animals and domestic dogs have been shown to harbour *T cruzi* and to act therefore as reservoir hosts. Human infection is by faecal contamination of the skin; a minute break in the skin or mucous membrane results in penetration by *T cruzi*. Intracellular amastigotes (2–3 μm) multiply in local histiocytes; these give rise to trypomastigotes which enter the circulation. The organisms are intensely antigenic, and the mechanism(s) by which they avoid the immune response is unclear. Many different zymodemes exist, and they vary in their ability to produce the mega-syndromes (Neva 1988). Also, some zymodemes of *T cruzi* seem to have the potential to depress specific humoral immunity (Brenière et al. 1989); this finding is obviously important in serodiagnosis.

In an acute infection, amastigote nests are present in the myocardium and smooth muscle. A ventricular aneurysm, pericarditis and acute cardiomyopathy are possible sequelae. The pathogenesis of the infection is very poorly understood (Neva 1988); a major advance would be a method of determining which infected individuals are likely to proceed to fully blown Chagas' disease.

Although autonomic nervous system involvement is common (this probably results from an autoimmune mechanism, and is the underlying cause of the mega-syndromes), clinical involvement of the CNS itself (first suggested by Carlos Chagas in the 1920s) is not in fact a major problem. In the acute form the brain and meninges are oedematous, and small inflammatory foci are scattered throughout the grey matter (Brown and Voge 1982; Manson-Bahr and Bell 1987b); perivascular cuffing is also present. Although *T cruzi* can sometimes be detected in CSF (Hoff et al. 1978), signs of meningoencephalitis are unusual

(Brown and Voge 1982). While parasitization of nerve cells is rare, ruptured pseudocysts in the cerebellum and basal ganglia result in death and disappearance of nerve cells. [Animal studies have demonstrated a diminution in the number of anterior horn cells in the spinal cord.] In the chronic form, various neurological syndromes with spastic paralysis, mental deficiency and cerebellar symptoms have been described (Okamura and Correa Netto 1963); a diminution in the number of Purkinje cells in the cerebellar cortex has also been demonstrated (Brandao and Zulian 1966).

Clinical Aspects

In an *acute* infection (which is most common in the first decade of life), fever, hepatosplenomegaly and lymphadenopathy are common manifestations; tachycardia may reflect cardiac involvement, and unilateral orbital oedema (Romaña's sign) occasionally heralds the disease, reflecting inoculation via the conjunctiva. A chagoma – a dusky, erythematous, indurated lesion – may be present at the portal of entry. Arrhythmias, cardiomegaly, and cardiac failure are signs of bad prognostic significance (Marsden 1989). A peripheral blood lymphocytosis may make differentiation from EBV infection difficult. In *chronic* infections, cardiomyopathy and subsequently bi-ventricular failure, arrhythmias and heart block should be differentiated from other cardiomyopathies. The mega-syndromes, although rarely lethal complications, cause a great deal of morbidity (Marsden 1989): dysphagia follows oesophageal, and constipation colonic (usually sigmoid) involvement.* Myositis, and endocrine and exocrine dysfunction may also occur (Marsden 1984).

Diagnosis

A parasitic diagnosis (i.e. demonstration of *T. cruzi*) is usually difficult in the chronic, although frequently straightforward in the acute phase of the disease. Serological tests are of value, but in an endemic area, these are often difficult to interpret and still leave much to be desired (Neva 1988); cross-reaction with leishmaniasis occurs. The ELISA is not yet widely used. Xenodiagnosis, which involves feeding uninfected reduviid bugs on the patient's blood and then examining their intestinal contents 25–30 days later, is also of value in diagnosis. The use of molecular probes to detect parasite material from the pooled intestinal content of infected insects used in xenodiagnosis, would greatly assist diagnosis (Neva 1988). Mouse inoculation and culture are other methods of diagnosis.

---

*The suggestion has been made that Charles Robert Darwin FRS (1809–1882) contracted Chagas' disease during his voyage in *HMS Beagle* (Kohn 1963; Medawar 1964). In *The Journal of a Voyage in HMS Beagle*, he wrote while staying in a village at the foot of the Argentine Andes: 'At night I experienced an attack (for it deserves no less a name) of the *Benchuca*, a species of *Reduvius*, the great black bug of the Pampas. It is most disgusting to feel soft wingless insects, about an inch long, crawling over one's body. Before sucking they are quite thin, but afterwards they become round and bloated with blood.' Certainly some of his symptoms in later life, many of them gastrointestinal in origin (which seem to have had a clear organic basis) could be attributed to chronic Chagas' disease, but the accuracy of this hypothesis will never be known.

Management

Treatment of a *T cruzi* infection has always posed major problems. However, two chemotherapeutic agents (nifurtimox and benznidazole) are now of proven value in the *acute* phase of the disease. Nifurtimox (a nitrofuran derivative) is administered orally (5–15 mg/kg body-weight daily (in 3 divided doses) for 60–120 days); side-effects include anorexia, weight-loss, neurotoxicity (peripheral neuropathy), psychoses and gastrointestinal symptoms. Haemolysis may occur in the presence of glucose-6-phosphate dehydrogenase deficiency. [Incidentally, this agent also shows some promise in late-stage African trypanosomiasis (Leech et al. 1988) (see above).] Benznidazole (a benzimidazole compound) is also given orally at a dose of 5 mg/kg body-weight daily for 30–60 days; side-effects include: general malaise, rashes (often photosensitive), nausea and a sensory neuropathy. The value of benznidazole given either alone or in combination with obioactin (a lymphokine hydrolysate from the spleen and serum of immune animals) was evaluated in a small clinical trial in Chile (Apt et al. 1986); there was a high rate of side-effects, and results were far from encouraging. Despite seemingly effective chemotherapy prolonged follow-up often reveals a positive xenodiagnosis; strains of *T cruzi* from Argentina and Chile seem more sensitive than those from Brazil (Marsden 1984). The value of these agents in *chronic* infections has not been properly assessed; it seems pointless to treat patients with advanced disease, which is unlikely to be reversible (Neva 1988). However, whether the use of toxic compounds in indeterminate disease is justified is problematic; there is very little controlled evidence upon which to answer this question. In longstanding chronic disease, symptomatic treatment is all that can be offered; cardiac failure, arrhythmias, and heart block should be treated on their merits, while balloon-dilatation and surgery can be used for oesophageal, and resection for colonic, involvement.

Possible lines for future research have been reviewed (Mar and Docampo 1986); these focus upon recent developments in the understanding of kinetoplast DNA and glycosomes, action of oxygen radicals, intermediary metabolism of purines, pyrimidines and folic acid, and microtubule formation. An in vitro study compared two analogues of *cis*-diamminedichloroplatinum (Osuna et al. 1987); the authors considered that the results gave encouragement for in vivo application. In vitro and in vivo studies in Argentina, using mice, indicate that clomipramine (a tricyclic antidepressant) could constitute a viable candidate for chemotherapy of *T cruzi* infection (Barioglio et al. 1987).

The Leishmaniases

This heading comprises a group of diseases which range from a generalized systemic illness (visceral leishmaniasis, Kala-azar) to ones with only localized cutaneous or mucocutaneous manifestations (Chulay and Manson-Bahr 1984 a,b; Chulay 1984; Peters and Killick-Kendrick 1987). The causative organism in cutaneous disease was first recognized by Cunningham (1985), and that responsible for Kala-azar by Leishman (1903) in a British soldier in India; Donovan

(1903) identified the parasite (subsequently named the Leishman–Donovan body) in splenic tissue. The responsible organisms are all conveyed by phleboto-mine sandflies (1.5–2.5 mm in length) which feed on a wide range of warm and cold-blooded animals, which in addition to man include: cats, dogs, various rodents, cattle, bats, birds and lizards. The leishmania which infect man usually possess canine (Chap. 11) or rodent reservoirs in which clinical manifestations range from an inapparent infection to visceral disease. Many species, and strains of organism are involved, and they produce several specific clinical entities (see below); the host immune mechanisms which are set into action after infection, and the genetics of susceptibility have been reviewed (Sypek and Wyler 1988).

Visceral Leishmaniasis (Kala-azar)

This disease is caused by *Leishmania donovani* (there are three subspecies which depend on the geographical location) and characterized by a febrile illness, hepatosplenomegaly, weight-loss, anaemia, leucopenia and hypergammaglobuli-naemia. The disease has a wide geographical spread: southern Europe and the Mediterranean littoral (Kinmond et al. 1989) and Islands, Middle-east, central Asia and northern China, the Indian subcontinent, sub-Saharan Africa, and much of South America. It has recently staged a comeback in India (Jayaraman 1988); this has largely resulted from a discontinuation of DDT spraying, which was formerly used in malaria control. Infection is conveyed by the sandfly; rarely conveyance by blood transfusion or sexual contact has been documented. The disease seems to be unduly common in individuals infected with HIV-1 and HIV-2 (Chap. 2).

Parasitology and Pathogenesis

Figure 12.5 summarizes the life-cycle of *L donovani*; following inoculation of promastigotes by the sandfly, a granuloma (consisting of histiocytes containing amastigotes) forms locally; meanwhile, amastigotes multiply within the reticu-loendothelial system. Figure 12.6 shows an example of an amastigote (2.3 μm) of *Leishmania* sp within a Kupffer cell. Reticuloendothelial components in the spleen, liver and bone-marrow contain parasites, and granulomas subsequently develop; many other organs are also involved. During the last few years, a great deal of work has been carried out on *Leishmania* sp (Peters and Killick-Kendrick 1987; Neva 1988); this has involved the structure and function of kinetoplast DNA, classification and evolutionary relationships of species, and antigenic analysis. The use of molecular probes to detect leishmanial DNA for diagnosis of infection, and differentiation between the many different species (which will prove to be of incalculable value in epidemiological studies), have also been investigated; however the use of these techniques in diagnosis is limited because at present they all require the use of radioisotopes (Neva 1988).

Clinical Aspects

The incubation period is usually 2–6 months; therefore the disease often presents months or years after the affected individual has left an infected area. Onset may

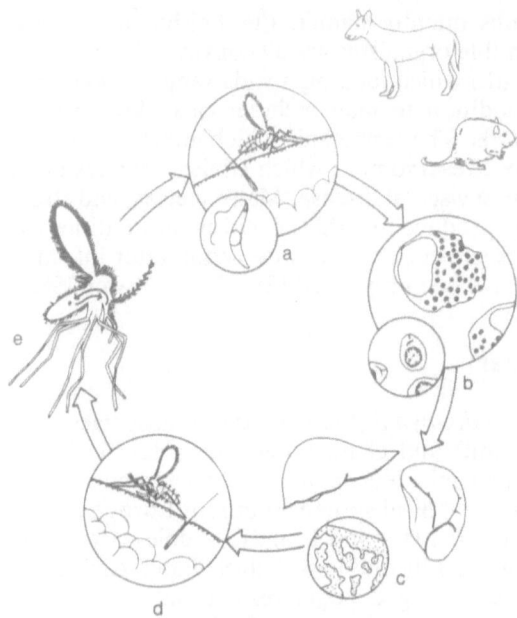

Fig. 12.5. Life-cycle of *Leishmania donovani*. (a) A promastigote is transmitted by the bite of an infected sandfly (reservoirs of infection exist in dog and gerbil populations); (b) after phagocytosis by a macrophage, transformation to the amastigote stage takes place; (c) fixed and wandering macrophages are infected throughout the reticuloendothelial system (spleen, bone-marrow, liver, etc.); (d) a sandfly becomes infected while sucking blood from an infected individual; (e) an amastigote transforms to a promastigote in the sandfly's intestine and migrates to the proboscis (from here the life-cycle can be completed).

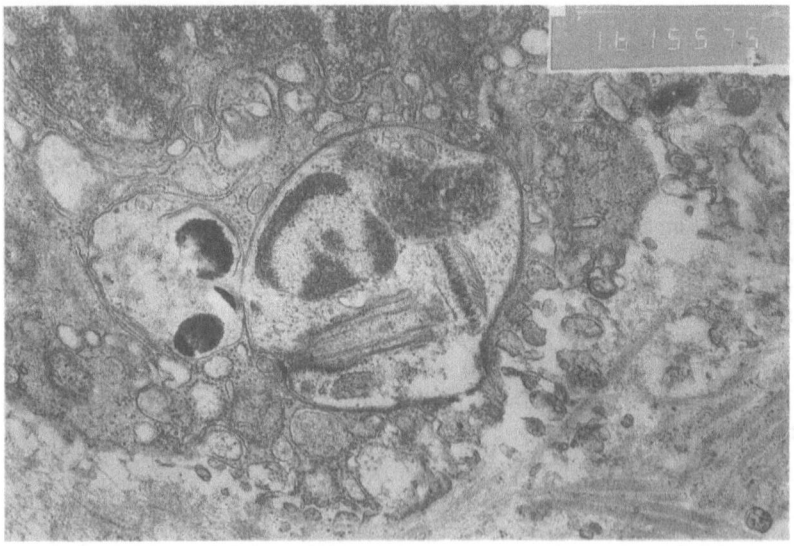

Fig. 12.6. Transmission electron-micrograph showing an amastigote of *Leishmania* sp in a Kupffer cell (× 21 000).

be acute or insidious. In addition to emaciation and evidence of anaemia, hepatosplenomegaly and frequently lymphadenopathy are usually present. Figure 12.7 shows an example of a young Englishman with Kala-azar acquired in Malta. The skin may become earthy-grey (the term Kala-azar is of Indian origin and refers to the 'black sickness'). Nasopharyngeal and laryngeal lesions present with mucosal swelling and hoarseness. Both acute bacterial and tuberculous pneumonia frequently complicate the disease; cancrum oris, uveitis, immune-complex glomerulonephritis and disseminated intravascular coagulation (DIC) are occasional events, and renal amyloidosis (presenting with a nephrotic syndrome) is a rare sequel. In India and far less frequently Africa and China, post-Kala-azar dermatitis (often involving the face) is a tiresome complication; the lesions appear at between a few months and 10 years after successful treatment.

The differential diagnostic list is a very long one and includes: malaria (especially hyperreactive malarious splenomegaly), African trypanosomiasis, *Schistosoma mansoni* infection, typhoid and brucellosis, tuberculosis, sarcoidosis, bacterial endocarditis, generalized histoplasmosis, Hodgkin's disease, chronic myeloid leukaemia and cirrhosis. The monoclonal hypergammaglobulinaemias can also be added to this list.

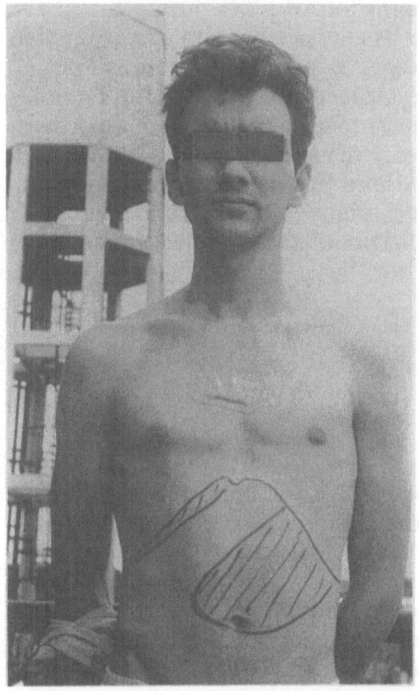

Fig. 12.7. A 21-year-old Englishman who presented with tiredness 21 months after a 2 week holiday in Malta (which was associated with anaemia – haemoglobin 8.2 g/dl); he was found to have splenomegaly. Bone-marrow aspirate contained numerous Leishman–Donovan bodies; serum IgG was 40.5 g/l (with a polyclonal rise); IgM was not elevated. Serology (IFAT) was mildly positive (1:60) for *Leishmania* sp. Total leucocyte count was 1.1×10^9/l and platelets 64×10^9/l. Treatment with sodium stibogluconate (700 mg daily for 21 days) was straightforward (see text).

Diagnosis

The disease, which is usually suspected first on clinical grounds – a consistent geographical history being obtained – is confirmed by visualization of the parasite. Splenic puncture (after checking the prothrombin time and platelet count) usually yields a positive result; the aspirate is injected into a culture medium, intraperitoneally into a hamster, and on to a microscope slide – amastigotes can be demonstrated by Giemsa or Leishman staining techniques. Bone-marrow smears give a slightly lower yield of positive results; amastigotes are demonstrable in 80%–85% compared with 98% of cases. A liver-biopsy specimen, lymph-node aspirate (Neva 1988) or buffy-coat smear (only in India) may also produce a definitive diagnosis. Serological tests are of value; the IFAT (which uses promastigotes as antigen) is positive in about 95% of cases of Kala-azar; although there may be a cross-reaction with other infections the titres are usually very much lower; recently, an ELISA (which also utilizes promastigote antigen) has proved equally valuable (Neva 1988). Formerly used tests, the formol-gel test (which merely detects high IgG and IgM concentrations) and the complement fixation test, now have very limited value in diagnosis. The leishmanin skin test is negative in acute Kala-azar, but becomes positive in 90% of patients between 6 weeks and one year after recovery; tuberculin sensitivity is similarly depressed reflecting a general depression of CMI during the active disease. Anaemia (of multifactorial origin) is usually present and a haemoglobin concentration of 6–8 g/dl is a common finding. Bone-marrow depression and hypersplenism are usually present, but at varying levels of severity. The Coomb's test may be positive. A leucopenia (with neutropenia, relative lymphocytosis, and absence of eosinophils) is usual; thrombocytopenia is common. Evidence of impaired hepatocellular function is reflected in a mild elevation of the serum transaminases and prolongation of the prothrombin time. Serum albumin is usually depressed, and polyclonal hypergammaglobulinaemia (most consisting of IgG) present.

Management

The spectrum of disease is broad and many mildly infected individuals recover spontaneously; however, the fully developed disease is uniformly fatal unless treated. Sodium stibogluconate (a pentavalent antimonial compound) continues to form the basis of chemotherapy (it has now been used for nearly half a century); the equivalent of 10 mg antimony per kg body-weight daily, has become the accepted dose – this is given for 10–20 days in India, China and Sudan, and 30 days in Kenya and other parts of East and Central Africa. This chemotherapeutic agent should be given slowly by the intravenous route using a 23–26 gauge needle. In a recent investigation in India, various dose regimens using the intramuscular route, have been compared (Thakur et al. 1988); cure rate correlated with the size of dose and length of treatment – when a 20 mg/kg dose was given for 40 days, this was 97%. However, with high dosage regimens it is usual to use the intravenous route (Neva 1988). Side-effects: general weakness, lethargy, nausea, anorexia, malaise, accompanied by minor abnormalities in liver-function tests, and ECG changes (usually T-wave inversion) are unusual. Over the last few years there has been an increased realization that the pentavalent antimonials are safer than had been previously considered; consequently higher dose regimens (e.g. 20 mg/kg daily for 20 days) are now more widely used (Neva 1988); with these higher dose regimens, arthralgias, myalgias and rarely leucopenia have been documented. In the rare event of relapse a further course at higher dosage and for a longer period (e.g. 20–30 mg antimony per kg body-weight for 60–90 days) usually produces a satisfactory cure. Alternative agents are pentamidine (isethionate or methane sulphonate); 4 mg/kg given intramuscularly three-times weekly for 4–6 months is usually effective, and does not produce the toxic-effects which occur when it is used for an AIDS-associated *Pneumocystis carinii* infection (Chap. 2). Amphotericin B and allopurinol have also been used, the latter usually in conjunction with a pentavalent antimony compound (Neva 1988). Recently, a good clinical response has been documented in 10 patients treated with sodium aurothiomalate (Singh et al. 1989); further evaluation in required. The suggestion has been made that itraconazole might be of value (Borelli 1987) and could form a useful substitute for the pentavalent antimonials. Rarely splenectomy has been undertaken in a resistant case; this is, however, highly undesirable in individuals living in a malarious area.

Other measures which should be taken into account are: blood transfusion in the early active disease, iron and vitamin supplements, and appropriate antibiotics for co-existent pneumonia, tuberculosis and other bacterial infections.

Cutaneous Leishmaniasis

This infection (Old World cutaneous leishmaniasis) produces well-circumscribed nodular and ulcerative skin lesions. *Leishmania tropica*, *L major* and *L aethiopica* are the aetiological agents involved (Chulay and Manson-Bahr 1984b; Peters and Killick-Kendrick 1987); the taxonomy of these is complex, and various species and strains produce different clinical results. Areas involved are the Mediterranean littoral, the Middle-east, the western parts of the Indian subcontinent, and sub-Saharan Africa.

Clinical Aspects

The incubation period is usually 2–8 weeks, and one as long as 3 years is exceptional; in the immunosuppressed it can be much longer. Any exposed area may be the site of infection. Following introduction of the organism a local CMI response ensues, and as the parasites are eliminated, epithelioid and giant cells appear; healing is by fibrosis. Clinical manifestations vary according to the species and strain of parasite; lesions may be single or multiple and of varying degrees of chronicity. They may consist of small papules, non-ulcerated plaques, or large ulcers with well-defined, raised, indurated margins. As the ulcer enlarges, serous fluid which forms a thick crust is produced. Satellite lesions are common. The resultant lesion, especially when involving the face, may be

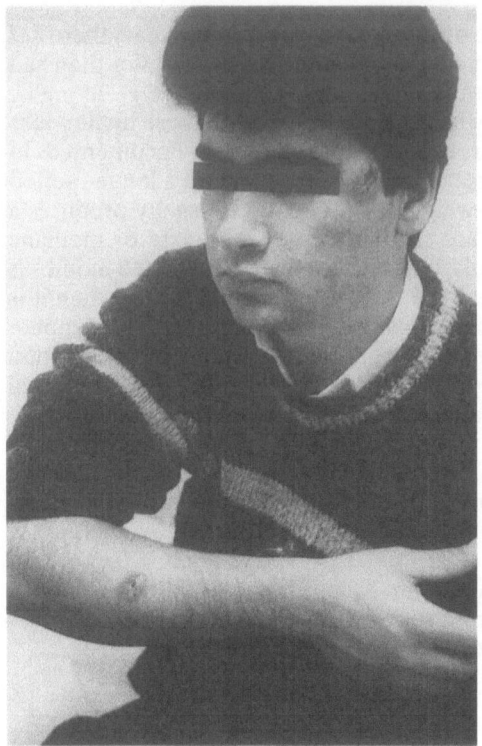

Fig. 12.8. A 16-year-old man from Cyprus with cutaneous leishmaniasis. A biopsy-specimen from the facial lesion showed scanty Leishman–Donovan bodies; culture produced a growth of promastigotes. Both lesions were successfully treated with paromomycin ointment.

disfiguring. Figures 12.8–12.10 show examples of cutaneous leishmaniasis. Lymphatic spread may occur in *L major* infections. An extremely chronic form, *leishmaniasis recidivans*, occasionally occurs in Iran and Iraq; this can persist for 20–40 years, and cutaneous tuberculosis is an important differential diagnosis; nasal destruction is an occasional sequel. Another variant is *disseminated cutaneous leishmaniasis* (DCL); this is usually caused by *L aethiopica* in Ethiopia and Kenya; immunologically this has similarities with lepromatous leprosy, although visceral spread does not occur.

Differential diagnoses include: tropical ulcer, tertiary syphilis, yaws, cutaneous tuberculosis, diphtheria, blastomycosis, basal-cell carcinoma, and other chronic nodules and ulcers. DCL should be differentiated from lepromatous leprosy.

Diagnosis

Demonstration of the causative organism is the only means of making a definitive diagnosis; an aspirate of exudate from the margin of the lesion (or scrape or biopsy) should be stained with Giemsa or Leishman (Neva 1988): varying

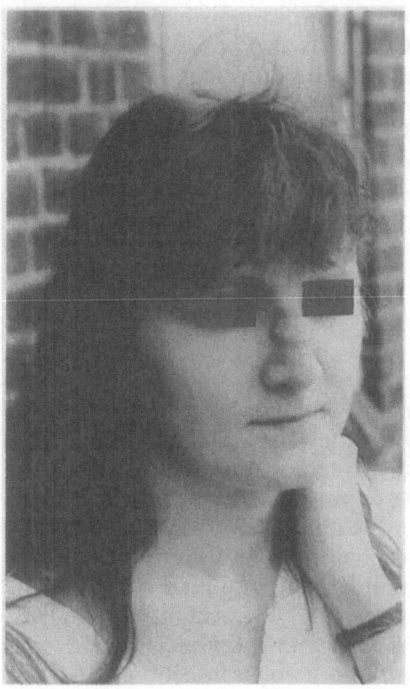

Fig. 12.9. A 23-year-old English woman with cutaneous leishmaniasis which she had contracted during a visit to Israel, Egypt and Greece. The diagnosis was confirmed histologically (amastigotes were present), and culture produced promastigotes of *Leishmania* sp. Response to intravenous sodium stibogluconate was satisfactory.

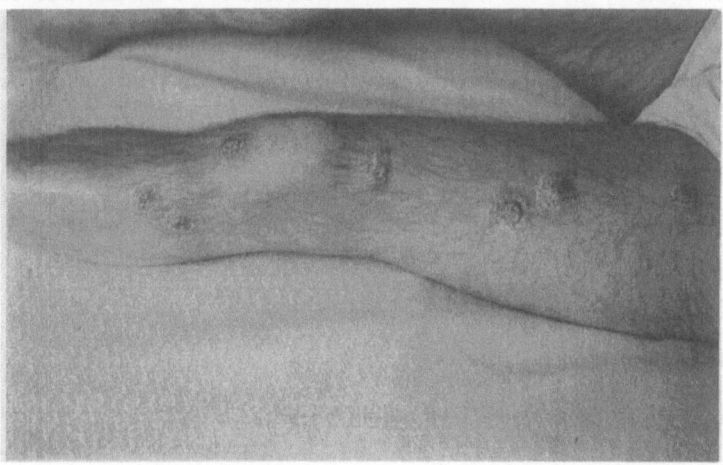

Fig. 12.10. Cutaneous leishmaniasis involving the left leg of a 53-year-old Englishman who had been working in Saudi Arabia for 4 years. Amastigotes of *Leishmania* sp were demonstrated in a biopsy, and culture produced a growth of promastigotes. He was treated successfully with intravenous sodium stibogluconate.

numbers of amastigotes are visible, which should be distinguished from *Histoplasma capsulatum* and *Toxoplasma gondii*. Culture is also possible. Serological tests in this disease, unlike Kala-azar, are of little or no value diagnostically (Neva 1988); results may be mildly positive in about 50% of infected individuals. The leishmanin skin test becomes positive within 3 months of the onset of the lesion(s) and remains positive for life; it is strongly positive in leishmaniasis recidivans, and negative in DCL. [Unfortunately the commercially produced antigen prepared by Burroughs Wellcome is no longer available because the commercial market proved too limited (Neva 1988).]

Management

Although the lesions are in most cases self-limiting (and provide subsequent life-long immunity) chemotherapy is advisable when they are large and/or multiple, and when the face is involved. Sodium stibogluconate is the usual chemotherapeutic agent; 10 mg/kg body-weight for 30 days or longer is usually necessary, and toxicity is unusual. Meglumine antimoniate, which has been widely used in new world cutaneous leishmaniasis (see below) has recently been shown to be of only limited use in *L major* infection in Algeria (Belazzoug and Neal 1986). Ketoconazole has given encouraging results (Neva 1988). Local infiltration with sodium stibogluconate or mepacrine has been used with some success. Paromomycin ointment has also given encouraging results in *L major* infections (El-On et al. 1986a); however further work is required. Recently, intradermal human recombinant gamma interferon (rIFN-γ) has given promising results (Harms et al. 1989). Local heat treatment (using an infra-red lamp) has also been advocated; this is only applicable to those patients who do not respond to conventional chemotherapy, e.g. DCL, and in whom the organism is heat-sensitive (Neva 1988). In leishmaniasis recidivans, injection of corticosteroids, emetine or transfer factor into the lesions may be necessary; a higher dose of antimony stibogluconate should be administered for a longer period of time. In DCL, pentamidine (given as a weekly injection of 4 mg/kg body-weight) seems superior to sodium stibogluconate. In vitro activity of chlorpromazine against *L major* has been documented (El-On et al. 1986b). Activity of methylbenzethonium chloride against this organism has also received attention in *in vitro* experiments (El-On and Messer 1986).

In endemic areas in Russia, Israel and Jordan vaccination using live, virulent promastigotes from cultures of *L major* has been used for many years; the resultant lesion is left to run its natural course.

Mucocutaneous Leishmaniasis

This disease (New World cutaneous leishmaniasis), which is characterized by ulcerative skin lesions, is caused by either the *L mexicana* complex or *L braziliensis* complex; with the latter species mucocutaneous lesions involving the mouth, nose and pharynx may be present (espundia). Collectively these diseases are often referred to as American cutaneous leishmaniasis (Chulay 1984; Peters and Killick-Kendrick 1987).

Clinical Aspects

The lesions are generally similar to those of Old World cutaneous disease. The incubation period varies from a few weeks to several months. An erythematous papule develops a raised and indurated margin, and subsequently ulcerates. Metastatic spread along lymphatics is common with some strains of *L braziliensis*. When mucosal lesions occur they usually appear several months after the initial cutaneous lesion has healed; chronic lesions may produce destruction of the nasal septum, palate, lips, pharynx and larynx. A form of DCL, similar to that encountered in Ethiopia, occasionally occurs in some areas.

In addition to the differential diagnoses listed in connection with Old World disease (see above) the following should be added: sporotrichosis, histoplasmosis, paracoccidioidomycosis and midline granuloma or Wegener's granulomatosis.

Diagnosis

Methods are similar to those used in Old World disease (see above); however, the organisms are fewer, and hence a more generous aspirate or biopsy is required (Neva 1988). Although negative early in the disease, serological tests are ultimately positive in 70%–80% of cases.

Management

The major difference from Old World cutaneous leishmaniasis, is that systemic chemotherapy is almost always indicated due to the risk of subsequent mucocutaneous disease. The pentavalent antimony compounds still dominate the scene; meglumine antimoniate has been widely used in Latin America as a result of general unavailability of sodium stibogluconate. However, the latter compound gives an excellent cure rate when used at a dose of 20 mg antimony per kg bodyweight for 20 days (Ballou et al. 1987); lower dosage regimens are relatively ineffective. A suitable regimen using meglumine antimoniate is: 14 mg antimony/kg body-weight daily for 10–15 days (Chulay 1984); in areas where mucocutaneous disease is common, a second 15-day course has been advocated after an interval of 15–20 days. Although espundia and DCL usually respond to chemotherapy, relapse is common. Intradermal gamma-interferon has proved effective in *L braziliensis* infection although results to date are less satisfactory than in Old World disease (Harms et al. 1989). Amphotericin B, nifurtimox and pentamidine have also been used.

The Filariases

Many filarial (nematode) helminths can infect man, but overt disease is divided into five major clinical entities: lymphatic involvement (*Wuchereria bancrofti* and

Brugia malayi), tropical pulmonary eosinophilia, *Onchocerca volvulus*, *Dracunculus medinensis* (guinea-worm), and *Loa loa* infection (Manson-Bahr and Bell 1987c). Adult worms live for many years, during which they continuously produce large numbers of microfilariae (immature larvae – which are present in blood, lymphatics and/or skin); these form the infective stage for the insect vector. As with most other parasites, there are marked strain differences which differ in their geographical distribution, and produce variable patterns of disease. Although the life-cycle of lymphatic filariasis has been known for over a century, many millions of people world-wide remain infected by these organisms. Clinical and laboratory aspects of the major filariases have been reviewed recently (Nanduri and Kazura 1989).

Lymphatic Filariasis

This infection has an interesting history: working in Amoy, China between 1875 and 1879, Manson (1877) demonstrated the man–mosquito cycle of *Wuchereria bancrofti*; this was the first clear documentation of insect-borne human disease. Elephantiasis, however, had been recognized for thousands of years, having been described in early Indian and Persian writings; it is also depicted in the thirteenth century *Mappa Mundi* ('map of the world') which is currently housed at Hereford Cathedral (Price 1989); the Latin script refers to the disease amongst the Sciopodes people, who are thought to have lived in Ethiopia.

Parasitology and Pathogenesis

One estimate is that 250 million people are infected with *W bancrofti* – which has a focal distribution throughout much of the tropics and subtropics between latitude 40° north and 30° south; the Middle-east is not affected. It was introduced to the Caribbean and southern America by the slave trade, and was described there by Sir Hans Sloane, amongst others, in the eighteenth century (Dunn 1972). *Brugia malayi*, a parasite closely related to *W bancrofti*, is limited to South and East Asia. *B timori* is limited to small volcanic islands of south-eastern Indonesia.

W bancrofti reaches maturity in the lymphatic vessels and nodes of man; the adults are white and threadlike (the female is about twice the size of the male and is 80–100 mm in length and 0.2–0.3 mm wide). Following the initial infection, the larvae (which are introduced by a mosquito-bite) migrate via the lymphatics to a lymph-node where they grow to maturity and mate; 6–12 months later, microfilariae appear in peripheral blood, and when taken up by a mosquito, the life-cycle – Fig. 12.11 – is complete. There is no evidence of a non-human reservoir. One form of *B malayi* (the subperiodic) has a reservoir in leaf monkeys; there is no good evidence, however, that domestic animals can be involved in either this or *B timori* infection, as they are with *B pahangi* (see below).

Host and parasite factors which are involved in infection are complex (Dennis 1984). The adult worms, and not the microfilariae, cause the pathological features of this infection; they live in lymph (inguinal, epitrochlear and axillary) nodes, and the major afferent lymphatics: testicular, epididymal, spermatic cord and abdominal (including the thoracic duct). Following an initial acute adeno-

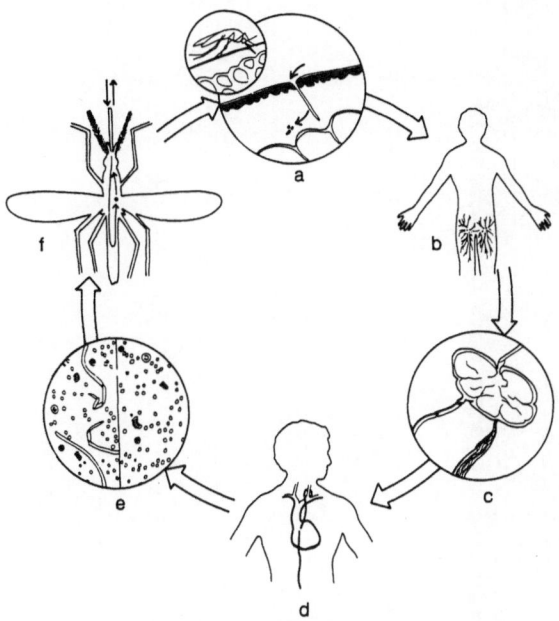

Fig. 12.11. Life-cycle of *Wuchereria bancrofti*. (a) A larva is introduced into the dermis by the bite of an anopheline or culicine mosquito; (b) migration to the regional lymph-nodes; (c) maturation of adult male (40 mm in length × 100 μm diameter) and female (80 mm × 300 μm) nematodes slowly takes place in the afferent lymph-vessels; (d) widespread dissemination of microfilariae (270 μm × 9 μm) which have been produced by the female adults; (e) appearance of microfilariae in peripheral blood; this shows a diurnal rhythm (they are demonstrable only during periods of rest, usually at night); (f) microfilariae penetrate the mosquito-intestine (after sucking blood from an infected individual), and migrate to the thoracic flight-wing muscles; here, infectious larvae (which later migrate to the mouth-parts) are produced (and the life-cycle can be completed).

lymphangitis, retrograde lymphatic inflammation occurs; dilatation of the channel is followed by endothelial thickening, and subsequently an obliterative lymphangitis. Lymphatic abscesses may form at the site(s) of dead or degenerating worms.

Clinical Aspects

Clinically, there is a great variation in the presentation in different individuals. An acute attack consists of localized pain, tenderness, swelling and erythema, and adenolymphangitis involving arms and/or legs; this may be accompanied by a generalized febrile systemic illness. These early presenting features may be recurrent. Orchitis, epididymitis and hydrocoele are frequent occurrences; *B malayi* and *B timori* do not, however, involve the genitalia. Filarial abscesses may also occur. Chronic disease resulting from lymphatic stasis gives rise to the classical clinical sequelae, which present about 10 years or more after the initial infection. Hydrocoele (Fig. 12.12) or chylocoele, and elephantiasis involving one or both lower limbs (upper limb involvement is more common in *B malayi* infection) follow repeated attacks of adenolymphangitis. As elephantiasis

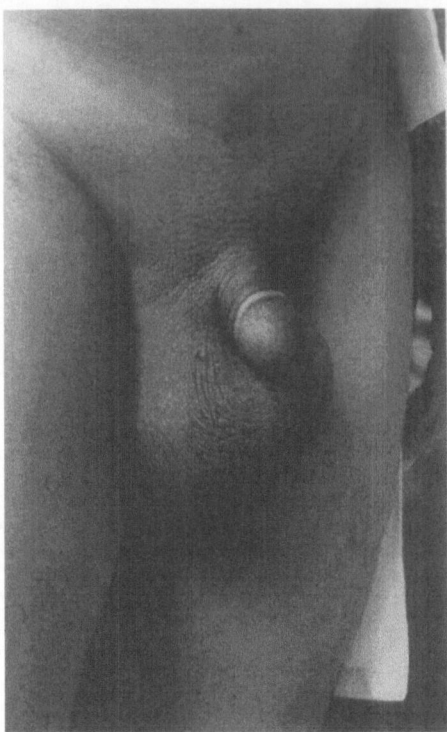

Fig. 12.12. A 24-year-old Indian student who presented with a right-sided hydrocoele; the fluid contained numerous microfilariae of *Wuchereria bancrofti*.

involves an increasing proportion of the limb(s) the swelling becomes firm, does not pit, and there is extensive hypertrophy and fibrous hyperplasia. Chyluria, which results from the rupture of abdominal lymphatics into the urinary tract, usually starts abruptly. *B malayi* and *B timori* infections tend to have a less severe clinical presentation; 'water bag' deformities rather than fibrous hyperplastic ones are produced, and these do not usually extend further than the knees or elbows. Differential diagnoses include other causes of lymphadenitis and lymphangitis, many genitourinary tract infections, numerous febrile illnesses in a tropical setting (including malaria and tuberculosis), and hereditary lymphangiectasia – Milroy's disease.

Diagnosis

Diagnosis is by identification of microfilariae in a nocturnal specimen of venous blood; when a concentration technique is used it is often possible to detect a microfilaraemia in a daytime specimen also. *B malayi* consists of nocturnally periodic and subperiodic types. *B timori* is nocturnally periodic. Microfilariae can also be detected in chylous urine and hydrocoele fluid. Biopsy of a lymph-node or vessel should be avoided. Serological tests for filariasis are not at present species specific; an indirect immunofluorescent or ELISA technique are usually used.

Management

Chemotherapy consists of a 21-day course of diethylcarbamazine (DEC) (2–3 mg three-times daily) which is an effective microfilaricide, but has limited activity against the adult worms; it also has no effect on the chronic manifestations of the disease. Side-effects following DEC administration consist of: (i) direct toxic-effects (these usually last for a few hours only and are mild); (ii) those resulting from antigen liberation from the dying microfilariae (these develop within 2 days of commencing treatment and are most common during treatment of *B malayi* and *B timori* infections); and (iii) acute attacks of adenolymphadenitis (some-times with abscess formation) which results from damage of adult worms. A low dose should be used initially (special care is required in areas where onchocercia-sis and loaiasis are common – see below) and the compound should be avoided both in pregnancy and in the presence of cardiac and renal disease. Metriphonate (10–15 mg/kg every 14 days for 5–16 doses) is also a good microfilaricide (Manson-Bahr and Bell 1987c). Aspiration may be required in the management of hydrocoele. Firm bandaging can reduce lymphoedema in elephantiasis. Reconstructive lymphatic surgery may be attempted for chyluria but is frequently unsuccessful.

Tropical Pulmonary Eosinophilia (TPE)

This condition, which is most commonly seen in southern India and Sri Lanka, consists of severe pulmonary disease resulting from dense parenchymal eosinop-hil infiltration, in the presence of (i) strongly positive filarial serology, and (ii) absence of macrofilariae in peripheral blood; a striking elevation of the perip-heral blood eosinophil count is usual. Pulmonary symptoms consist of dyspnoea and a paroxysmal cough, which is most marked nocturnally; there is little or no sputum production. Coarse rhonchi are present on examination. A chest-radiograph shows an increase in bronchovascular markings with fine diffuse miliary mottling. Peripheral eosinophil count is usually $>3.0 \times 10^9/l$; serum IgE is elevated; filarial serology is strongly positive. Although *W bancrofti* and *B malayi* have been recovered, most cases are probably caused by animal filariae including *B pahangi*. Differentiation from Löffler's syndrome (which is caused by migra-tory intestinal helminths including *Ascaris lumbricoides* and *Strongyloides stercoralis*), allergic aspergillosis, autoimmune vasculitis, drug allergies etc. is important. Response to DEC is usually rapid and excellent; a corticosteroid 'cover' is advisable.

Onchocerciasis

This infection, which involves populations living in vast tracts of land in Africa, Central and South America, and parts of the Arabian peninsula, is caused by *Onchocerca volvulus*, which is transmitted by black flies (the *Simulium damno-sum* complex); close proximity to fast-flowing rivers and streams constitutes a favourable site for these vectors. As with the other filariases the spectrum of clinical manifestation ranges from trivial symptoms to serious disease; in this case the major manifestations are ophthalmic lesions ('river blindness'), dermatitis and subcutaneous nodules (Connor et al. 1987). In a heavily infected area severe morbidity may affect 15% or more of the local population; ophthalmic and skin involvement are the main problems.

Parasitology and Pathogenesis

Adult worms measure 23–50 mm × 250–450 μm (female) and 16–42 mm × 125–200 μm (male) in size; the unsheathed microfilariae (which should be distinguished from *Mansonella streptocerca* and *M ozzardi*) measure 220–360 × 5–9 μm. Figure 2.13 shows an example of an adult *O volvulus*. The importance of an animal reservoir is unclear; in Africa, the gorilla is known to be infected. Maturation of larvae to adults (which survive for up to 15 years) occurs in subcutaneous tissue (in Africa the pelvic region is most commonly infected, while in South America the upper part of the body is usually involved) and after copulation millions of microfilariae (which can live for up to 2 years) are produced, and these concentrate in the eyes and lymph nodes. Microfilariae are taken up by the fly vector and after a period of 7–9 days the larvae, which are introduced into the human host, emerge. Although they can produce disfiguring nodules, the adult worms are essentially benign; it is the microfilariae which after several months of active life die and produce inflammatory lesions (which subsequently fibrose) and cause significant tissue damage. Nodules (which contain tightly coiled female worms) form in the deep dermis and subcutaneous tissue, often over bony prominences. Microfilariae produce (i) an eosinophilic reaction (which may increase after diethylcarbamazine administration – see below), and (ii) granuloma formation. In some geographical areas, associated lymphadenopathy occurs (e.g. in the Arabian peninsula, where the disease presents as hyperpigmented skin lesions and is termed 'sowda'); this may occasionally obstruct lymphatic flow and give rise to changes ('hanging groins')

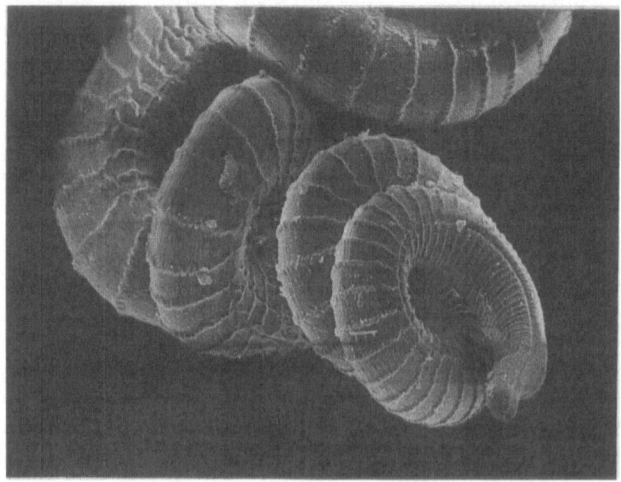

Fig. 12.13. Scanning electron micrograph of an adult *Onchocerca volvulus* (× 100).

comparable with elephantiasis (see above). As with all helminthic infections, the immunological bases of immunity are poorly worked out; CMI response to *O volvulus* antigen varies in different individuals; eosinophils are important in the host attack on the microfilariae. 'Sowda' (see above) is associated with the presence of very few microfilariae and probably represents a hyperreactive immunological response. The degree of protection offered by the immune system in an infected individual is questionable; a heavily infected person who is cured by chemotherapy does not appear to be substantially protected against re-infection (Connor et al. 1984).

Clinical Aspects

Clinically, this disease is not uniform geographically; whereas for example, blindness caused by sclerosing keratitis (see below) is common in the African savannah it is unusual in forest areas; 'hanging groins' (see above) are common only in disease in Africa; skin lesions are generally less marked in southern America compared with Africa; 'Sowda' (see above) is most common in Yemen. Worm load is important in symptomatology; expatriates with light infections may, for example, merely have a localized disfiguring rash; ophthalmic lesions and nodules are rare. Dermatitis usually presents with pruritus over the affected area; a papular rash over the buttocks and legs, altered pigmentation, and the sequelae of scratching (including secondary infection) are important; skin in a young individual appears prematurely aged. Depigmentation can produce confusion with leprosy; however, sensory change is absent. Nodules vary in size from 5 mm to 10 cm in diameter. The site of the dermal or subcutaneous nodules reflects the regions of the body most heavily infected (see above) and whereas in Africa, the pelvis, anterior superior iliac crest, femoral trochanter, sacrum and coccyx are common sites, in southern America, most are around the head and upper part of the body.

Ophthalmic changes are numerous and include (Connor et al. 1984): the mere presence of microfilariae in the anterior chamber (revealed by slit-lamp examination), punctate keratitis (an ill-defined 'fluffy' opacity approximately 0.5 mm in diameter may be present surrounding dead corneal microfilariae), sclerosing keratitis (the entire cornea is opaque and vascularized), anterior uveitis (synechiae formation produces severe complications and accounts for much blindness in Central America), choroidoretinitis, optic neuritis and atrophy, and glaucoma. Epilepsy resulting from skull erosion by *O volvulus* nodules is an occasional complication in Central America and Sudan (Chap. 8). Treatment (see below) is sometimes complicated by an acute arthritis and tenosynovitis. Differential diagnoses include many dermatological conditions including: scabies, contact dermatitis, prickly heat, eczema, tertiary yaws, vitiligo, leprosy and streptocerciasis.

Diagnosis

A definitive diagnosis is made by microscopical demonstration of microfilariae emerging from a skin-snip (taken from standard sites, e.g. buttock, iliac crest, scapula or calf); when examined 1–3 hours later microfilariae can be seen emerging into the surrounding normal saline. A quantitative count can be made by weighing the snip and counting the microfilariae which have emerged. In heavily infected individuals and after DEC treatment, microfilariae can be demonstrated in blood, urine, sputum, lacrimal fluid and CSF. Adult female worms can be visualized in an excised nodule; fragments of worms can also be identified in an aspirate of a nodule. Slit-lamp examination (see above) is a simple non-invasive procedure. The Mazzotti test (which should only be used for the diagnosis of light infections) consists of producing pruritus by administration of a single dose of 50 mg DEC; erythema, oedema and papules may also be produced, and in a heavy infection systemic symptoms (including ocular complications) and a marked eosinophilia may be produced. Several serological tests (including an ELISA) have been used but these currently lack species specificity; there iŝ also a degree of cross reaction with *Strongyloides stercoralis* (Chap. 5).

Management

Management is unsatisfactory because most chemotherapeutic agents (e.g. DEC and ivermectin) are microfilaricidal and do not exert a lethal effect on adult worms; those agents (e.g. suramin) which are macrofilaricidal are relatively toxic. Also, chemotherapy does not reverse scarring and long-standing changes to the eyes, skin or lymphoid tissues. DEC (which is dependent on a T-cell response) is given orally as 50 mg (first day), 50 mg tds (second day), 100 mg tds (third day) and 250 mg tds (from the fourth to twenty-first day); some physicians consider that a shorter course is equally effective (Manson-Bahr and Bell 1987c). A corticosteroid cover is often recommended because this prevents most of the side-effects (dermatological manifestations, joint pains, swollen lymph-nodes, headache, oedema of the eyelids and accentuation of eye lesions, and hypotension and sudden death) which usually develop 30 minutes to 24 hours after starting treatment. Microfilariae will again be detectable 3–12 months after treatment.

Suramin has micro- and macro-filaricidal properties. A test-dose (100 mg is initially given intravenously) is followed by weekly doses of 200, 400, 600, 800, 1000, and 1000 mg in a 70 kg adult. Side-effects include: an exfoliative dermatitis, tenderness of palms and soles, polyuria, albuminuria (with granular casts), aphthous ulceration, diarrhoea, various systemic manifestations, as well as exacerbation of the eye lesions and, rarely, sudden death. Local reactions resulting from death of the adult worms can also be troublesome. As with DEC, the complications can be reduced by a corticosteroid 'cover'. For a complete cure, a DEC course followed by suramin is sometimes given.

Mebendazole (1 g bd for 3–4 weeks) reduces the microfilarial count for at least 1 year (Cook 1990). Ivermectin (given as a single oral dose of 100–200 μg/kg) can be given at yearly intervals and is associated with a lower incidence of serious side-effects (especially ophthalmic ones) than DEC (Goldsmith 1988; Taylor et al. 1989); however, minor evidence of toxicity occurs in up to one-third of patients (Rothova et al. 1989). In Senegal, a double-blind comparison of ivermectin and DEC showed the former agent to be safer and more effective (Diallo et al. 1986). A combination of mebendazole and levamisole has been used (Manson-Bahr and Bell 1987c). Flubendazole (another benzimidazole compound) has also been tried. Metriphonate is an effective microfilaricide but has no advantages over DEC. The benzodiazepine derivative midazolam has been tested in vitro and certainly possesses anti-*O volvulus* activity (Laukamm-Josten 1987). Nodulectomy has been widely used in South America; by reducing the adult worm load, microfilaraemia is diminished and the prevalence of ophthalmic involvement significantly reduced. In prevention, mass chemotherapy is not an option because the available chemotherapeutic agents are unsatisfactory (see above). Recent experimental work has been directed to the production of an anti-microfilarial vaccine (Tamashiro et al. 1989).

Dracontiasis

This disease, which causes a great deal of morbidity in endemic areas, is caused by *Dracunculus medinensis* which burrows into the subcutaneous and connective tissues of man (Muller 1971, 1984). It is confined to rural areas of West Africa, western India, and scattered foci in the Middle-east; it often has a seasonal incidence. The World Health Organisation is currently attempting to eradicate this disease by providing sieved drinking water (free of *Cyclops* sp) in all villages in the affected areas (Hopkins 1988); the last WHO success in the eradication of a human disease concerned smallpox on 26 October 1977.

Parasitology and Pathogenesis

Human infection occurs when *Cyclops* sp (containing *D medinensis* larvae) are ingested in contaminated fresh drinking water; larvae, when released, penetrate the intestine and migrate to connective tissues – especially the axillary and inguinal regions. After mating, the diminutive male worms (about 2.5 cm in length) die. The adult female worm takes about 1 year to mature in human tissues (when it measures up to 70 cm in length × 0.2 cm diameter); a blister then forms at its anterior end, which after bursting through the skin results in an ulcer with about 5 cm of the worm extruded (this usually occurs after the affected limb (or other part of the body) has been immersed in fresh water). Many thousands of larvae (one adult female contains up to 3 million) are then released from the end of the worm which after ingestion by *Cyclops* sp completes the life-cycle. There is no animal reservoir. There seems to be little or no acquired immunity to infection.

Clinical Aspects

Clinically, the most frequent presentation is with a small, painful blister at the site of the emergence of the worm; however, a female worm lying in subcutaneous tissue may be palpable, or there may (in about one third of cases) be various allergic symptoms – consisting of urticaria, fever, giddiness, dyspnoea and gastrointestinal symptoms. The blister forms over a period of 3–5 days during which time there is local itching and a severe burning pain; although larvae are present the blister fluid is initially bacteriologically sterile. If uncomplicated, the surrounding epithelium grows over the ulcer and when the worm has been spontaneously expelled, or extracted, the ulcer heals completely. However, secondary infection is common and a local cellulitis occurs in nearly 50% of cases. If the female worm bursts into the tissues, an abscess may form; this often gives rise to an intra-articular abscess involving most frequently the knee or ankle joint; a spinal extradural abscess is a further possibility (Chap. 8).

Diagnosis

When the ulcer has appeared (and burst) the diagnosis is usually clinically obvious. The larvae can be identified easily with low-powered microscopy, after having been obtained by applying cold water to the ulcer. Immunodiagnosis using a *D medinensis* fluorescent antibody technique is of no practical use. In an active infection, calcifications (resulting from one or more dead adult *D medinensis*) may be demonstrable in a radiograph usually involving the lower limbs (Fig. 12.14).

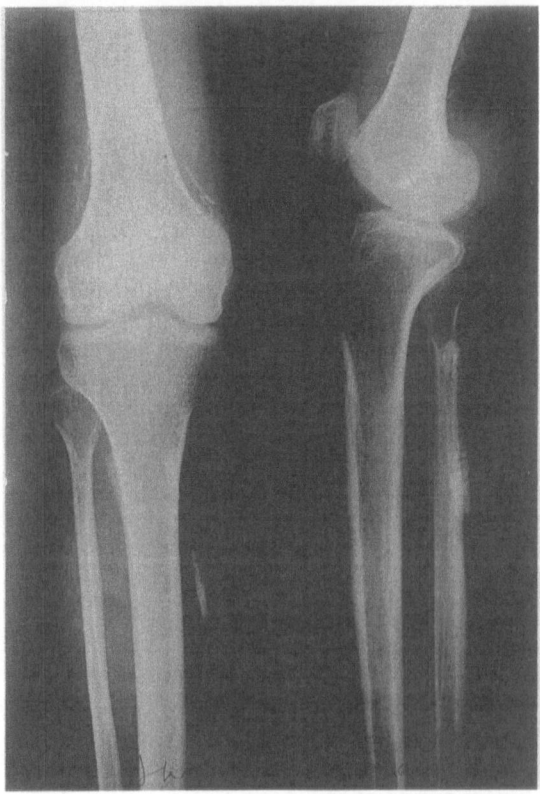

Fig. 12.14. Lower-limb radiograph which shows extensive calcifications produced by a dead (inactive) female *D medinensis*.

Management

Traditional treatment consists of winding the adult worm on a matchstick (a few cm daily) after it has emerged; sterile dressings and antiseptics should be used to prevent secondary infection. Initially this procedure is facilitated by placing the affected part in cold water; this produces a flaccid worm and is followed by the release of many eggs. Surgical extraction is widely practised in India if the course of the worm is entirely superficial. During the last 10–15 years several chemotherapeutic agents have been used with partial success (adult doses or dose/body weight are given): (i) metronidazole (400 mg daily for 10–20 days); (ii) niridazole (25 mg/kg body-weight for 10 days); (iii) thiabendazole (50 mg/kg daily for 3 days); and (iv) mebendazole (400–800 mg daily for 6 days). None of these chemotherapeutic agents affects the pre-emergent worm or the larvae contained therein.

Loaiasis

Loaiasis is caused by the filarial nematode *Loa loa* which is conveyed by tabanid flies (deer flies) (genus: *Chrysops*). Compared with the other four filarial infections covered in this chapter, the major symptoms are relatively trivial: transient subcutaneous ('Calabar') swellings, and conjunctival invasion with worm migration. The disease has a limited geographical distribution, most cases being located in the rain forest regions of West and Central Africa; this is determined by the distribution of the insect vectors.

Parasitology and Pathogenesis

The adult worms measure 50–70 × 0.5 mm (female), and 30–35 × 0.3–0.4 mm (male). The microfilariae (230–300 × 6–8 μm) have a diurnal periodicity and are most plentiful in human peripheral blood between 0800 and 1700 hours. There is no known animal reservoir. The clinical manifestations of infection differ between visitors to an endemic area and local residents. In the former, allergic symptoms, hypergammaglobulinaemia, an elevated IgE concentration and marked eosinophilia are more pronounced (Nutman et al. 1988); the ratio of CD4/CD8$^+$ T-cells is also significantly increased. The hyperresponsive state encountered in expatriates with a *Loa loa* infection is associated with (i) specific dysregulation of the immune response to parasite antigen, and (ii) non-specific immune activation.

Clinical Aspects

Calabar swellings are the most common clinical features of infection; these are subcutaneous (non-pitting and itchy), usually located on a wrist, or the dorsum of a hand or forearm – frequently following trauma – and are caused by a host hypersensitivity response to antigenic material liberated by a developing or mature worm. They occur from one to several years after infection, and recur for

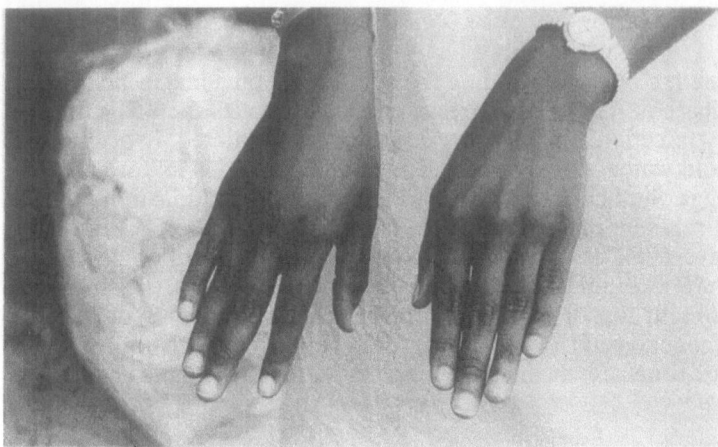

Fig. 12.15. A Calabar swelling on the dorsum of the right hand of a 20-year-old Nigerian medical student; a daytime peripheral blood-film contained numerous microfilariae of *Loa loa*; peripheral blood eosinophil count was $1.6 \times 10^9/l$; filaria FAT was positive at $1 \geqslant 512$. She was treated successfully with diethylcarbamazine.

a year or so. The usual duration of a swelling is a few hours or at most days; they may be accompanied by urticaria, fever and irritability. Figure 12.15 shows an example of a Calabar swelling. If the worms die in the subcutaneous tissue, a local abscess may ensue. The adults or larvae can cross the conjunctiva, and may cause oedema of the eyelids with local itching and discomfort; this is a frequent clinical presentation in West Africa. Other filariae can also produce intraocular disease (Beaver 1989); in a review of 56 cases of supposed human intraocular filariasis, only six were proved definitively to be caused by *Loa loa*. Many infected individuals are completely asymptomatic, but transient fever, tiredness and arthritic pains have been attributed to infection. The major complication of infection is meningoencephalitis (Chap. 8); this occasionally proves fatal. The precise role, if any, of this infection in endomyocardial fibrosis and nephrotic syndrome in endemic areas is undetermined; the peripheral blood eosinophilia may be profound and this has been implicated in endocardial damage (Spry 1988; Willmot 1980).

Diagnosis

A daytime peripheral blood smear is used for diagnosis; microfilariae may be plentiful or only detected after the use of a concentration technique. An eosinophilia is usually present and may be gross. Calcified worms are occasionally visualized on a radiograph, in subcutaneous tissue. Serological tests (IFA or ELISA) are non-specific, and cross-reaction with the other filariases makes specific diagnosis impossible by these techniques; if a microfilaraemia is present they are in any case unnecessary.

Management

Treatment is with DEC, starting with a low dose (see above), but a corticosteroid 'cover' should usually be provided. If onchocerciasis is present concurrently, a severe cutaneous reaction may ensue. Mebendazole (which is partially effective in onchocerciasis – see above) has also been evaluated in loaiasis (1 g bd for 21 days) (Burchard and Kern 1987); the microfilarial count in peripheral blood was unchanged. Ivermectin (which has microfilaricidal properties in an *O volvulus* infection – see above) has also been evaluated in loaiasis (Richard-Lenoble et al. 1988); although encouraging results were produced, further studies are required. Wandering subconjunctival adult worms can be removed surgically.

References

Apt W, Arribada A, Arab F, Ugarte JM, Luksic I, Solé C (1986) Clinical trial of benznidazole and an immunopotentiator against Chagas' disease in Chile. Trans R Soc Trop Med Hyg 80:1010

Ballou WR, McClain JB, Gordon DM, Shanks GD, Andujar J, Berman JD, Chulay JD (1987) Safety and efficacy of high-dose sodium stibogluconate therapy of American cutaneous leishmaniasis. Lancet ii:13–16

Barioglio SR de, Lacuara JL, Oliva PP de (1987) Effects of clomipramine upon motility of *Trypanosoma cruzi*. J Parisitol 73:451–452

Beaver PC (1989) Intraocular filariasis: a brief review. Am J Trop Med Hyg 40:40–45

Belazzoug S, Neal RA (1986) Failure of meglumine antimoniate to cure cutaneous lesions due to *Leishmania major* in Algeria. Trans R Soc Trop Med Hyg 80:670–671

Bittencourt AL (1976) Congenital Chagas' disease. Am J Dis Child 130:97–103

Borelli D (1987) A clinical trial of itraconazole in the treatment of deep mycoses and leishmaniasis. Rev Infect Dis 9:S57–S63

Brandão HJS, Zulian R (1966) Nerve cell depopulation in chronic Chagas' disease in a qualitative study in the cerebellum. Rev Inst Med Trop São Paulo 8:281–286

Brenière SF, Carrasco R, Antezana G, Desjeux P, Tibayrenc M (1989) Association between *Trypanosoma cruzi* zymodemes and specific humoral depression in chronic chagasic patients. Trans R Soc Trop Med Hyg 83:517

Brown WJ, Voge M (1982) Neuropathology of parasitic of parasitic infections. Oxford University Press, Oxford, p 240

Bruce D (1895) Preliminary report on the tsetse fly disease or nagana, in Zululand. Bennett and Davis, Durban

Burchard GD, Kern P (1987) Failure of high dose mebendazole as a microfilaricide in patients with loaiasis. Trans R Soc Trop Med Hyg 81:420

Castellani A (1903) On the discovery of a species of trypanosoma in the cerebrospinal fluid of cases of sleeping sickness. Proc R Soc 71:501–508

Chagas C (1909) Nová trypanozomiaze humana. Estudos sobre a morfolojia e o cielo evolutivo do *Schizotrypanum cruzi* n. gen., n. sp., ajente etiolojico de nova entidade morbida do nomen. Mem Inst Osw Cruz 1:159–218

Chulay JD (1984) Cutaneous leishmaniasis of the new world. In: Strickland GT (ed) Hunter's tropical medicine, 6th edn. Saunders, Philadelphia, pp 589–593

Chulay JD, Manson-Bahr PEC (1984a) Visceral leishmaniasis (Kala-azar). In: Strickland GT (ed) Hunter's tropical medicine, 6th edn. Saunders, Philadelphia, pp 578–585

Chulay JD, Manson-Bahr PEC (1984b) Cutaneous leishmaniasis of the old world. In: Strickland GT (ed) Hunter's tropical medicine, 6th edn. Saunders, Philadelphia, pp 585–589

Connor DH, Gibson DW, Taylor HR, Mackenzie CD, Meyers WM, Neafie RC (1984) Onchocerciasis. In: Strickland GT (ed) Hunter's tropical medicine, 6th edn. Saunders, Philadelphia, pp 667–680

Cook GC (1988) Chemotherapy of parasitic infections. Curr Opin Infect Dis 1:423–438

Cook GC (1990) 'Exotic' parasitic infections: recent progress in diagnosis and management. J Infect 20:95–102

Cunningham DD (1885) On the presence of peculiar parasitic organisms in the tissue of a specimen of Delhi boil. Sci Mem Med Off Army India 1:21–31

Dennis DT (1984) Bancroftian filariasis. In: Strickland GT (ed) Hunter's tropical medicine, 6th edn. Saunders, Philadelphia, pp 649–659

Diallo S, Aziz MA, Lariviere M, Diallo JS, Diop-Mar I, N'Dir O, Badiane S, Py D, Schulz-Key H, Gaxotte P, Victorius A (1986) A double-blind comparison of the efficacy and safety of ivermectin and diethylcarbamazine in a placebo controlled study of Senegalese patients with onchocerciasis. Trans R Soc Trop Med Hyg 80:927–934

Donovan C (1903) On the possibility of the occurrence of trypanosomiasis in India: Br Med J ii:79

Duggan AJ, Hutchinson MP (1966) Sleeping sickness in Europeans: a review of 109 cases. J Trop Med Hyg 69:124–131

Dunn RS (1972) Sugar and slaves: the rise of the planter class in the English West Indies, 1624–1713. University of North Carolina Press, Williamsburg, VA, p 359

Dutton JE (1902) Preliminary note upon a trypanosome occurring in the blood of man. Thompson Yates Lab Rep 4:455–468

El-On J, Messer G (1986) *Leishmania major*: antileishmanial activity of methylbenzethonium chloride. Am J Trop Med Hyg 35:1110–1116

El-On J, Livshin R, Evan-Paz Z, Hamburger D, Weinrauch L (1986a) Topical treatment of cutaneous leishmaniasis. J Invest Dermatol 87:284–288

El-On J, Rubinstein N, Kernbaum S, Schnur LF (1986b) *In vitro* and *in vivo* anti-leishmanial activity of chlorpromazine alone and combined with N-meglumine antimonate. Ann Trop Med Parasitol 80:509–517

Garattini S (1988) Remedies for tropical diseases. Lancet i:1338

Goldsmith RS (1988) Recent advances in the treatment of helminthic infections: ivermectin, albendazole and praziquantel. In: Leech JH, Sande MA, Root RK (eds) Parasitic infections. Churchill Livingstone, New York and Edinburgh, pp 327–347

Harms G. Zwingenberger K, Chéhadé AK, Talhari S, Racz P, Mouakeh A, Douba M, Näkel L, Naiff RD, Kremsner PG, Feldmeier H, Bienzle U (1989) Effects of intradermal gamma-interferon in cutaneous leishmaniasis. Lancet i:1287–1292

Hayes MM, Cox HW (1984) Complement reversal of immunosuppression induced with plasma of rats infected with *Trypanosoma brucei rhodesiense*. J Parasitol 70:864–870

Hoff R, Teixeira RS, Carvalho JS, Mott KE (1978) *Trypanosoma cruzi* in the cerebrospinal fluid during the acute stage of Chagas' disease. New Engl J Med 298:604–606

Hopkins DR (1988) Dracunculiasis eradication: the tide has turned. Lancet ii:148–150

Hudson KM, Terry RJ (1979) Immunodepression and the course of infection of a chronic *Trypanosoma brucei* infection in mice. Parasite Immunol 1:317–326

Jayaraman KS (1988) Leishmaniasis resurgent in India. Nature 333:590

Jennings FW (1987) Chemotherapy of late-stage trypanosomiasis: the effect of the nitrothiazole compounds. Trans R Soc Trop Med Hyg 81:616

Kinmond S, Galea P, Simpson EM, Parida SK, Goel KM (1989) Kala-azar in a Scottish child. Lancet ii:325

Köberle F (1974) Pathogenesis of Chagas' disease. In:Trypanosomiasis and leishmaniasis with special reference to Chagas' disease. Associated Scientific Publishers, Amsterdam, pp 137–152. (Ciba Foundation symposium 20)

Kohn LA (1983) Charles Darwin's chronic ill health. Bull Hist Med 37:239–256

Laukamm-Josten U (1987) The paralyzing effect of midazolam on *Onchocerca volvulus* microfilariae in vitro. Am J Trop Med Hyg 37:152–156

Leech JH, Sande MA, Root RK (eds) (1988) Parasitic infections. Churchill Livingstone, New York and Edinburgh, p 364

Leishman WB (1903) On the possibility of the occurrence of trypanosomiasis in India. Br Med J i:1252–1254 and ii:1376–1377

Manson P (1877) *Filaria sanguinis hominis*. Med Rep Imperial Customs, China, 13th issue:30–38

Manson-Bahr PEC, Bell DR (eds) (1987a) African trypanosomiasis. In: Manson's tropical diseases, 19th edn. Baillière Tindall, London, pp 54–73

Manson-Bahr PEC, Bell DR (eds) (1987b) American trypanosomiasis (Chagas' disease). In: Manson's tropical diseases, 19th edn. Baillière Tindall, London, pp 74–86

Manson-Bahr PEC, Bell DR (eds) (1987c) Filariasis. In: Manson's tropical diseases, 19th edn. Baillière Tindall, pp 353–406

Mar JJ, Docampo R (1986) Chemotherapy for Chagas' disease: a perspective of current therapy and considerations for future research. Rev Infect Dis 8:884–903

Marsden PD (1984) American trypanosomiasis. In: Strickland GT (ed) Hunter's tropical medicine, 6th edn. Saunders, Philadelphia, pp 565–573

Marsden PD (1989) American trypanosomiasis. Br Med J 299:969–970

McCann PP, Bitonti AJ, Bacchi CJ, Clarkson AB (1987) Use of difluoromethylornithine (DFMO, eflornithine) for late-stage African trypanosomiasis. Trans R Soc Trop Med Hyg 81:701

Medawar PB (1964) Darwin's illness. Ann Intern Med 61:782–787

Molyneux DH, Raadt P de, Seed JR (1984) African human trypanosomiasis. In: Gilles HM (ed) Recent advances in tropical medicine 1. Churchill Livingstone, Edinburgh, London, pp 39–62

Muller R (1971) Dracunculus and dracontiasis. Adv Parasitol 9:73

Muller R (1984) Dracontiasis. In: Strickland GT (ed) Hunter's tropical medicine, 6th edn. Saunders, Philadelphia, pp 687–689

Nanduri J, Kazura JW (1989) Clinical and laboratory aspects of filariasis Clin Microbiol Rev 2:39–50

Nantulya VM, Musoke AJ, Rurangirwa FR, Barbet AF, Ngaira JM, Katende JM (1982) Immune depression in African trypanosomiasis: the role of antigenic competition. Clin Exp Immunol 47:234–242

Neva FA (1988) Recent advances in the diagnosis and management of leishmaniasis and American trypanosomiasis. In: Leech JH, Sande MA, Root RK (eds) (1988) Parasitic infections. Churchill Livingstone, New York and Edinburgh, pp 243–258

Nutman TB, Reese W, Poindexter RW, Ottesen EA (1988) Immunologic correlates of the hyperresponsive syndrome of loiasis. J Infect Dis 157:544–550

Oka M, Ito Y, Furuya M, Osaki H (1984) *Trypanosoma gambiense*: immunosuppression and polyclonal-cell activation in mice. Exp Parasitol 58:209–214

Okamura M, Correa Netto A (1963) Etiopatogenia do megacolo Chagasico. Rev Hosp Clin Fac Med Univ São Paulo 18:351–360

Osuna A, Ruiz-Perez LM, Lopez MC, Castanys S, Gamarow F, Craciunescu DG, Alonso C (1987) Anti-trypanosomal action of cis-diamminedichloroplatinum (II) analogs. J Parasitol 73:272–277

Pehrson P-O, Wahlgren M, Bengtsson E (1982) Intracranial calcifications probably due to congenital Chagas' disease. Am J Trop Med Hyg 31:449–451

Pepin J, Milord F, Guern C, Mpia B, Ethier L, Mansinsa D (1989a) Trial of prednisolone for prevention of melarsoprol-induced encephalopathy in Gambiense sleeping sickness. Lancet i:1246–1250

Pepin J, Milord F, Mpia B, Meurice F, Ethier L, DeGroof D, Bruneel H (1989b) An open clinical trial of nifurtimox for arseno-resistant *Trypanosoma brucei gambiense* sleeping sickness in central Zaire. Trans R Soc Trop Med Hyg 83:514–517

Peters W, Killick-Kendrick R (eds) (1987) The leishmaniases in biology and medicine, 2 vols. Academic Press, London, p 941

Price EW (1989) Mappa Mundi and tropical medicine. Trans R Soc Trop Med Hyg 83:574

Raseroka BH, Ormerod WE (1985) Protection of the sleeping sickness trypanosome from chemotherapy by different parts of the brain. E Afr Med J 62:452–458

Raseroka BH, Ormerod WE (1986) The trypanocidal effect of drugs in different parts of the brain. Trans R Soc Trop Med Hyg 80:634–641

Richard-Lenoble D, Kombila M, Rupp EA, Pappayliou ES, Gaxotte P, Nguiri C, Aziz MA (1988). Ivermectin in loiasis and concomitant *O. volvulus* and *M. perstans* infections. Am J Trop Med Hyg 39:480–483

Robertson M (1913) Notes on the life history of Trypanosoma gambiense. Repts Sleep Sickn Comm R Soc 13:119

Rothova A, Lelij A van der, Stilma JS, Wilson WR, Barbe RF (1989) Side-effects of ivermectin in treatment of onchocerciasis. Lancet i:1439–1441

Schmidt H, Bafort JM (1985) African trypanosomiasis: treatment-induced invasion of brain and encephalitis. Am J Trop Med Hyg 34:64–68

Scott EMD (1988) Remedies for tropical diseases. Lancet ii:108

Singh MP, Mishra M, Khan AB, Ramdas SL Panjiyar S (1989) Gold treatment for Kala-azar. Br Med J 299:1318

Spencer HC (1984) African trypanosomiasis. In: Strickland GT (ed) Hunter's tropical medicine, 6th edn. Saunders, Philadelphia, pp 553–565

Spry CJF (1988) Eosinophils: a comprehensive review and guide to the scientific and medical literature. Oxford University Press, Oxford, p 450

Stephens JWW, Fantham HB (1910) On the peculiar morphology of a trypanosome from a case of sleeping sickness and the possibility of its being a new species (*T. rhodesiense*). Proc R Soc Lond (Biol) 83:28–33

Sypek JP, Wyler DJ (1988) Host defense in leishmaniasis. In: Leech JH, Sande MA, Root RK (eds) Parasitic infections. Churchill Livingstone, New York and Edinburgh, pp 221–242

Tamashiro WK, Ibrahim MS, Moraga DA, Scott AL (1989) *Dirofilaria immitis*: studies on anti-microfilarial immunity in Lewis rats. Am J Trop Med Hyg 40:368–376

Taylor HR, Semba RD, Newland HS, Keyvan-Larijani E, White A, Dukuly Z, Greene BM (1989) Ivermectin treatment of patients with severe ocular onchocerciasis. Am J Trop Med Hyg 40:494–500

Thakur CP, Kumar M, Kumar P, Mishra BN, Pandey AK (1988) Rationalisation of regimens of treatment of Kala-azar with sodium stibogluconate in India: a randomised study. Br Med J 296:1557–1561

Traub N, Hira PR, Chinta C, Mhango C (1978) Congenital trypanosomiasis: report of a case due to *Trypanosoma brucei rhodesiense*. E Afr Med J 55:477–481

Turner M (1980) How trypanosomes change coats. Nature 284:13

Weinberg JR, Wright PA, Cook GC (1989) Tropical pyomyositis associated with *Trypanosoma brucei rhodesiense* infection in a Europid. Trans R Soc Trop Med Hyg 83:77–79

Willmott S (ed) (1980) The eosinophil in tropical disease. Trans R Soc Trop Med Hyg 74[Suppl]:1–63

Subject Index

Ascaris lumbricoides – cont.
  clinical aspects 55–6
  diagnosis 56
  life-cycle of 55
  management 56
  parasitology 54–5
  pathogenesis 54–5
Ascaris suum 54
Azathioprine in malaria-associated nephrotic
    syndrome 22

Babesia sp 7, 8
Bacterial meningitis 96, 144
Balantidium coli 104, 112
Benzimidazoles
  in hydatid disease 161, 221
  see also Albendazole; Cambendazole;
    Flubendazole; Mebendazole;
    Thiabendazole
Benznidazole in *T cruzi* infection 238
Bephenium hydroxynaphthoate in small-
    intestinal nematode infections 62
Bilharzia disease 127
Biliary tract, parasites of 68–9
Biomphalaria 123
Biomphalaria arabica 122
Bithionol
  in biliary tract infection 69
  in paragonimiasis 159
Blastocystis hominis 63, 78, 85, 104
Borrelia burgdorferi 223
Brown-Séquard syndrome 196
Brugia malayi 248–51
Brugia pahangi 209, 215, 248, 251
Brugia timori 248–51
Burkitt's lymphoma 171
Busk, George 58

Calabar swellings in *Loa loa* infection 257
Cambendazole
  in *Strongyloides stercoralis* infection 60, 98
Campylobacter jejuni 82
Candida albicans 82
Canine-associated parasitic infections 207–28
Capillaria hepatica 151, 155, 209, 212, 213
Capillaria philippinensis 41, 60
Capillariasis 60
Cardiomyopathy 112, 237
Cell-mediated immunity (CMI) 37–9, 41, 80,
    172, 175
Cellulose acetate precipitation (CAP) 151
Central nervous system (CNS) parasitoses 141–
    65
  cestode infections 159–61
  nematode infections 151–6
  protozoan infections 141–51
  taxonomic classification of major protozoan
    and helminthic infections 142
  trematode infections 156–9
Cerebral abscess, caused by *E histolytica* 150–1

Cerebral malaria 5, 7, 18–19, 141–7
  chemotherapeutic regimens for use in 145–6
  clinical and laboratory indices 146
  clinical aspects 144
  diagnosis 145
  differential diagnoses 144, 146
  management 145–6
  mortality rate in 146
  parasitology 142–4
  pathogenesis 142–4
  prognosis 146
Cestode infections
  canine-associated 215–22
  involving CNS 159–61
  involving small-intestine 57–60
Chagas' disease 112, 235–8
Cheyletiella sp 209, 222
Chilomastix mesnili 104
Chloramphenicol in malaria 17
10-(4'-chlorophenyl)-3-methylflavin in malaria
  21
Chloroquine
  in malaria 3, 10–14, 16–17, 19–22, 145
  in *P carinii* infection 36
Chloroquine sulphate in cerebral malaria 145
Chlorproguanil in malaria 10, 14
Chlorpromazine in cutaneous leishmaniasis
  246
Choroidoretinitis in *T gondii* 173–4, 178, 183
Cinchona 2
Ciprofloxacin in malaria 20
Clindamycin
  in cryptosporidiosis 85
  in malaria 16, 17, 20
  in *P carinii* infection 36, 37
  in *T gondii* infection 182–4
Clonorchis sinensis 56, 68–70, 209, 215
Clonorchis sp 68
Coccidia 1, 32, 42, 63, 77–90
  see also Small-intestinal coccidiosis
Coccidiosis of the small-intestine. *See* Small-
    intestinal coccidiosis
Coenuriasis 159–60, 222
Coenurus cerebralis 199
Colonic disease, complications of 115–6, 103–
    19, 129
Colonic schistosomiasis. *see* Schistosomiasis
Colorectal disease in AIDS 115–16
Colorectal helminths 113–16
Colorectal parasitic infections 103–19
Colorectal helminths 113–15
Colorectal protozoa 104–12
Contracaecum 57
Coombs negative haemolytic anaemia 173
Cor pulmonale 132
Cortex peruanus 2
Corticosteroids
  in *Angiostrongylus cantonensis* infection 153
  in cutaneous leishmaniasis 246
  in *Gnathostoma spinigerum* 153
  in loaiasis 259